Contents

Preface   xv

Acknowledgments   xvii

About the Authors   xix

Chapter One
Key Concepts of Advanced Cardiac Life Support   1

Introduction   2

Key Elements of Cardiac Resuscitation   3

Cerebral Resuscitation: The Fundamental Goal   3
Treat the Patient—Not the Rhythm   4
Basic-to-Advanced Life Support: A Continuum   5
Time: A Critical Factor   5
Manage Conditions That May Lead to a Cardiac Arrest   5
Care Does Not Stop After Successful Resuscitation   6
Apply the Chain of Survival to All Situations   6
Use Judgment about Futile Resuscitation Attempts   6
The Phased-Response Approach: A Standardized Structure   7

Ethical Considerations in Cardiac Resuscitation   8

Advance Directives and Surrogates   8
Do-Not-Resuscitate and No-CPR Orders   9

Chapter Two
Systematic Approach to Emergency Cardiac Care: The Primary and Secondary Surveys   12

Introduction   13

Preliminary, Presurvey Actions 13

Assess the Scene for Safety Hazards 14

Assess for Unresponsiveness 15

Call for Help 16

Position the Patient 17

Position the Members of the Resuscitation Team 18

Primary Survey 18

A = Airway: Open the Airway 18

B = Breathing: Assess for Breathlessness and Provide Ventilation 19

C = Circulation: Assess for Pulselessness and Provide Chest Compressions 21

D = Defibrillation: Defibrillate Ventricular Fibrillation and Pulseless
Ventricular Tachycardia 21

Secondary Survey 23

A = Airway: Perform Endotracheal Intubation 24

B = Breathing: Assess Endotracheal Tube Placement
and Effectiveness of Ventilation 25

C = Circulation: Establish an IV Line, Attach the ECG,
and Administer Cardiac Medications 26

D = Differential Diagnosis: Consider the Etiology
of the Cardiac Arrest or Rhythm 27

Chapter Three
Airway Management, Ventilation, and Oxygen Therapy 32

Introduction 33

Airway Management 33

Airway Assessment 34

Basic Airway Management Techniques 35

Manual Airway Maneuvers 35

Basic Mechanical Airway Adjuncts 37

Advanced Airway Management Techniques 43

Endotracheal Intubation 44

Alternative Orotracheal Intubation Techniques 59

Digital Intubation 59

Transillumination (Lighted Stylet) Intubation 61

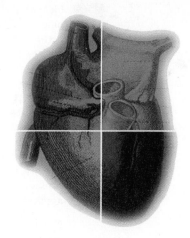

Advanced Cardiac Life Support

Joseph J. Mistovich, M.Ed, NREMT-P
Chairperson, Department of Health Professions;
Associate Professor, Youngstown State University, Youngstown, Ohio

Randall W. Benner, M.Ed, NREMT-P
Program Director, Emergency Medical Technology; Instructor,
Department of Health Professions, Youngstown State University, Youngstown, Ohio

Gregg S. Margolis, MS, NREMT-P
Associate Director of Education; Program Director, Paramedic Education,
Center for Emergency Medicine, Pittsburgh, Pennsylvania

Howard A. Werman, M.D., *Medical Editor*

PRENTICE HALL
Upper Saddle River, New Jersey 07458

Library of Congress Cataloging-in-Publication Data
Mistovich, Joseph J.
    Advanced cardiac life support; a manual for course preparation and
review / Joseph J. Mistovich, Randall W. Benner, Gregg S. Margolis, Howard
A. Werman, medical editor.
        p.   cm.
    includes index.
    ISBN 0-8359-5050-6
    1. Cardiovascular emergencies.   2. Cardiovascular emergencies—
–Case studies.   I. Benner, Randall W.   II Margolis, Gregg S.
III. Werman, Howard A.   IV. Title.
        [DNLM: 1. Heart Arrest—therapy.   2. Heart Arrest—therapy—
–examination questions.   3. Life Support Care.   4. Life Support Care—
examination questions.   5. Resuscitation.   6. Resuscitation—
–examination questions.   WG 205 M678a 1998]
RC675.M57   1998
616.1'025—dc21
DNLM/DLC
for Library of Congress

Publisher: *Susan Katz*
Managing development editor : *Lois Berlowitz*
Project editor: *Sandy Breuer*
Editorial/production supervision: *Janet McGillicuddy*
Managing production editor: *Patrick Walsh*
Director of production/manufacturing: *Bruce Johnson*
Prepress/manufacturing buyer: *Ilene Sanford*
Editorial assistant: *Carol Sobel*
Electronic page make-up: *Stephen Hartner*
Creative director: *Marianne Frasco*
Interior design: *Marianne Frasco*
Cover design: *Bruce Kenselaar*
Interior photographer: *Carl Leet*
Cover image: *John Lund*

© 1998 by Prentice-Hall, Inc.
A Simon & Schuster Company
Upper Saddle River, New Jersey 07458

Printed in the United States of America
10 9 8 7 6 5 4 3 2 1

ISBN 0-8359-5050-6

PRENTICE-HALL INTERNATIONAL (UK) Limited, *London*
PRENTICE-HALL of Australia Pty. Limited, *Sydney*
PRENTICE-HALL Canada, Inc., *Toronto*
PRENTICE-HALL Hispanoamericana, S.A., *Mexico*
PRENTICE-HALL of India Private Limited, *New Delhi*
PRENTICE-HALL of Japan, Inc., *Tokyo*
SIMON & SCHUSTER Asia Pte. Ltd., *Singapore*
EDITORA PRENTICE-HALL do Brasil, Ltda., *Rio de Janeiro*

Alternative Airway Adjuncts   63

Esophageal Obturator Airway (EOA)   63
Esophageal Gastric Tube Airway (EGTA)   66
Other Airway Adjuncts   67

Translaryngeal and Transtracheal Airways   70

Transtracheal Catheter Ventilation   71
Cricothyrotomy   73
Tracheostomy   74

Ventilation Techniques   74

Mouth-to-Mouth and Mouth-to-Nose Ventilation   74
Mouth-to-Mask Ventilation   75
Bag-Valve Devices   76
Flow-Restricted, Oxygen-Powered, Manually Triggered Ventilation Device   80
Automatic Transport Ventilator (ATV)   81

Suction   83

Oropharyngeal Suctioning   83
Tracheobronchial Suctioning   83

Oxygen Therapy   85

Equipment   85

Chapter Four
Gaining Intravenous Access   93

Introduction   94

IV Cannulas   96

Peripheral IV Lines   96

Techniques for Cannulating Peripheral Veins   98

Cannulating an Arm or Leg Vein   98
Cannulating an External Jugular Vein   99

Complications   99

Chapter Five
Dysrhythmia Recognition   102

Introduction   103

Basic Electrophysiology   103

Pacemakers   104
The Cardiac Conduction System   104
Myocardial Working Cells   105

The Electrocardiogram   105

Monitoring Systems   107

Analyzing the ECG   108

Rate   108
Regularity   110
The QRS Complex   110
The P Waves   111
The P-R Interval   111

The Normal ECG and Sinus Rhythms   111

Normal Sinus Rhythm   111
Sinus Tachycardia   113
Sinus Bradycardia   114
Sinus Dysrhythmia   115

Abnormal ECGs   116

Fibrillatory Dysrhythmias   116
Reentry Dysrhythmias   119
The Absence of Rhythm: Asystole   122
The Blocks   122
Ectopic Beats   127

Chapter Six
Electrical Therapy   140

Introduction   141

Defibrillation   141

Importance of Defibrillation   142
Components of a Defibrillator   142

Transthoracic Resistance to Energy Flow   143

Procedure for Defibrillation   146

Defibrillation and Asystolic Hearts   148

Current-Based Defibrillation: "Smart Defibrillators"   148

Automated External Defibrillation   148

Components of an Automated External Defibrillator   148

Types of AEDs   149

Procedure for Defibrillation with an AED   149

Coordination of ACLS with AEDs   151

Emergency Synchronized Cardioversion   153

Indications for Synchronized Cardioversion   153

Procedure for Synchronized Cardioversion   153

Special Situations Involving Electrical Therapy   155

Defibrillation of Hypothermic Patients   155

AED Use in Pediatric Patients   155

Defibrillation of Patients with Automatic Implantable
Cardioverter/Defibrillator (AICD)   156

Interruption of CPR   156

Monitor/Defibrillator and AED Maintenance   156

Emergency Cardiac Pacing   157

Components of a Cardiac Pacemaker   157

Indications for Emergency Cardiac Pacing   158

Transcutaneous Pacing Equipment   158

Procedure for Transcutaneous Pacing   159

Standby Pacing   160

Complications of Transcutaneous Pacing   160

Contraindications to Transcutaneous Pacing   160

Other Pacing Techniques   162

Chapter Seven
Pharmacological Therapy   166

Introduction: Cardiovascular Pharmacology   167

Organization of this Chapter   168

PART ONE: OXYGEN   168

PART TWO: **SYMPATHOMIMETICS** 171

Epinephrine 171
Norepinephrine 174
Isoproterenol 176
Dopamine 177
Dobutamine 179
Amrinone 180

PART THREE: **SYMPATHOLYTICS** 181

Beta Blockers 182

PART FOUR: **ANTIDYSRHYTHMICS** 183

Rhythm Control 184

Lidocaine 184
Procainamide 187
Bretylium Tosylate 189
Magnesium Sulfate 191

Rate Control 192

Atropine Sulfate 192
Adenosine 196
Calcium Channel Blockers: Verapamil and Diltiazem 197
Digitalis Glycosides 200
Other Drugs for Rate Control 202

PART FIVE: **ANALGESICS AND ANTIANGINAL AGENTS** 203

Morphine Sulfate 203
Nitroglycerin 205

PART SIX **DIURETICS** 206

Furosemide 206

PART SEVEN: **ANTIHYPERTENSIVES** 207

Sodium Nitroprusside 207
Other Antihypertensive Drugs 208

PART EIGHT: **THROMBOLYTICS** 208

Thrombolytic Therapy 209

PART NINE: OTHER CARDIOVASCULAR DRUGS 211

Sodium Bicarbonate 211
Calcium Chloride 213

Chapter 8
Acute Coronary Syndromes 222

Introduction 223

The Heart as a Pump 223

The Right-Side Pump 224
The Left-Side Pump 224
The Cardiac Output 225

Pathophysiology of an AMI 226

Who Is at Risk? 230
General Presentation of an Acute Myocardial Infarction 230

Assessment of the AMI Patient 231

General Presentation 232
The ABCs 232
Vital Signs 233
ECG Tracings 233
History 236
Conclusions 236

Management of AMI: Prehospital, Emergency Department,
and Hospital Considerations 237

Alleviation of Pain and Apprehension 237
Prevention and Management of Dysrhythmias 237
Limiting the Size of the Infarction 238
Initiation of Thrombolytic Therapy 238

Management of Specific AMI Presentations 238

Management of the Uncomplicated AMI 239
Management of AMI Complicated by Dysrhythmia 249
Management of AMI with Hemodynamic Alteration 252

Chapter Nine
Acute Stroke   261

Introduction   262

Acute Stroke and Transient Ischemic Attack (TIA)   262

Etiology of an Acute Stroke   262
Etiology of a Transient Attack (TIA)   263
Clinical Presentation of an Acute Stroke or TIA   263

Initial Assessment of the Patient with an Acute
Stroke or TIA   265

Airway   265
Vital Signs   265
Respiratory Effort   266
Circulatory Status   266
Neurological Assessment   267
Differential Diagnosis for the Acute Stroke/TIA Patient   270

Treatment Strategies for the Acute Stroke Patient   271

General Considerations in Initial Care of Acute Stroke   272
Special Considerations in the Management of the Acute Stroke Patient   275
Overall Goals of Acute Stroke/TIA Management   279

Chapter Ten
Putting it All Together: The Algorithms   283

Introduction   284

Classification of Therapeutic Interventions   284

Key Considerations in the Algorithm Approach
to Emergency Cardiac Care   285

Algorithms for Patients in Cardiac Arrest   286

Universal Algorithm   286
Ventricular Fibrillation/Pulseless Ventricular Tachycardia (VF/VT) Algorithm   288
Pulseless Electrical Activity (PEA) Algorithm   292
Asystole Algorithm   294

Postresuscitation Patient Management   296

Postresuscitation Interventions   296
Other Interventions and Considerations   297

Algorithms for Patients Not in Cardiac Arrest   298

Bradycardia Algorithm   299
Tachycardia Algorithm   302

Chapter Eleven
Case Studies: Application Exercises   315

Some Questions and Answers about the ACLS Course   316

Why did you come to the course?   316
What should you get out of the course?   316
But, I will *NEVER* have to run a code where I work!   317
So what is case-based teaching?   317

The Core Cases   318

Respiratory Arrest with a Pulse   318
Witnessed Ventricular Fibrillation, Adult Cardiac Arrest   321
Adult Ventricular Fibrillation/Pulseless Ventricular Tachycardia   323
Pulseless Electrical Activity   327
Asystole   329
Acute Myocardial Infarction   331
Bradycardia   335
Unstable Tachycardia   337
Stable Tachycardia   339

Chapter Twelve
Special Resuscitation Situations   347

Introduction   348

Traumatic Cardiac Arrests   348

Approach to the Traumatic Cardiac Arrest Patient   349
Treatment of the Traumatic Cardiac Arrest Patient   350

Cardiac Arrest and Pregnancy   351

Treatment of the Pregnant Cardiac Arrest Patient   352

Lightning Strikes   353

Treatment of the Patient in Cardiac Arrest from a Lightning Strike   354

Hypothermia and Near Drowning   354

Hypothermia and Near Drowning in Association with Arrest   354

Basic-Life-Support Treatment   355

Advanced-Life-Support Treatment   356

Toxicologic Cardiac Emergencies and Arrest   358

Chapter Thirteen
Special Treatment Considerations   363

Introduction   364

Cerebral Resuscitation   365

Cerebral Perfusion Pressures   365
Oxygenation   365
Hyperventilation   366
Metabolic Acidosis Correction   367
Temperature Regulation   367
Glucose Requirements   367
Sedation and Anticonvulsant Therapy   367
Brain Resuscitation after Cardiopulmonary Arrest   368

Advanced Monitoring Interventions for Cardiac
Arrest Patients   368

Arterial Cannulation   368
Cannulation of the Pulmonary Artery   368
Arterial Puncture   369

Adjuncts for Artificial Circulation   369

Alternative Techniques to Compressions   369
Mechanical Devices for CPR   370
Invasive CPR   370

CPR Assessment   371

Appendix: Recommendations of the American College of Cardiology
and the American Heart Association on Practice Guidelines
for the Management of Patients with Acute Myocardial Infarction   375

Review Questions: Answers and Rationales   385

Index   413

Preface

Management of acute cardiovascular emergencies requires rapid and decisive actions by the health care team. Standardized procedures must be established so that an effective continuum of cardiac care can be provided from the prehospital environment and emergency department through the more definitive care that is provided in the cardiac care unit. The educational background and clinical experience of emergency cardiac care providers is very diverse. To accommodate the needs of this varied group of providers, *Advanced Cardiac Life Support* presents comprehensive information regarding cardiac care procedures in a condensed format.

Advanced Cardiac Life Support contains thirteen chapters that provide the core information necessary to prepare a candidate for the American Heart Association's ACLS Provider course. The information is presented in a logical manner that allows the reader to progress from a foundation of basic core knowledge to more complex case management material. The first nine chapters are the core knowledge-building chapters. This basic information is presented in the text to help the reader comprehend and master the algorithms and case studies presented in the later chapters. As the chapters progress, the information, cases, and algorithms become more complex, requiring integration of the knowledge gained from the previous chapters. Review questions at the end of each chapter allow the reader to use the text as an ACLS review manual as well as for the purpose of self-assessment.

Below are key features of the text.

Presentation The material is presented in a logical order that lends itself to continuous reinforcement of previously learned information. The key information required to build a suitable knowledge base for comprehension of algorithms and cases is covered prior to any of the complete algorithms or the case studies in which the reader must integrate this information.

In this text, the algorithms (which are sometimes presented in a single group) are separated and introduced in different chapters. The chapter where each algorithm is presented is the chapter where the information learned so far has prepared the reader to understand the algorithm and where the algorithm is relevant to the chapter topic. This provides the reader the opportunity to work through the technical information with adequate background information and in a logical sequence.

Case Studies A brief Case Study is presented at the beginning of each chapter (with a Case Study Follow-up at the end of the chapter) to reinforce the material presented in the chapter. While each case is specific and relevant to the information in that chapter, it is also built on information that was presented in the previous chapters. As an example, the Chapter 5 "Dysrhythmias" case study focuses on dysrhythmia recognition but also incorporates respiratory and intravenous therapy concepts from the previous two chapters. This cumulative approach to the case studies allows the reader to review previous material while applying it to a practical scenario. In Chapter 11, the core case studies from the ACLS course are presented with page references to earlier chapters to help the reader integrate and apply the information that has been learned as well as to preview the core case studies in preparation for the ACLS course.

Review Questions Each chapter ends with a set of multiple-choice or short-answer items that can be used as self-assessment and review. The answers, with rationales, are provided in the back of the text. This feature makes the book especially useful for those who need to review when repeating an ACLS course.

Reinforcement A key feature of this text is the inclusion of four distinct levels of reinforcement of information. This systematic reinforcement will aid the reader in mastering the information and in attaining a level of comfort with the knowledge necessary to successfully complete the ACLS course, and more importantly, provide efficient emergency cardiac care.

Following are the four levels of information reinforcement provided in this text:

- Initial introduction of information in a logical progression
- Algorithms that are introduced at points of relevancy to chapter topics
- Case studies that address new information in each chapter while also reinforcing information from prior chapters
- Review questions that allow the students to assess their own understanding of the information and determine the need for remediation

The methods of teaching the concepts of emergency cardiac care in this textbook have evolved from the authors' many years of classroom instruction of hundreds of students in ACLS courses. We have pulled together our experience as educators and clinicians and have compiled what we believe to be the most logical and comprehensive approach to ACLS. We wish you success in your educational and clinical endeavors and hope that you find this textbook a useful resource in expanding your knowledge and developing your skills in emergency cardiac care.

JJM

RWB

GSM

Acknowledgments

A special thanks to our contributing writers: Craig A. Soltis, MD, FACEP, Associate Director, Department of Emergency Medicine, Salem Community Hospital, Salem, Ohio; Medical Director, Emergency Medical Technology Program, Youngstown State University, Youngstown, Ohio and James W. Drake, BS, NREMT-P, Limited Service Faculty, Youngstown State University, Youngstown, Ohio.

Thanks also to Dr. Howard A. Werman, Associate Professor, Department of Emergency Medicine, The Ohio State University School of Medicine, Columbus, Ohio. Dr. Werman carefully reviewed all the material every step of the way in the development of this text. His reviews, insight, and suggestions were greatly appreciated and significantly contributed to this textbook

We also wish to specially thank the following individuals:

Susan Katz, Publisher, for her integrity, professionalism, and inspiration. She is an exceptional business associate, and most importantly a true friend and a great coach.

Sandy Breuer, Project Editor, for keeping this entire project together. She is an amazing person with intuition that continues to astonish us. She is a true pleasure to work with and has contributed more to this textbook than any of us will ever realize.

Lois Berlowitz, Managing Development Editor, for her calm sense of organization. She kept us all in line and moving along with her encouraging words and finesse in enforcing deadlines.

Janet McGillicuddy, Editorial/Production Supervision, for her diligent and tireless efforts in fitting all the pieces together. Her commitment, perseverance, and guidance is greatly appreciated.

Stephen Hartner, Electronic Page Make-up, for working magic with paging the textbook. He is truly an expert at his work.

Carol Sobel, Editorial Assistant, for fielding the extraneous items with such grace and keeping all of our schedules on track. She is a true pleasure to work with.

Judy Streger and Judy Stamm, Marketing/Sales, for taking such a personal approach to understanding the textbook and truly believing in us and the products that they sell.

Pat Walsh, Managing Production Editor, for his contribution of expertise and skill in producing this text.

Helen Verdream, Secretary, Department of Health Professions, Youngstown State University, for her encouragement and support on a daily basis, and for doing all the extra things that make our work a little easier. Also, just for being a great listener when we need to vent.

Dr. John J. Yemma, Dean of the College of Health and Human Services, Youngstown State University, for providing Joe Mistovich and Randy Benner with the necessary encouragement and support of the University administration to pursue such scholarly activities.

Floyd Jackson, Director of Media Services, Youngstown State University, for his support in providing a photographer, facilities, and equipment to shoot and process the photographs contained in this textbook.

Carl Leet, Photographer, Youngstown State University, for his professional photography, flexibility, and great sense of humor.

We wish to thank the following people and organizations for their assistance in creating the photo program for the textbook: **Salem Community Hospital, Salem, Ohio;** Dr. Craig A. Soltis, Pam Hershey, Lori Robbins, Bev Richey, and Robin Weyant.

Lane LifeTrans Paramedic Service, Austintown, Ohio: Randall Pugh, Supervisor; Tod Filmer, Todd Claypoole, Joe Wrenn, and Jeff Krikland.

Cardinal Fire District, Canfield, Ohio: Robert Tieche, Chief; and Robert Tieche, Jr.

YSU Students: Robert Ariza and Susan Fabrizio.

ACLS Reviewers

The authors thank the following reviewers for their comments and suggestions during the development of this text.

Brenda M. Beasley RN, BS, EMT-P
  EMS Progam Director
  Calhoun Community College
  Decatur, AL

Terry Bitterlich NREMT-P
  Safety Training, Ltd.
  Albuquerque, NM

Jerry Brungardt BS, NREMT-P
  Director of Allied Health
  Northeast Community College
  Norfolk, NE

Douglas K. Cline BSW, NREMT-P
  Lead EMS Instructor
  Chapel Hill Fire Department
  Chapel Hill, NC

Garry L. DeJong NREMT-P
  Flight Paramedic
  Albuquerque Fire Department
  Albuquerque, NM

Rudy Garrett
  Paramedic Training Coordinator
  Somerset-Pulaski Co, EMS
  West Somerset, KY

Tonnie Glick RN, MED, CCRN, CRRN
  Program Director
  Union County College Paramedic Program
  Cranford, NJ

Paul R. Hinchey BA, EMT-P
  Paramedic Curriculum Chairperson
  Westchester Community College
  Valhalla, NY

Lindi Kempfer MS, EMT-P
  EMS Educator
  Methodist Hospital of Indiana
  Indianapolis, IN

David J. Kuchta RN, NREMT-P, BSAS
  Advance Life Support Coordinator
  Division of Emergency Medical Services
  Mississippi State Department of Health
  Jackson, MS

Baxter Larmon
  Associate Professor of Medicine
  UCLA School of Medicine
  Los Angeles, CA

Danny Marcum RN, NREMT-P
  Flight Nurse Health Net III
  Cabell-Huntington Hospital
  Huntington, WV

Lori L. Moore MPH, EMT-P
  EMS Director
  International Association of Fire Fighters
  Washington, DC

Judith Rafkin RN, CEN
  Peninsula Regional Medical Center
  Salisbury, MD

Suzann E. Schmele NREMT-P
  Department of Emergency Medicine
  School of Medicine
  Oregon Health Sciences University
  Portland, OR

Randy L. Smith MS, NREMT-P
  National Director EMS Education
  Rural/Metro Corporation
  Scottsdale, AZ

Richard G. Stump
  Betsy Johnson Memorial Hospital
  Carey Area EMS
  Dunn, NC

Paul A. Werfel NREMT-P
  Paramedic Program Director
  SUNY Health Science Center
  Stony Brook, NY

Sonya Young RN, NREMT-P
  EMS Coordinator/Emergency Dept.
  Good Samaritan Hospital
  Cincinnati, OH

About the Authors

Joseph J. Mistovich, M.Ed, NREMT-P

Joseph Mistovich is the Chairperson of the Department of Health Professions and an Associate Professor at Youngstown State University in Youngstown, Ohio. He has twelve years of experience as an educator in emergency medical services and multidisciplinary allied health courses, including advanced cardiac life support. He is an Ohio Affiliate ACLS Faculty for the American Heart Association and an active ACLS, BCLS, and PALS instructor.

Mr. Mistovich received his Master of Education degree in Community Health Education from Kent State University in 1988. He completed a Bachelor of Science in Applied Science degree with a major in Allied Health in 1985 and an Associate in Applied Science degree in Emergency Medical Technology in 1982 from Youngstown State University. He is also certified as a Nationally Registered Emergency Medical Technician-Paramedic.

Mr. Mistovich has over fifteen years of experience providing advanced life support in the prehospital environment and continues to function as a paramedic on a part-time basis. He is a co-author of *Prehospital Emergency Care*, 5th edition. He has made many presentations at local, state, and national conferences.

Randall W. Benner, M.Ed, NREMT-P

Randall Benner, Instructor in the Department of Health Professions at Youngstown State University, has over ten years of experience as an educator in emergency medical services and as a field paramedic. He serves as the Director of the Emergency Medical Technology Program at YSU and is responsible for all levels of emergency medical education. In addition, he actively functions as a paramedic on an advanced life support unit.

Mr. Benner has served as a contributing author for a variety of EMS textbooks and instructor resource materials. He also serves as a medical content reviewer for emergency medical services and allied health publications. He is a contributing author to the revision of the United States Department of Transportation National Standard EMT-Intermediate and Paramedic curricula. He serves on several local, state, and national EMS committees. Mr. Benner is completing his Ph.D program in curriculum and instructional design at Kent State University.

Gregg S. Margolis, MS, NREMT-P

Gregg Margolis is the Associate Director of Education at the Center for Emergency Medicine in Pittsburgh, Pennsylvania. He is responsible for the development, coordination, management, and supervision of all levels of emergency medical education and is the Program Director of the Center's Paramedic Education Program. Mr. Margolis holds a Bachelor's degree in Physiology, a Master's degree in Health Care Supervision and Management, and is currently pursuing a doctorate in education. Mr. Margolis is an active

American Heart Association Advanced Cardiac Life Support Instructor and Affiliate Faculty member. He has taught and coordinated hundreds of ACLS courses. He remains clinically active as a Flight Paramedic with STAT MedEvac in Pittsburgh.

Chapter One

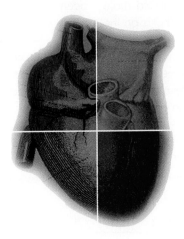

Key Concepts of Advanced Cardiac Life Support

When cardiac arrest occurs and circulation ceases, it may mean the end of life. Sometimes, however, a spontaneous rhythm, cardiac output, and cerebral perfusion can be restored before the brain is permanently damaged. The goal of both basic and advanced cardiac life support is to restore the cardiac rhythm and myocardial contractility as quickly as possible so that the patient can, ultimately, regain both physical and mental health.

This chapter presents an overview of key concepts of advanced cardiac life support. The topics to be covered are:

- Key Elements of Cardiac Resuscitation
- Ethical Considerations in Cardiac Resuscitation

The key icon marks each key element of cardiac resuscitation.

CASE STUDY SCENARIOS

"Medic 107—respond code 3 to 2234 West Chalmers for a 48-year-old male patient who is pulseless and apneic. YFD is on the scene. This is a confirmed nonbreather. AED has been initiated. Time out 0923 hours."

"Express team alert—emergency department. Express team alert—emergency department. You have a 65-year-old female patient in cardiac arrest. Down time of 12 minutes. The patient is intubated and two IV lines have been established. Current rhythm is ventricular fibrillation. Defibrillation and drug therapy initiated."

"Code blue—coronary care unit. Code blue—coronary care unit for a 62-year-old male post-MI patient in pulseless ventricular tachycardia."

Introduction

Scenarios like the above are encountered by health care practitioners in both the out-of-hospital and hospital environment on a daily basis. For many patients in the out-of-hospital environment, cardiac arrest may be the first indication that the patient has been suffering some type of coronary artery disease. Unfortunately, a large number of these patients do not survive, and therefore they never get a chance to receive medical treatment to correct the condition. However, through organized resuscitative efforts by well-trained health care practitioners in both the out-of-hospital and hospital environment, survival rates may be significantly improved.

To maximize the effectiveness of the resuscitation effort, the following knowledge areas and skills must be mastered:

- Basic and advanced airway management to include endotracheal intubation
- Ventilation and oxygen therapy techniques
- Ability to recognize and manage the following cardiovascular conditions:
  - bradycardia
  - tachycardia
  - acute myocardial infarction (MI)
  - hypotension
  - cardiogenic shock
  - pulmonary edema
  - stroke
- Ability to recognize and manage lethal dysrhythmias including:
  - ventricular fibrillation (VF, or V-fib)/pulseless ventricular tachycardia (VT, or V-tach)
  - pulseless electrical activity (PEA)
  - asystole/agonal
- Electrical therapy to include defibrillation, cardioversion, and transcutaneous pacing
- Intravenous therapy techniques and invasive monitoring

- Ability to recognize and manage the following nonlethal dysrhythmias:
  - artifact
  - bradycardias
  - tachycardias
  - atrial dysrhythmias
  - sinus rhythm
  - pacemaker rhythms
  - morphologic electrocardiogram (ECG) changes associated with myocardial ischemia and acute MI
- Ability to determine the actions, indications, dose, administration, precautions, and contraindications of the cardiovascular medications used in resuscitation of patients suffering a cardiovascular crisis
- Ability to recognize special considerations and provide early management for the patient suffering from:
  - stroke
  - traumatic cardiac arrest
  - drowning and near-drowning
  - hypothermia
  - cardiac arrest when pregnant
  - electrocution and lightning strikes
  - drug overdose
  - electrolyte imbalances

The topics listed above will all be addressed in the course of this book. However, there are several key elements that you should become acquainted with before you begin and that you should keep in mind throughout your preparation for advanced cardiac life support verification—as well as throughout your career as an ACLS practitioner.

Key Elements of Cardiac Resuscitation

Certain elements are crucial to the efficiency of resuscitation efforts for patients suffering cardiac arrest or cardiovascular or cardiopulmonary compromise. These key elements must be considered for every patient, since the patient's survival may depend on them (Table 1-1).

Cerebral Resuscitation: The Fundamental Goal

When performing basic and advanced cardiac life support, it is important to remember the most fundamental goal of resuscitation: Restart the heart *to restore cerebral perfusion.*

Resuscitating a patient to the point where he is neurologically intact, or at least near his neurologic capacity prior to cardiac arrest, is the ultimate goal of resuscitation. Restarting hearts alone is not an adequate concept of cardiac resuscitation. For this reason, Peter Safar introduced the concept of cardio-pulmonary-cerebral resuscitation (CPCR), where as much emphasis is placed on cerebral resuscitation as on cardiac resuscitation. Cerebral resuscitation involves concerns such as cerebral perfusion pressures, oxygenation, temperature control, and drug therapies, which will be discussed in Chapter 13.

TABLE 1-1 KEY ELEMENTS OF CARDIAC RESUSCITATION
Cerebral resuscitation is the fundamental goal.
Treat the patient—not the rhythm.
Basic-to-advanced life support is a continuum of care.
Time to CPR and time to defibrillation are critical factors.
Manage conditions that may lead to cardiac arrest.
Care does not stop after successful resuscitation.
Apply the chain of survival to all situations.
Use judgment about futile resuscitation attempts.
The phased-response approach provides a standardized structure.

Treat the Patient—Not the Rhythm

Whether in or out of the hospital, a patient in cardiac arrest is a highly charged and dramatic situation (Figure 1-1). In a circumstance like this, it is easy to lose the ability to think calmly, to see the whole picture, and to proceed in a systematic fashion.

A common error is to develop tunnel vision and concentrate on one skill, such as getting the patient intubated or starting an IV, and not focus on other important aspects of patient care like chest compressions, dysrhythmia recognition, and defibrillation. Do not treat the rhythm without considering the probable etiology (cause) of the cardiac arrest and the rhythm itself. Ask yourself, "Why is this patient in cardiac arrest?" "Why is the patient in this rhythm?" You must focus on treating possible causes of the problem, such as hypoxia caused by an airway obstruction. You must constantly concentrate on ensuring an adequate airway, providing effective

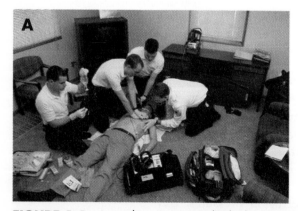
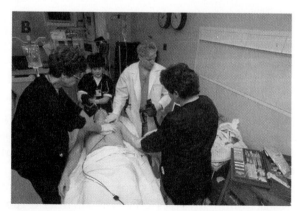

FIGURE 1-1 A cardiac arrest is a high-drama situation. Make an effort to remain calm, think clearly, and consider the big picture. "Treat the patient—not the rhythm." (A) an out-of-hospital cardiac arrest; (B) a hospital cardiac arrest.

ventilation and oxygenation, providing effective artificial circulation, administering the appropriate medications, and defibrillating the appropriate rhythms—never allowing yourself to focus on just one of these skills.

Basic-to-Advanced Life Support: A Continuum

A clear line of demarcation where basic life support stops and advanced life support begins no longer exists. Many first responders are now providing defibrillation by automated external defibrillator. Emergency Medical Technician-Basics in many states are now taught to perform endotracheal intubation or use other advanced airway devices. The continuum begins with basic cardiac life support (BCLS), assuring an open airway and CPR, which is vital to resuscitation—and which must be performed anywhere along the continuum of care that it is needed. Advanced cardiac life support (ACLS) is at the other end of the continuum with medication administration, continued defibrillation, cardiac pacing, and other more advanced techniques. Between basic and advanced cardiac life support is intermediate cardiac life support, which is defined on a case-by-case basis.

The key is to develop a response team of trained individuals who can provide basic life support and defibrillation at the earliest possible time, followed by providers with more advanced cardiac life support techniques. This applies to both the hospital and out-of-hospital environment.

Time: A Critical Factor

Time is one of the most critical factors that will determine the success of resuscitation and patient outcome. With each passing minute, the chances of successfully resuscitating a *neurologically intact* patient decline.

Time to CPR is one crucial variable. Irreversible brain damage is likely to occur 4 to 6 minutes following cessation of blood flow. If performed promptly, CPR will extend the time during which successful resuscitation is possible; however, CPR alone usually does not lead to successful resuscitation.

Time to defibrillation is another crucial variable. With each minute that passes by, the success rate of defibrillation declines. After 10 minutes, it is likely that the patient will have deteriorated from a rhythm that could have been defibrillated to a rhythm that cannot be defibrillated. Likewise, even if the rhythm is still one that can be defibrillated, the myocardium has become too hypoxic and acidotic and thus is no longer conducive to successful defibrillation. In addition, it is likely that the brain has suffered significant irreversible damage. The survivability of a patient in ventricular fibrillation who has not been defibrillated within 10 minutes following cardiac arrest approaches zero. This is why early defibrillation takes precedence even over chest compressions and ventilation.

Two other factors that are considered time critical are early definitive airway management by endotracheal intubation to prevent potential aspiration, and early administration of epinephrine to augment cerebral and coronary perfusion.

Manage Conditions That May Lead to a Cardiac Arrest

"Treat the patient and not the rhythm" is a concept that applies to a possible prearrest as well as to an arrest situation. Identify conditions that are likely to cause the patient to deteriorate to cardiac arrest and manage them—for example, MI or chest pain. The ability to recognize these prearrest conditions and provide rapid emergency care is critical.

Care Does Not Stop After Successful Resuscitation

Once the pulse is regained and the patient resuscitated, the battle is not over. You must be prepared to handle the postarrest patient as efficiently as you managed the patient while in cardiac arrest. Without proper care, the patient can easily suffer from hypoperfusion, become hypoxic, or even deteriorate back into cardiac arrest.

Apply the Chain of Survival to All Situations

The basic concepts of the chain of survival, as recognized by the American Heart Association, apply to patients in out-of-hospital and hospital environments (Figure 1-2). The continuum of care must not be jeopardized as the patient is moved from the out-of-hospital to the hospital setting. It is a team effort on the part of out-of-hospital, emergency-department, and critical-care team members.

The chain of survival has four distinct but interrelated links:

- **Early access**—recognition of the cardiac event, activating the appropriate response and resources, and seeking the necessary equipment
- **Early CPR**—performance of basic life support skills as early as possible
- **Early defibrillation**—providing defibrillation of ventricular fibrillation and pulseless ventricular tachycardia at the earliest possible point
- **Early ACLS**—rapid advanced-cardiac-life-support intervention following initiation of basic life support and early defibrillation

A break in any link of the chain of survival will reduce the chances for successful resuscitation. The components of each link may vary, depending on the setting and whether the cardiac arrest event occurs out of the hospital or in the hospital.

Use Judgment about Futile Resuscitation Attempts

Some patients have simply reached the end of their life and need to die with dignity. Resuscitation can be very demeaning and undignified to these patients and health care providers alike. Be decisive and use good judgment in determining when to start and when to stop resuscitation efforts. Be familiar with and follow your local guidelines, policies, procedures, or protocols. **Out-of-hospital and hospital personnel need to have considered when to start and stop resuscitation BEFORE care is needed.**

Chain of Survival

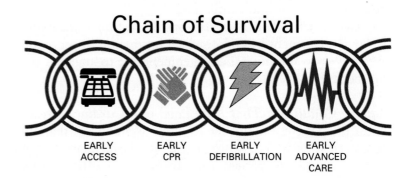

EARLY
ACCESS

EARLY
CPR

EARLY
DEFIBRILLATION

EARLY
ADVANCED
CARE

FIGURE 1-2 The chain of survival.
American Heart Association

The Phased-Response Approach: A Standardized Structure

The American Heart Association has developed a phased-response approach to cardiac arrests occurring in or out of the hospital (Table 1-2). This approach provides a standardized structure that should be applied during every cardiac arrest event.

Phase 1: Anticipation

This phase involves either the response of out-of-hospital care personnel or team anticipation of the cardiac arrest patient's arrival in the emergency department. Initial data should be analyzed, the team assembled, team leadership identified, duties and responsibilities assigned, equipment prepared and checked, and team members positioned.

Phase 2: Entry

The team leader identifies himself as the resuscitation begins or continues. Initial vital signs are obtained, patient transfer occurs, baseline laboratory values are ascertained, a brief history is gathered, and vital signs are repeated.

Phase 3: Resuscitation

Resuscitation efforts should adhere to and focus on the ABCs: airway, breathing, and circulation. The team leader must be decisive and provide direction to the team; however, he must also be open to and seek suggestions from the other team members. Orders must be precise and clearly stated. The team leader's voice, inflection, and attitude can set the stage for the whole resuscitation.

Team members must seek clarification of any orders that are unclear or questionable. Team members must state aloud when procedures are completed or medications have been administered.

Phase 4: Maintenance

In this phase, the patient is stabilized and secured. Attention should be continuously directed to maintaining the airway, breathing, and circulation.

TABLE 1-2 THE PHASED-RESPONSE APPROACH	
Phase 1	Anticipation
Phase 2	Entry
Phase 3	Resuscitation
Phase 4	Maintenance
Phase 5	Family Notification
Phase 6	Transfer
Phase 7	Critique Process

Phase 5: Family Notification
If possible, the family should be advised that resuscitation efforts have begun and be updated as appropriate. The family is, of course, notified of the outcome of the resuscitation. The outcome that is relayed may be positive or negative. Be prepared to deliver the message with empathy, sensitivity, and honesty.

Phase 6: Transfer
The patient transfer must be as smooth a transition as possible. Patient care is assumed by a team of equal or higher qualifications and expertise. It is essential that proper information is transferred before and with the patient.

Phase 7: Critique Process
A critique of the resuscitation should be conducted regardless of the patient outcome and length of resuscitation time. This is an educational process that provides critical feedback on the team's efforts. It also may be a time for defusing and grieving.

Ethical Considerations in Cardiac Resuscitation

Cardiac resuscitation must be initiated unless an attempt to resuscitate is clearly futile according to the physician in charge or under your local guidelines and protocols or there is a binding legal directive not to proceed.

Every patient who is deemed competent and capable of making a rational decision has the legal right to refuse medical care, including basic and advanced cardiac resuscitation. For the competent patient to refuse care it is not required that the patient be suffering from a terminal illness, nor that family members agree with the decision, nor that approval be obtained from the physicians or hospital administrators.

When the patient is unable to make an informed or rational decision at the time medical intervention is needed—for example, when the patient is already in cardiac arrest and unresponsive—the physician must rely on any advance directives (wishes the patient had previously expressed, either orally or in writing) or decisions rendered by a legal surrogate (such as a relative who has been given a power of attorney to make health care decisions for the patient).

Advance Directives and Surrogates
When a person anticipates that he may, at some future time, lose the ability to make an informed or rational decision regarding his own medical care or resuscitation, he may make his wishes known in advance of such an event. This is known as an advance directive. The most common advance directives occur in conversations with family, friends, or health care providers. However, for obvious reasons, oral directives are considered less trustworthy than directives that are written, and unwitnessed written directives are considered less trustworthy than witnessed written directives.

Most states have passed legislation that provides some way for citizens to help ensure that their wishes will be followed, or their best interests taken into consideration, if they become unable to make such decisions themselves. Some states recognize "living wills." In a living will, a person can state his desires regarding care in the event he becomes terminally ill and incapable of making decisions regarding his medical care. In other states, a person is permitted to designate a surrogate, or proxy—usually a close relative or friend—who holds a "durable power of attorney" to make health care decisions for the person if he becomes unable to do so for himself. In contrast to the living will, a durable power of attorney for health care applies to any medical situation, not just terminal illness.

For an advance directive to be effective, of course, the health care team must know about it. The optimal situation is when a legal document is present and can be verified before treatment begins. This is why persons who have such advance wishes and legal documents must make an effort to discuss them with and to provide copies to their physicians, medical facilities, and out-of-hospital services that are likely to treat them.

Very often, of course, this will not have happened when you are in a situation where care and resuscitation decisions have to be made, especially in the out-of-hospital setting. In these circumstances, you must rely on your own judgment and common sense as well as on local protocols and, when possible, orders from the physician or medical director in charge. Some states (such as Ohio) have passed legislation stating whether advance directives can be applied in an emergency situation. Be aware if there are laws of this sort in your state. If there is any doubt, initiate full advanced cardiac life support resuscitation.

Do-Not-Resuscitate and No-CPR Orders

Patients with serious illnesses, whether they are in or out of the hospital, often discuss do-not-resuscitate or no-CPR orders with their physician. These orders stipulate to what extent resuscitation, if any, should be conducted if the patient deteriorates to cardiac arrest. However, such stipulations should *not* be taken to imply that other forms of patient care or management must be limited or discontinued. Although no-CPR orders may exist, it is important to recognize that other medical treatments may be appropriate and acceptable, such as administration of antidysrhythmics or fluids. Oxygen is considered a standard comfort measure and should be administered to all patients who require it.

As yet, the terminology regarding no-resuscitation orders has not been standardized. A variety of terms are in use and may be confusing. The term *do not resuscitate (DNR)* implies that resuscitation would be successful if performed. Since resuscitation efforts often are not successful, the term *do not attempt resuscitation (DNAR)* may be more reflective of the chances of successfully resuscitating a patient. The term *no CPR* may be used to indicate that CPR should not be initiated or continued on the patient in the event of cardiac arrest. However, all three terms—*do not resuscitate (DNR), do not attempt resuscitation (DNAR),* and *no CPR*—have essentially the same meaning and are often used interchangeably.

DNR, DNAR, or no-CPR orders must not be confused with other kinds of advance directives such as living wills. Just because a living will or other advance directive exists, it does not necessarily mean that the patient wants CPR or resuscitation withheld. For example, a living will may stipulate that the patient does not want long-term efforts such as prolonged use of a ventilator, but may not prohibit short-term resuscitation efforts such as CPR and defibrillation. Living wills and other sorts of advance directives must be interpreted by a physician and must not be automatically used as, or in place of, a DNR, DNAR, or no-CPR order.

Initiation or cessation of patient resuscitation in both the out-of-hospital and hospital setting often poses ethical dilemmas. As stated earlier, it is imperative that you follow the guidelines or protocols for resuscitation established by the prehospital medical director or hospital ethics committee, legal counsel, and medical directors.

SUMMARY

To maximize the effectiveness of the resuscitation effort, it is essential to master the knowledge and skills relevant to basic and advanced airway management, ventilation and oxygenation, management of cardiovascular compromises, electrical therapy, IV therapy and invasive monitoring, recognition and management of lethal dysrhythmias, recognition and management of nonlethal dysrhythmias, administration of cardiovascular medications used in resuscitation, and recognition and early management for a variety of special resuscitation situations.

Certain key elements must be considered for every patient suffering cardiac arrest or cardiovascular or cardiopulmonary compromise. These include cerebral resuscitation; treating the patient, not the rhythm (keeping the big picture of patient care in mind, including airway, ventilation, oxygenation, medications, and defibrillation of appropriate rhythms); consideration of ACLS as part of a continuum of basic-to-advanced life support; consideration of time as a critical factor in successful resuscitation; management of conditions that may lead to cardiac arrest; continuation of care after successful resuscitation; applying the chain of survival to all situations; using judgment about futile resuscitations; and applying the phased-response approach to all cardiac arrest events.

It is important to be aware that patients may have given advance directives on their wishes regarding resuscitation. These advance directives may be oral or written, informal statements or legal documents. There may also be do-not-resuscitate or no-CPR orders that the patient has discussed with his physician or has presented as a written legal document. Use judgment and follow state and local guidelines or protocols regarding advance directives. If there is any doubt, initiate full resuscitation.

REVIEW QUESTIONS

1. One of the major goals of patient management during resuscitation is to
   a. determine the etiology of the cardiac arrest and the ECG rhythm.
   b. focus on the ECG rhythm and treat it according to the algorithm.
   c. provide medications prior to any electrical therapy or advanced airway management.
   d. administer as many medications as possible via the endotracheal route to enhance absorption.

2. The most critical factor that influences successful defibrillation is the
   a. energy level at which defibrillation is performed.
   b. amount of transthoracic resistance.
   c. time delay to defibrillation.
   d. ability to administer medications prior to defibrillation.

3. Which of the following is **not** a link in the chain of survival?
   a. early access
   b. early CPR
   c. early prevention
   d. early ACLS

4. A patient has the legal right to refuse medical care only if
   a. the patient is suffering from a terminal illness.
   b. the family is in agreement with the decision.
   c. the physician agrees and acquires approval from the hospital administrator.
   d. the patient is deemed competent and capable of making a rational decision.

5. You encounter a patient in cardiac arrest. The family presents a do-not-resuscitate (DNR) order. There is a question regarding the validity of the order. You should immediately
   a. contact the patient's family physician to verify the order.
   b. begin full advanced cardiac life support resuscitation until the order can be clarified.
   c. begin and continue basic life support until the family physician is contacted.
   d. consult the family regarding the validity of the order.

Chapter**Two**

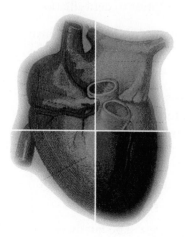

Systematic Approach to Emergency Cardiac Care: The Primary and Secondary Surveys

Emergency care providers are accustomed to the familiar assessment steps often known as the ABCDs, or the primary and secondary survey. These steps have been adapted to provide a systematic approach to assessing and managing a patient who is in cardiac arrest or suffering from a cardiopulmonary emergency.

Following the simple mnemonics of the primary and secondary survey for emergency cardiac care will ensure that the necessary basic and advanced care procedures are conducted in an organized and efficient sequence. It will counteract the tendency of some health care professionals to skip vital basic procedures and proceed directly to more advanced and dramatic skills such as placement of an endotracheal tube or a central line. It will also provide each member of the resuscitation team with a clearer understanding of his or her role in the resuscitation effort. Topics for this chapter are:

CASE STUDY

At the hospital, you are summoned to a patient's room by a woman who calmly informs you that she does not know whether her husband, the patient, is sleeping soundly or dead. As you enter the room, you find the 58-year-old male patient lying motionless in bed. He is ashen gray. You quickly ask the wife, "How long has he been like this?" as you step to the patient's side. The wife states, "Oh, only a few minutes, I think. He looked as if he was resting so peacefully."

How would you proceed to assess and care for this patient? This chapter will describe the systematic assessment of a patient in cardiac arrest or suffering a cardiorespiratory emergency. Later, we will return to the case and apply the procedures learned.

- Preliminary, Presurvey Actions
- Primary Survey
- Secondary Survey

Introduction

A systematic approach to providing care for patients suffering cardiac arrest or a cardiorespiratory emergency will assure a more organized resuscitation attempt. Also, it will lessen each health care practitioner's confusion as to his or her exact responsibility and the progression of the resuscitation.

A simple approach using an "ABCD" mnemonic for both a primary and secondary survey has been developed.[1] This approach provides standard guidelines that can easily be applied to all prearrest, actual arrest, and postarrest situations. In addition, if you ever reach a point where you are not sure what direction you should take next, you can step back and repeat the ABCDs to ensure that all necessary care is being provided.

Even before you conduct the primary and secondary surveys, there are some preliminary actions that must be performed. The results of these preliminary actions may determine how you will proceed in your resuscitation efforts. The preliminary actions are followed by a basic primary survey that does not involve invasive techniques, which in turn is followed by a more advanced secondary survey that requires invasive techniques of management. Both the primary and the secondary survey use the mnemonic ABCD, but the letters stand for something slightly different in each survey (Figure 2-1).

The remainder of this chapter will discuss the specifics of the preliminary actions, the primary survey, and the secondary survey for emergency cardiac care.

Preliminary, Presurvey Actions

Before providing any noninvasive or invasive care—before the "A" of the primary survey—you must take a few preliminary steps. You must assess

[1] American Heart Association, *Textbook of Advanced Cardiac Life Support,* 1994: 1-4–1-10.

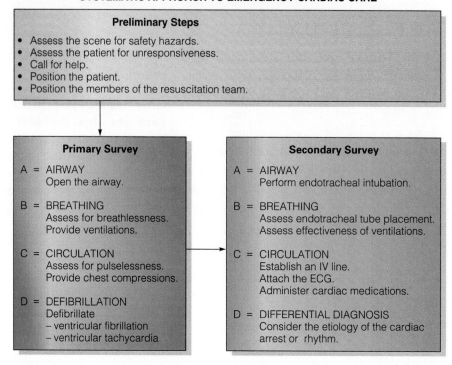

FIGURE 2-1 Systematic approach to emergency cardiac care.

your own safety before you approach the patient, and you must assess the patient's level of responsiveness, call for help, position the patient, and position the members of the resuscitation team as they enter the scene or resuscitation room.

Assess the Scene for Safety Hazards

Ensure your own safety before approaching any emergency scene. Of course, assessing the scene for safety hazards is more appropriate for out-of-hospital care providers than for those providing emergency cardiac care in a controlled environment. However, the environment that is thought to be controlled can just as easily become uncontrolled and hazardous. Do not become complacent, regardless of the environment you are in.

The cardiac arrest or cardiorespiratory patient is typically a highly charged scene; therefore it is easy for the health care provider to become totally engrossed in what care he or she is going to provide, develop tunnel vision while approaching the scene, and not use all of his senses to identify potential scene safety hazards. Many violent altercations have erupted, literally over patients in cardiac arrest. Health care providers can easily walk into these scenes when they are too hasty in approaching the patient.

It is not just violent scenes that may injure health care providers. A patient may be in cardiac arrest due to inhalation of a hazardous material. Health care providers hastily approaching this scene may succumb to the same hazardous fumes that overcame the patient. In some situations, the scene should not be approached.

The out-of-hospital environment is very uncontrolled and unforgiving, with a myriad of potential hazards. The basic principle is: If the scene is not safe, either make it safe without jeopardizing your own life, or retreat until it is made safe by law enforcement, fire service, or other appropriate agencies.

Similar safety issues may confront those providing care in a controlled environment such as a hospital emergency department. It is very possible for a patient to come into the emergency department in cardiac arrest and have a loaded gun or other weapon on his person. Similarly, a patient from a hazardous-material scene may have not been properly decontaminated and will pose similar hazards to the emergency department resuscitation team members.

Also assess the scene for clues to and evidence of the nature of the emergency, such as pill bottles, unusual odors, and mechanisms of traumatic injury.

Always remember the necessity of taking infection-control precautions for personal protection. Gloves, mask, and eye protection must be used to reduce the risk of infectious disease transmission through contact with body fluids.

Assess for Unresponsiveness

When you first come in contact with the patient, you must determine the level of responsiveness. You do this by gently shaking the person and shouting, "Are you OK?" If you suspect that the patient has suffered some type of trauma that may have injured the spinal column, do not shake and shout. Obviously, shaking can further destabilize the spinal column and shouting may cause the patient to move his head or body. Instead, "touch and talk" to the possible spine-injured patient.[2]

You must keep the suspected trauma patient's cervical spine in a neutral, in-line position with the remainder of the spine as straight as possible. Ideally, bring the head and neck into a neutral in-line position and maintain manual stabilization. Do this by bringing the nose in line with the umbilicus and keeping the head and neck neutral without any extension or flexion (Figure 2-2). Keep in mind that any manipulation of the cervical spine, and certainly any shaking, may cause or aggravate a spinal cord injury.

If the non-trauma patient responds to your shaking or shouting, or the trauma patient responds to your talking and touching, it is obvious that he

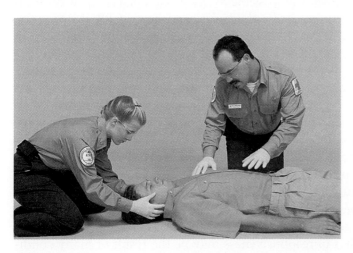

FIGURE 2-2 For the possible spine-injured patient, touch and talk to establish unresponsiveness. Maintain manual stabilization of the head and spine.

[2] American Heart Association, *Textbook of Advanced Cardiac Life Support,* 1994: 1-5.

or she is not in cardiac arrest. If there is no response, then you must proceed to assess the airway, breathing, and circulation. Remember also that a patient may make some response to shaking and shouting, or talking and touching, yet may still require airway management and ventilatory support.

Call for Help

Once unresponsiveness is confirmed, the first rule is to summon help immediately. In the out-of-hospital setting, a bystander who happens to be a health care professional may be the only one at the scene at the time of the incident—or a trained first responder may be the first person to arrive at the scene. That person must activate an advanced-life-support response by making radio contact with EMS or by dialing 911 or the appropriate emergency access number.

It is imperative to call for advanced cardiac life support (ACLS) in any potential cardiac arrest situation, either before or at the same time as basic cardiac life support (BCLS) measures are initiated. It is critical to the patient's chances for survival to get equipment and personnel to the scene for defibrillation, advanced airway management, and drug therapy as quickly as possible. Basic cardiac life support may maintain minimal perfusion of oxygenated blood until these advanced cardiac life-support measures can be initiated, but basic cardiac life support alone is unlikely to achieve a successful resuscitation. Delaying the call for advanced cardiac life support while basic cardiac life support is initiated is likely to be a fatal error. Even with CPR, the patient should optimally receive defibrillation and other advanced measures within 4 to 6 minutes and is unlikely to survive if these measures are not initiated before 10 minutes from the time of collapse.

In the hospital setting, it may be necessary to shout out or push a wall button to activate the resuscitation team. Immediate response with a "crash cart" and additional resuscitation team members is necessary. It may or may not be necessary to leave the patient's side when summoning additional help. In either case, it is your responsibility to be familiar with the method established to initiate the ACLS resuscitation team.

After summoning help, it is just as important for the care provider to return to the patient as quickly as possible to assess and open the airway, begin positive pressure ventilation, assess the pulse, and begin CPR if necessary. Out-of-hospital survival is directly related to decreasing the time interval from the onset of the cardiac arrest to the return of spontaneous and effective circulation. Although this is primarily achieved through defibrillation and other advanced care, don't forget that basic-life-support measures will provide the critical circulation of oxygenated blood until advanced care can begin.

The layperson has been taught to "phone first," then perform the steps of CPR when dealing with an unresponsive adult and no other help is available. As described above, the trained health care provider is also generally advised to call for help first. However, health care providers may sometimes face a dilemma because of their ability to provide care beyond the basic level, which their experience and judgment tells them may be more useful to the patient than immediately getting to the phone. The trained health care provider will know that unresponsiveness may be the result of many conditions other than cardiac arrest. For example, clues in the surrounding environment may suggest a drug overdose, head injury, or a choking incident. If you suspect an obstructed airway as the cause of unresponsiveness, then you must assess the airway and employ the foreign body airway obstruction maneuver immediately. You must use judgment, be decisive, and provide the most appropriate care possible given the patient situation.

Several special situations may arise when you are alone when you encounter a patient you suspect is in cardiac arrest. One special situation may be that you have access to a defibrillator, often an automated external defibrillator. In this situation, you should not delay defibrillation to seek additional help. Instead, perform the following steps after establishing unresponsiveness:

1. Call out for help.
2. Manually open the airway with a head-tilt, chin-lift or jaw-thrust maneuver.
3. Deliver two breaths to ensure a clear and open airway.
4. Assess the carotid pulse to confirm pulselessness.
5. Retrieve, apply, and operate the defibrillator.

Do not initiate chest compressions until after you have delivered the first set of three defibrillations. Only then, conduct one minute of CPR before reassessing the pulse and delivering another set of three defibrillations if the patient remains pulseless and in a shockable rhythm. The benefit of early defibrillation by far outweighs the consequent delay in initiating or continuing CPR.

Another special situation for you, as a lone care provider, may be that the nearest phone or nursing station is so far away it will take more than a few minutes to get to it. A delay in the initiation of CPR of 1 to 2 minutes to access EMS or obtain a defibrillator is acceptable for a patient who you suspect is in ventricular fibrillation. However, if an extended period of time would elapse while you activate EMS or obtain a defibrillator, then you must decide whether to initiate CPR or to leave the patient to seek help.

Suppose, for example, that you are in a desolate or remote area when you witness a cardiac arrest and there is no quick way to call for help. This patient is most likely in ventricular fibrillation. In this situation, it may be most appropriate to establish an airway and positive pressure ventilation, deliver several precordial thumps, and provide CPR for approximately 10 to 15 minutes. You would realize that CPR and precordial thumps alone are very unlikely to convert the rhythm and restore circulation, but under the circumstances they are somewhat more likely to help the patient than the arrival of advanced cardiac life support after a very long delay. It is most reasonable to continue CPR for about 10 to 15 minutes. If the resuscitation is unsuccessful after that period of time, then CPR can be stopped. The traditional recommendation to continue CPR until exhausted is unrealistic, since most fit individuals may be able to perform CPR for more than one hour.

Position the Patient

The patient in cardiac arrest must be placed on a firm surface. In the out-of-hospital setting, the patient is likely to be placed initially on the floor and then on a long backboard for transport. If resuscitation is to be conducted with a patient in a bed, a firm board or other support device must be placed under the posterior thorax. CPR boards are typically used for this purpose.

Resuscitation cannot be attempted on a patient who is in a prone, lateral, sitting, or semi-sitting position. The prone patient or patient lying on his side must be immediately rolled as a unit to a supine position, while the patient who is in a sitting or semi-sitting position must first be placed on the floor or other hard, flat surface. If a mechanism of injury exists that is consistent with possible cervical spine injury, such as a motor vehicle crash, diving accident, or a fall, it is necessary to take special precautions when moving the patient. The goal is to maintain the head, neck, and trunk of the body in a straight line.

If you are alone, kneel next to the patient and place one hand on the back of the head and neck. With the other hand, roll the patient over into a supine position. If two or more people are available to provide the move, position one person at the head of the patient to maintain the head and neck in a neutral in-line position. No traction or pulling force should be applied. Instead, simple manual stabilization by holding the head and neck in place is required. Other rescuers, directed by the person at the head, will roll the patient over as a unit. The patient's head, neck, and body must be maintained in a neutral in-line position throughout the resuscitation effort.

Position the Members of the Resuscitation Team

If you are working alone, your best position is at the level of the patient's shoulders. This gives you access to the chest and airway during CPR without the need to move your knees.

As other members of the resuscitation team arrive, it is important to place them in key positions to facilitate the best possible care to the patient. The person controlling the airway should be placed at the head of the patient. Chest compressions should be provided by a person who is beside the patient at the level of the thorax. The person operating the defibrillator must be able to see the oscilloscope and all members of the team to avoid accidental shocks to team members. The person establishing intravenous access must be positioned at the arm and not interfering with the chest compressor or defibrillator operator. Proper positioning can identify team member responsibility and provide for optimal safety of the resuscitation team. Excuse unnecessary personnel to reduce confusion and improve safety during the resuscitation attempt.

Primary Survey

The primary survey is a systematic approach to the patient that uses basic skills to open and maintain the airway, assess and assist ventilation, assess for pulselessness, initiate chest compressions, and provide defibrillation for ventricular fibrillation or pulseless ventricular tachycardia. The mnemonic ABCD is used to facilitate an organized approach to the patient and to counteract any desire to perform more invasive or advanced skills without first performing the vital basic skills of resuscitation (Table 2-1).

A = Airway: Open the Airway

Open and inspect inside the mouth for blood, vomitus, secretions, or other foreign materials. Immediately suction any blood, vomitus, or secretions. Remove foreign bodies with your gloved fingers covered in gauze. If you encounter heavy vomitus, turn the patient on his side and sweep the vomi-

TABLE 2-1 PRIMARY SURVEY FOR EMERGENCY CARDIAC CARE

Assessment	Critical Actions
A Airway	Suction any vomitus, secretions, or blood from the mouth. Remove any foreign material. Open the airway with manual maneuvers.
B Breathing	Assess for breathlessness. Provide positive pressure ventilation.
C Circulation	Assess for pulselessness. Provide chest compressions.
D Defibrillation	Assess for ventricular fibrillation or pulseless ventricular tachycardia. Defibrillate.

tus from the mouth until it is clear. Loose dentures may become completely dislodged and occlude the airway. Therefore, if the dentures are loose, remove them; if the dentures are firmly in place, leave them. If not loose, dentures provide a firm structure that enhances your ability to establish and maintain a good seal with a mask when performing bag-valve-mask or mouth-to-mask ventilation. However, dentures should be removed when intubation is attempted.

Open the airway using a manual maneuver. The head-tilt, chin-lift maneuver is the standard method of opening the airway. However, if a cervical spine injury is suspected, the head and neck must be maintained in an in-line neutral position. Use the jaw-thrust or chin-lift maneuver for the trauma patient with suspected neck or spine injury (Figure 2-3).

B = Breathing: *Assess for Breathlessness and Provide Ventilation*
Once the airway is opened and cleared of any foreign materials, place your ear close to the patient's nose and mouth while looking in the direction of

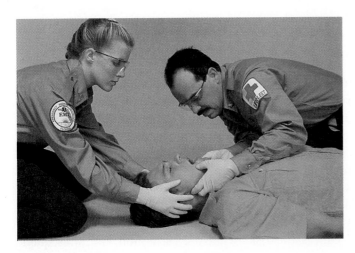

FIGURE 2-3 Use a head-tilt, chin-lift maneuver to open the airway of a medical patient, a jaw-thrust maneuver to open the airway of a trauma patient. Inspect and clear any foreign materials from inside the mouth.

FIGURE 2-4 Look, listen, and feel to assess breathing.

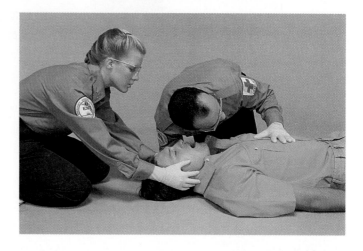

the patient's chest. To assess for adequate breathing, you will look, listen, and feel (Figure 2-4).

- **Look** at the patient's chest for spontaneous rise and fall or any other respiratory movement.
- **Listen** for any evidence of air moving out of the patient's nose or mouth.
- **Feel** for any air movement out of the nose or mouth.

Opening the airway may be the only intervention needed to resume spontaneous ventilation in some patients. However, most patients will require some type of positive pressure ventilation with supplemental oxygen. Airway management and effective ventilation are vital to the resuscitation effort. If an airway cannot be established or adequate ventilation performed, all other resuscitation efforts will be futile.

Once you have established that the patient is not breathing, you must consider the following:

- Absence of air movement, which may signify an airway obstruction
- Whether noninvasive or invasive maneuvers are necessary to dislodge the obstruction
- Which ventilation device will provide the most effective positive-pressure ventilation
- Which ventilation device can deliver high concentrations of oxygen
- The rate and volume necessary to adequately ventilate the patient
- Methods to determine whether the ventilation is effective or not

If possible and immediately available, insert an oropharyngeal airway and begin positive pressure ventilation with a pocket mask. The pocket mask should have a one-way valve to allow the patient's exhalation to be vented away from the mask and ventilator. An oxygen inlet port is also desirable. This basic ventilation device should be a standard piece of equipment in all patient care areas and on all crash carts.

Deliver two slow ventilations, each over a period of 1.5 to 2 seconds allowing for adequate exhalation between ventilations. Delivering the ventilations slowly, as described, rather than quickly or abruptly, decreases the esophageal opening pressure and reduces the risk of gastric distention and subsequent regurgitation and aspiration. In addition, cricoid pressure (direct posterior pressure placed on the anterior portion of the cricoid ring) should be applied to reduce the risk of gastric distention, regurgitation, and aspiration. Cricoid pressure should not be used, however, if there is suspicion of cervical injury.

With the first two ventilations, it is necessary to determine whether the ventilations were effective or not. If resistance was met or the chest did not rise or fall with the first ventilation, reposition the head with a manual airway maneuver before attempting the second ventilation. If resistance is still met, an airway obstruction may exist. Also, suspicion of airway obstruction is based on the history of events prior to the cardiac arrest, such as eating food.

Next you must determine what methods to employ to remove the obstruction: manual foreign body airway obstruction maneuvers or more advanced techniques like laryngoscopy and the use of McGill forceps. This will be determined by your level of training, experience, and available equipment. Remember, chest compressions without effective ventilations are useless. Refer to Chapter 3 for a more detailed discussion on airway management and ventilation techniques and equipment.

C = Circulation: *Assess for Pulselessness and Provide Chest Compressions*

According to the primary survey's systematic approach to the patient, once the airway has been opened, breathlessness established, and two ventilations delivered, you should next check the patient's carotid pulse. Check the pulse on the side of the patient that is closer to you for 5 to 10 seconds. An unresponsive patient who is not breathing and is pulseless is in full or complete cardiac arrest and needs cardiopulmonary resuscitation immediately.

You must initiate chest compressions along with effective positive pressure ventilation (Figure 2-5). Continuously assess for effectiveness of chest compressions and ventilations. The team leader will direct the initiation and cessation of compressions and ventilations.

D = Defibrillation: *Defibrillate Ventricular Fibrillation and Pulseless Ventricular Tachycardia*

A key concept of advanced cardiac life support is to provide defibrillation to the patient in ventricular fibrillation or pulseless ventricular tachycardia as

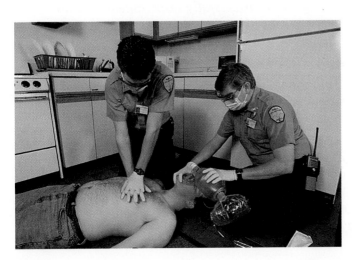

FIGURE 2-5 Initiate chest compressions and positive pressure ventilation.

FIGURE 2-6 Provide defibrillation of ventricular fibrillation or pulseless ventricular tachycardia as soon as possible.

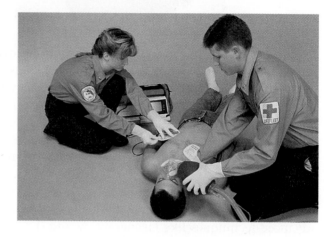

quickly as possible (Figure 2-6). In reality, a cascade of events leads to successful resuscitation of a cardiac arrest patient, but studies show that time to defibrillation is one of the most pivotal components in determining survival. Early defibrillation takes priority over airway management, ventilation, and chest compressions. Your goal should be to get a defibrillator to the patient as quickly as possible and provide defibrillation. As discussed earlier, that is one reason why the layperson is instructed to "phone first" after establishing unresponsiveness in the adult patient.

Two methods of external defibrillation are currently available. Many first responder units use automated or semi-automated external defibrillators (AEDs). These devices, which automatically determine the rhythm of the patient and the need to defibrillate, are relatively easy to use and can deliver defibrillations quickly to the patient. The manual defibrillator is used by more highly trained personnel and requires the operator to determine the rhythm and need for defibrillation. Regardless of the type of defibrillator being used, it is imperative to deliver three "stacked" shocks (three shocks in quick succession, without pausing to recheck for pulselessness) in the shortest time possible prior to any basic or advanced care.

When determining the importance of defibrillation, consider the following points, which have been confirmed in a number of clinical and epidemiological studies: [3, 4]

> *Most adults who have been successfully resuscitated from nontraumatic cardiac arrest (greater than 90% in most studies) were in ventricular fibrillation.*
>
> *The success of defibrillation is directly related to time to defibrillation.*
>
> *The patient in ventricular fibrillation or pulseless ventricular tachycardia has an estimated probability of 70% to 80% of surviving*

[3] Eisenberg, M. S., B. T. Horwood, R. O. Cummins, R. Reynolds-Haertle, T. R. Hearne, "Cardiac Arrest and Resuscitation: A Tale of 29 Cities," *Annals of Emergency Medicine,* 1990: 19:179-186.

[4] Eisenberg, M. S., R. O. Cummins, S. Damon, M. P. Larsen, T. R. Hearne, "Survival Rates from Out-of-Hospital Cardiac Arrest: Recommendations for Uniform Definitions and Data to Report," *Annals of Emergency Medicine,* 1990: 19:1249-1259.

upon succumbing to cardiac arrest at time zero. With each minute that passes, the probability of successfully defibrillating the patient to a perfusing rhythm decreases by about 2% to 10%.

If 10 minutes have passed since the collapse of the patient and you have not been able to defibrillate him, his chance of surviving is near zero.

Instruction in defibrillation has been implemented at various levels of training. This has been done to decrease the time to defibrillation of the patient.

For a detailed discussion of defibrillation, see Chapter 6.

Secondary Survey

The secondary survey is conducted immediately following conclusion of the primary survey. Like the primary survey, it also uses a systematic approach and the mnemonic ABCD, however with different definitions of each component (Table 2-2). The secondary survey concentrates on more advanced and invasive care, compared to the basic care provided in the primary survey. The steps in the secondary survey should be performed almost simultaneously.

The resuscitation team leader is the facilitator who directs patient care. Each team member should understand his role and perform his duties without specific direction from the team leader. If not enough trained personnel are available, the team leader may need to step in and perform the most essential steps of resuscitation.

It is recommended that endotracheal intubation precede intravenous access. This is because the endotracheal tube can provide a secure airway and serve as a drug route for some of the initial cardiac medications which can be administered via the trachea. In most situations, especially in the

TABLE 2-2 SECONDARY SURVEY FOR EMERGENCY CARDIAC CARE	
Assessment	**Critical Actions**
A Airway	Reassess basic manual maneuver effectiveness. Consider advanced airway care, most likely endotracheal intubation.
B Breathing	Assess ventilation effectiveness following endotracheal intubation or other advanced airway maneuvers.
C Circulation	Establish an intravenous line. Attach the continuous ECG monitor and identify the rhythm and rate. Assess blood pressure using noninvasive technique. Administer the appropriate drug therapy.
D Differential Diagnosis	Determine the etiology of the cardiac arrest or cardiac rhythm.

out-of-hospital environment, endotracheal intubation takes precedence over intravenous therapy.

A = Airway: Perform Endotracheal Intubation

Continue manual airway maneuvers while the patient and equipment are prepared for endotracheal intubation. Select the appropriate laryngoscope handle and blade, proper-sized endotracheal tube, a stylet, lubrication, 10 ml syringe, suction machine, and securing device. The specific equipment is dependent on the characteristics of the patient: short neck, fat neck, or anatomically challenged. Check all equipment while the patient is being hyperventilated. Use body substance isolation precautions, such as gloves and eye protection, when performing intubation. Perform the intubation without interrupting ventilations for greater than 30 seconds. If the attempt reaches 30 seconds, remove the laryngoscope and immediately resume hyperventilation for a period of 30 to 60 seconds. Reattempt the intubation following adequate oxygenation and hyperventilation.

An endotracheal tube isolates the trachea and is considered a definitive method to establish and maintain an airway. With an endotracheal tube in place, the airway is said to be "protected," since the distal cuff blocks any vomitus or secretions from traveling down the trachea and into the lungs (Figure 2-7). Endotracheal intubation should be performed at the earliest possible point to definitively secure the airway.

Other advanced airway adjuncts exist, such as the esophageal tracheal Combitube® (ETC) and the pharyngeotracheal-lumen (PtL®) airway; however, none is considered to be an adequate substitute for an endotracheal tube.

Cricoid pressure can be used to reduce the risk of gastric distention, regurgitation, and aspiration prior to and during the attempt at endotracheal intubation. Applying cricoid pressure also moves the glottic opening slightly posterior, facilitating visualization and tube placement during the intubation technique. Some studies have shown an increase of 10% in the success rate of intubation when cricoid pressure is performed.

If bag-valve-mask or pocket-mask ventilation appears to be effective in ventilating the patient, and there is no evidence of vomitus, regurgitation, or

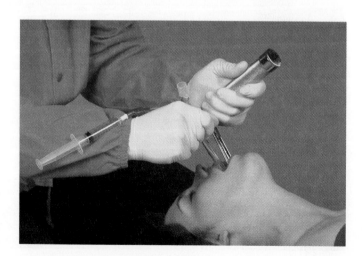

FIGURE 2-7 Protect the airway by inserting an endotracheal tube.

gastric distention, endotracheal intubation can be delayed while other interventions are performed.

For a detailed discussion of endotracheal intubation, see Chapter 3.

B = Breathing: Assess Endotracheal Tube Placement and Effectiveness of Ventilation

If the patient has been intubated with an endotracheal tube, you must assess for proper tube placement. During the first ventilation after tube placement, immediately inspect the chest for rise and auscultate over the epigastrium for sounds in the stomach. If sounds are heard over the epigastrium or the chest does not rise with the ventilation, the tube has probably been misplaced in the esophagus. Immediately remove the tube and begin hyperventilating the patient.

If no sounds are heard over the epigastrium and the chest rises with the ventilation, the tube has been placed in the trachea. However, it is still possible that the tube may have been advanced too far into one of the mainstem bronchi, thereby directing air into only one lung. To check for this possibility, auscultate for equal bilateral breath sounds over the midaxillary line at about the fourth or fifth intercostal space. Absent or decreased breath sounds on the left may indicate a right mainstem intubation. (Because of the lesser angle of the right mainstem bronchus, right mainstem intubation is far more common than left mainstem intubation.) Deflate the cuff and pull back on the tube 1 to 2 cm and reassess bilateral breath sounds. Repeat this procedure until equal breath sounds are heard bilaterally. One should also consider the unlikely possibility that a pneumothorax or fluid in the pleural cavity is the cause of inequality in breath sounds.

Other methods to assess tube placement are chest x-ray, end-tidal CO_2 detector, and endotracheal tube aspirator. The most reliable method is to visualize tube placement in the glottic opening with the laryngoscope if there is any doubt as to whether the tube is properly placed. If doubt of proper tube placement still exists, remove the tube, hyperventilate for 30–60 seconds, and continue ventilation with a bag-valve-mask or pocket mask device.

Continue to assess effective ventilation by watching the chest rise and fall and auscultating the chest (Figure 2-8). After every move of the

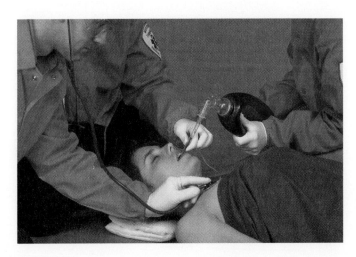

FIGURE 2-8 Ventilate the patient and assess for proper tube placement by watching for chest rise and auscultating the chest.

patient, such as from the ambulance stretcher to the emergency department bed, tube placement must be reassessed by auscultation over the epigastrium and chest.

If the patient is not intubated, continue to assess for effective ventilation by watching for adequate chest rise and fall. Monitor the stomach for evidence of gastric distention which, when present, may indicate the need to reposition the head and intubate the patient quickly.

C = Circulation: *Establish an IV Line, Attach the ECG, and Administer Cardiac Medications*

An intravenous line should be initiated, using a large bore catheter in the most accessible vein available, which is usually the antecubital vein (Figure 2-9). The solution of choice is 0.9% normal saline, which is an isotonic volume expander. There is a risk of causing pulmonary edema with large amounts of volume administered, but in the amounts given in this situation this has not been found to be a significant or frequent problem. Normal saline is relatively inexpensive and has a longer shelf life than many other solutions.

The use of glucose-containing solutions, such as D_5W, has been associated with poor neurologic outcomes in postresuscitation patients and those with other types of intracranial pathology. Therefore, the use of D_5W and other glucose-containing solutions should be avoided.

When administering medication by the intravenous route, elevate the arm and deliver a 20 to 30 ml bolus of fluid following injection of the medication. This will facilitate quicker entry into the central circulation.

Certain medications can be administered down the endotracheal tube. Lidocaine (Xylocaine), epinephrine, atropine, and naloxone (Narcan) can be given endotracheally. The mnemonic LEAN provides an easy method to remember the restricted number of drugs that are acceptable for endotracheal administration (Table 2-3).

To administer medication by the endotracheal route, it is necessary to thread a long catheter—a 35 cm intracatheter works well—down the endotracheal tube. The catheter should extend beyond the tip of the tube. Stop chest compressions, inject 2 to 2.5 times the regular dose of medication into the catheter and down the tube, and follow it with a 10 ml flush down the catheter. Attach the bag-valve or other ventilation device and

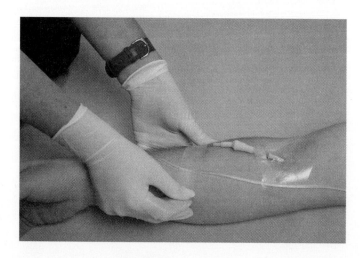

FIGURE 2-9 Initiate an intravenous line in the antecubital vein.

TABLE 2-3	RESUSCITATION MEDICATIONS ADMINISTERED BY THE ENDOTRACHEAL ROUTE	
L	lidocaine (Xylocaine)	
E	epinephrine	
A	atropine	
N	naloxone (Narcan)	

deliver 3 to 4 forceful ventilations to distribute the medication. A heparin lock with a 20 gauge needle pierced through the wall of the endotracheal tube may be used if an intracath or commercial catheter device is not available. The medications will be aerosolized during ventilation. Drug absorption, with endotracheal administration, is questionable; therefore, drugs should be administered endotracheally only in situations where an intravenous line is not available and only until an IV is available.

Attach the ECG monitor to allow for continuous monitoring of the cardiac rhythm. In order to detect any changes, it is important to constantly assess the rhythm both before and following any medication administration, defibrillation, or other intervention. Any change in rhythm necessitates a pulse check. If a pulse is found, the blood pressure is measured.

For more detailed discussions of intravenous access and medications, see Chapters 4 and 7.

D = Differential Diagnosis: Consider the Etiology of the Cardiac Arrest or Rhythm

At this point, the team leader must consider the actual cause of the cardiac arrest or specific rhythm. Just treating rhythms and not the patient as a whole will not necessarily lead to successful resuscitation of the patient, especially if the underlying cause of the cardiac arrest or rhythm is something other than coronary artery disease. A reversible cause to the condition should be sought in an attempt to regain spontaneous circulation.

Examine the rhythm and explore potential etiologies of that rhythm. As an example, might the severe symptomatic bradycardia be due to organophosphate poisoning in the migrant worker brought into the emergency department? Might the pulseless tachycardia be due to a tension pneumothorax in the patient found in cardiac arrest at the bottom of the steps? Could the sinus tachycardia be due to occult gastrointestinal bleeding in the nursing home patient? or due to dehydration in the patient with the flu? These are the types of questions that must be considered when evaluating the patient.

The desire is to treat the patient as a whole, and not just the rhythm, as a part of comprehensive patient care. Decisions on patient management may be based on the questions and answers regarding cardiac arrest and rhythm etiology. Do not develop tunnel vision and treat only the rhythm when, in fact, the rhythm may have a reversible etiology. This will only lead

CASE STUDY FOLLOW-UP

Preliminary Presurvey Actions

You have been called into a hospital room by the wife of a 58-year-old male patient to check if he is in just a deep sleep or in cardiac arrest. As you enter the room, there are no apparent safety hazards. You note the patient is ashen gray and motionless. You move to his side, shake him, and shout, "Mr. O'Brien, Mr. O'Brien, are you okay?" but there is no response. You reach for the button on the wall to call for a "code-blue." The express team will bring a monitor/defibrillator, crash cart with the intubation and intravenous equipment and drugs, and a CPR board.

Primary Survey

You move to Mr. O'Brien's head and open his airway with a head-tilt, chin-lift maneuver. You note vomitus in his mouth as you open it. Two members of the resuscitation team, Mary and John, arrive with the monitor/defibrillator, crash cart, and CPR board. You immediately instruct Mary to suction the vomitus from the airway. Once it is clear, you position your ear close to Mr. O'Brien's nose and mouth and look toward his chest. You inspect for chest rise and fall while listening and feeling for air movement. You do not detect any respiratory movement and indicate this to Mary.

Mary inserts an oropharyngeal airway and, using a pocket mask, delivers two ventilations over a 4-second period while you check for a carotid pulse for 5 seconds. You state, "No pulse—start chest compressions." John, who has been in position beside Mr. O'Brien, slides the firm CPR board under him, finds the correct landmark on his chest, and begins compressions.

You move the crash cart with the monitor/defibrillator into position next to Mr. O'Brien. You turn on the monitor, switch the lead indicator to paddles, stop CPR, and perform a "quick-look" after applying the defib pads to the chest. The oscilloscope shows coarse ventricular fibrillation. You immediately charge the paddles to 200 joules, inspect around the patient, and yell, "I'm clear, you're clear, everybody's clear," then deliver the first shock. The oscilloscope still shows ventricular fibrillation. With the paddles

to an unsuccessful resuscitation. Always perform a complete physical exam and patient history to identify possible reversible causes of the cardiac arrest or dysrhythmia. For more information on rhythm recognition and assessment, see Chapter 5, Dysrhythmia Recognition, and Chapter 10, Case Studies: Application Exercises.

SUMMARY

Within this chapter we have covered a systematic assessment and management approach to the patient who is in cardiac arrest or suffering from a cardiorespiratory emergency. By using the mnemonic ABCD, it is easy to remember an organized, appropriate, and efficient approach to assess and manage the patient. It is imperative that the care move from the basic procedures in the primary survey to the more advanced care in the secondary survey.

Much more information will be provided in the following chapters regarding airway management and ventilation, oxygen therapy, electrical therapy, ECG interpretation, and drug therapy. Resuscitation required in specific cases and conditions will also be discussed.

It is important to apply this standard approach to every patient suffering cardiac arrest or a cardiorespiratory emergency. This will provide you

(continued)

still on the chest, you charge to 300 joules, clear the patient a second time, and deliver the shock. Mr. O'Brien remains in ventricular fibrillation, so you charge to 360 joules, clear the patient, and deliver the third shock. You watch the oscilloscope as John checks the carotid artery for a pulse. The patient remains pulseless. You instruct John to resume chest compressions as Mary resumes ventilations.

Secondary Survey

Two other team members, Heather and Matt, arrive. Matt prepares intubation equipment for Mary as Heather spikes a 500 ml bag of normal saline and prepares equipment to gain intravenous access. Matt applies cricoid pressure as Mary performs the laryngoscopy and inserts the endotracheal tube. She assesses, finds indications of proper tube placement, and secures the tube in place. She resumes bag-valve ventilation with oxygen attached to the reservoir and set at 10 lpm.

You attach the electrodes to Mr. O'Brien's chest and set the lead selector to Lead II. Heather establishes an intravenous line with a 14-gauge angiocath in the antecubital vein. Once the IV line is secure, you call for the administration of 1 mg of epinephrine intravenously. Heather calls back the order and administers the drug by IV bolus. She elevates Mr. O'Brien's arm and gives a 30 ml bolus of fluid.

Sixty seconds go by and you stop compressions to reassess the rhythm. It is still ventricular fibrillation. You clear yourself and the team, charge the defibrillator to 360 joules, and deliver the shock. John indicates "No pulse" and continues chest compressions. You continue to alternate medications with defibrillation as Mr. O'Brien remains in ventricular fibrillation.

You begin to try to determine the cause of the arrest and start looking for clues as to why the patient will not convert. Is it severe lactic acidosis? Is it profound hypoxia? How long was Mr. O'Brien in cardiac arrest before his wife noticed?

You continue to attempt to resuscitate the patient and alter the management based on your differential diagnosis and suspected etiology.

and the entire resuscitation team a guideline to ensure that the best possible emergency cardiac care is afforded to the patient.

REVIEW QUESTIONS

1. Unresponsiveness should be assessed
   a. after opening the airway.
   b. after the initial pulse check.
   c. after assessing the scene for safety hazards.
   d. after delivery of the first two ventilations.

2. You are summoned by the waiter to assist a woman who suddenly becomes cyanotic while eating her dinner at a local restaurant. As a trained health care provider, it would be most appropriate to
   a. establish unresponsiveness, open the airway, and attempt to ventilate.
   b. immediately begin the foreign body airway obstruction removal maneuvers.
   c. go to the phone and dial 911 to get a defibrillator to the scene immediately.
   d. establish unresponsiveness, open the airway, and begin chest compressions.

3. A patient found at the bottom of one flight of steps is unresponsive. You should next
   a. perform a head-tilt, chin-lift maneuver to open the airway.
   b. establish manual in-line stabilization and open the airway using a jaw thrust maneuver.
   c. take manual stabilization of the head and perform a head-tilt, chin-lift to open the airway.
   d. keep the head and neck in a neutral position and begin ventilation.

4. When conducting the primary survey, it is appropriate to
   a. perform basic airway management, ventilations, chest compressions, and initial defibrillation.
   b. establish an intravenous line, administer medications, and intubate the patient.
   c. perform chest compressions, initiate intravenous therapy, administer medications, and defibrillate.
   d. establish an airway by endotracheal intubation, suction, perform hyper-ventilation, and initiate chest compressions.

5. The most important variable related to successful defibrillation is
   a. antiarrhythmic medication administration.
   b. successful endotracheal intubation.
   c. time to defibrillation.
   d. establishing an airway.

6. The recommended order in which you should proceed during the secondary survey is
   a. perform endotracheal intubation, establish an intravenous line, and administer medications.
   b. establish an intravenous line, perform endotracheal intubation, and administer medications.
   c. attach the ECG monitor, administer medications, and perform endotra-cheal intubation.
   d. determine a differential diagnosis, establish an intravenous line, and administer drugs.

7. Which of the following drugs is **not** appropriate for endotracheal adminis-tration?
   a. Narcan   c. bretylium
   b. epinephrine   d. atropine

8. What intravenous solution is preferred for use in a cardiac arrest patient?
   a. lactated Ringer's
   b. normal saline
   c. 5% dextrose in water
   d. 45% normal saline and 5% dextrose

9. What is the appropriate dose for medications being administered endotracheally?
    a. 1 to 2 times the standard IV dose
    b. the standard IV dose
    c. 2 to 2.5 times the standard IV dose
    d. half the standard IV dose

10. The differential diagnosis is conducted as part of the
    a. preliminary actions prior to patient interventions.
    b. secondary survey after medication administration has been initiated.
    c. primary survey following the initiation of chest compressions.
    d. interval between the primary and secondary survey.

Chapter**Three**

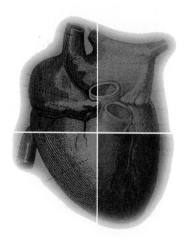

Airway Management, Ventilation, and Oxygen Therapy

The most important skills that you will perform in an acute emergency are airway management and ventilatory support, no matter what level of care is being provided to a patient. Without a patent airway and adequate ventilation and oxygenation, all other interventions will be futile. Some patients may require basic airway management, whereas others may require more advanced or surgical airway interventions. Likewise, ventilatory support may involve very basic equipment to more advanced ventilatory devices. The care you will be able to provide and equipment you can use will depend on your level of training and experience.

The topics to be covered in this chapter are:

- Airway Assessment
- Basic Airway Management Techniques

CASE STUDY

You are frantically summoned by Mr. Brookley to come immediately to check on his wife. He states, "She was talking with me and suddenly fell back in bed, began gasping, and became unconscious." As you walk into the room, you notice Mrs. Brookley, who is approximately 75 years of age, lying back in bed and beginning to appear ashen gray and cyanotic. Heavy vomitus is streaming from her mouth as you approach the bed. Her husband pleads, "Please do something for her," as you signal for help and ask him to leave the room.

How would you proceed to assess and manage the airway and ventilation for this patient? This chapter will describe the assessment and management of a patient with airway and ventilatory compromise. Also, oxygen therapy will be reviewed. Later we will return to the case and apply the procedures learned.

- Advanced Airway Management Techniques
- Alternative Orotracheal Intubation Techniques
- Alternative Airway Adjuncts
- Translaryngeal and Transtracheal Airways
- Ventilation Techniques
- Suction
- Oxygen Therapy

Introduction

Airway management is one of the most fundamental skills you will need when caring for patients suffering from acute medical illnesses. Without a patent airway, all other interventions will be futile. Airway management may be as simple as performing a head-tilt, chin-lift maneuver or as complex as performing a surgical cricothyrotomy to relieve an airway obstruction. The key objective is to intervene rapidly to reverse any real or potential obstruction and to establish and maintain a patent airway.

Assessing the adequacy of ventilation and oxygenation is another basic skill you must master to deal with acute medical crises. Your ability to determine the severity of respiratory compromise and the need for positive pressure ventilation when spontaneous breathing is inadequate or absent will be of utmost importance. Administration of supplemental oxygen to a patient suffering from any type of cardiac or respiratory compromise is also a fundamental skill. Several methods of providing positive pressure ventilation and oxygen therapy will be discussed in this chapter.

Airway Management

In order to have adequate ventilation and oxygenation, the airway must be open. Therefore, airway assessment is the first component of the initial assessment of the patient. Upper airway obstruction may result from displacement of the tongue; from food, blood, vomitus, or foreign objects; or from edema associated with epiglottitis, burns, trauma, or anaphylaxis.

A patient with an altered mental status can easily suffer from an upper airway occlusion as a result of relaxation of the submandibular muscles that provide direct control of the tongue and indirect control of the epiglottis. As the muscles relax, the tongue is displaced posteriorly and occludes the airway at the level of the pharynx, while the relaxed epiglottis causes occlusion at the level of the larynx.

Airway Assessment

An alert patient who is talking or crying is assumed to have an open airway. Therefore, you can form a general impression of airway status upon your initial approach to the alert patient. If the patient has an altered mental status and is not alert, you should assume that the patient has lost his gag and cough reflex and cannot effectively control his own airway. Aggressive and rapid intervention will be necessary to reverse or prevent occlusion of the airway or aspiration of foreign material into the trachea and lungs.

In a patient with an altered mental status, you will have to open the patient's mouth to assess for airway occlusion. Use a crossed-finger technique to open the mouth (Figure 3-1). Inspect inside the mouth for any evidence of secretions, blood, vomitus, or other potential obstructions. You may need to immediately apply suction or finger sweeps to remove the material to clear a potential or actual occlusion and prevent aspiration of foreign material into the lungs. If the patient is breathing, a noisy airflow during inspiration may indicate a significant airway obstruction. When assessing the upper airway, listen for the following sounds that may indicate significant airway obstruction:

- **Sonorous sounds** or **snoring** occurs when the upper airway is partially occluded by the tongue or other tissue in the pharynx.
- **Crowing** is a sound similar to that of a cawing crow that indicates laryngeal muscular spasm and narrowing of the tracheal opening.
- **Gurgling** indicates the presence of fluids or fluidlike substances such as blood or vomitus in the upper airway. Gurgling signals the need for immediate suction to remove the substance.

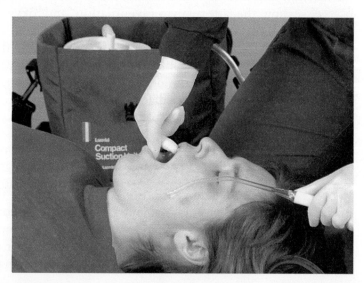

FIGURE 3-1 Use a crossed-finger technique to open the mouth.

- **Stridor** is a harsh, high-pitched sound heard upon inspiration, usually associated with laryngeal edema.

Central cyanosis, an indicator of significant hypoxia, is a late sign of airway obstruction. Retractions of the suprasternal notch, supraclavicular spaces, and intercostal spaces may also be signs of airway obstruction in the patient who appears to be breathing spontaneously. This patient should be treated as if a complete airway obstruction is present.

If airway obstruction is caused by foreign material in the mouth and upper airway, you need to remove it as rapidly as possible by suction or by sweeping the substance clear from the mouth. If no spine injury is suspected, you may need to place the patient in the recovery (lateral recumbent) position to facilitate the removal of the material and prevent possible aspiration.

If the airway is obstructed by a foreign body, initially attempt to manage it with basic foreign-body-obstruction maneuvers. If unsuccessful, you may need to employ advanced techniques, such as direct laryngoscopy and removal of the foreign body by Magill forceps.

If the airway is obstructed by the tongue or epiglottis, relieve the obstruction by manually positioning the head. Insert a mechanical airway if the manual maneuver is insufficient in establishing or maintaining the airway.

Endotracheal intubation is the preferred method of advanced airway management. The airway is considered to be "protected" once the endotracheal tube is properly placed. Less-preferred devices used to manage the airway are the pharyngeo-tracheal lumen (PtL®) airway, the esophageal-tracheal Combitube® (ETC), the esophageal obturator airway (EOA), and the esophageal gastric tube airway (EGTA). These devices are recommended only if endotracheal intubation is not available or not successful.

In the event you cannot achieve a patent airway by employing a manual maneuver or by inserting a mechanical device, you may have to proceed to a surgical airway. Transtracheal catheter ventilation (also called needle cricothyrotomy) and cricothyrotomy are the two methods to consider. These procedures are rarely performed and are used only in specific situations and after attempts at manual and mechanical airway control methods have failed.

Basic Airway Management Techniques

Basic airway management techniques include the use of manual maneuvers and simple airway adjuncts to establish and maintain an open airway. Use the necessary body substance isolation precautions, such as gloves and eye protection, when managing a patient's airway.

Manual Airway Maneuvers

The two manual maneuvers are the head-tilt, chin-lift and jaw-thrust technique. The head-tilt, chin-lift maneuver is most commonly used. However, if a spinal injury is suspected, the jaw-thrust maneuver is performed while the head and neck are maintained in a neutral in-line position.

Head-Tilt, Chin-Lift Maneuver

Loss of tone of the submandibular muscles in the patient with an altered mental status causes the tongue to be displaced posteriorly, partially occluding the airway at the level of the pharynx. The epiglottis indirectly loses support and creates an airway occlusion at the level of the larynx. By lifting the mandible forward, the tongue is displaced anteriorly away from the hypopharynx and the epiglottis is pulled up away from the glottic opening, relieving the obstruction at both the pharynx and larynx.

Perform the head-tilt, chin-lift maneuver by placing the palm of one hand on the patient's forehead and the tips of the fingers of the other hand under the bony part of the mandible. Avoid compression of the soft tissues under the mandible, which might obstruct the airway. Lift the mandible while tilting the head backward (Figure 3-2).

Jaw-Thrust Maneuver

The jaw-thrust maneuver, like the head-tilt, chin-lift maneuver, moves the mandible forward, causing the tongue to be pulled away from the hypopharynx. Unlike the head-tilt, chin-lift maneuver, however, the jaw-thrust maneuver does not tilt the head backward. In the spine-injured patient, the head and cervical spine must be maintained in a neutral in-line position to prevent or reduce the chances of further injury to the spinal column and spinal cord. The jaw-thrust maneuver is the preferred method used to open the airway, since the head and neck are not flexed or extended during the maneuver. The jaw thrust should be employed if the head-tilt, chin-lift maneuver is unsuccessful in opening the airway or if a cervical spine injury is suspected.

ADULT

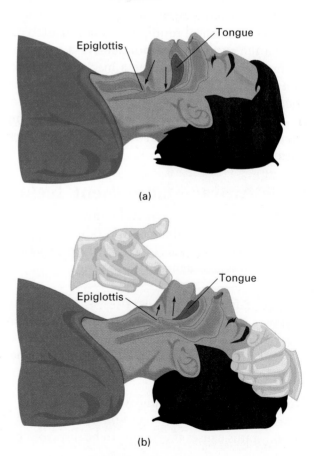

(a)

(b)

FIGURE 3-2 The head-tilt, chin-lift maneuver.

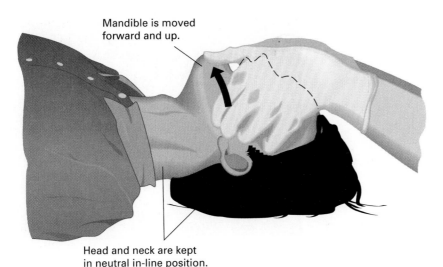

Mandible is moved forward and up.

FIGURE 3-3 The jaw-thrust maneuver.

Head and neck are kept in neutral in-line position.

To perform a jaw thrust, position yourself at the head of the patient. Place one hand at each side of the patient's head. While maintaining the head in a neutral in-line position, place one hand at each side of the patient's head. Grasp the angles of the mandible with the index, middle, and ring fingers. With the thumbs on the chin, move the mandible forward. Retract the lower lip with the thumb if necessary to open the mouth (Figure 3-3).

Either the head-tilt, chin-lift or the jaw-thrust maneuver must be performed prior to insertion of any type of airway adjunct. An airway occlusion may be relieved simply by manual positioning. However, it may be necessary to insert an airway adjunct to maintain airway control.

Basic Mechanical Airway Adjuncts

The simple airway adjuncts that require minimal skill to insert are the oropharyngeal airway and the nasopharyngeal airway. Both adjuncts extend down to the level of the hypopharynx. It must be emphasized that neither manual maneuvers nor simple airway adjuncts protect the airway or prevent aspiration of substances into the trachea and lungs. The following general principles apply to both oropharyngeal and nasopharyngeal airway adjuncts:

- The adjunct can become obstructed by secretions or vomitus. For an adjunct to be effective, it must be kept clear of any foreign material.
- The adjunct must be properly sized to avoid potential complications from its use.
- The adjunct does not protect the airway. Aspiration of blood, secretions, vomitus, or other foreign substances can occur with the adjunct properly in place.
- Both adjuncts require the patient to have an altered mental status. The oropharyngeal airway requires that the patient have a complete loss of gag reflex. Careful and continuous monitoring of the mental status is necessary when either device is used. Recovery of the gag reflex as a result of improved mental status while an airway adjunct is in place is likely to cause vomiting and aspiration.

FIGURE 3-4 Oropharyngeal airways.

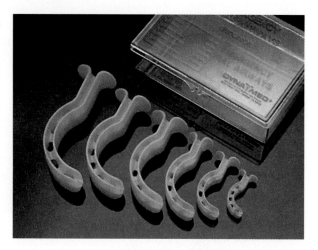

Oropharyngeal Airway

Also known as the oral airway, the oropharyngeal airway is semicircular, typically disposable, and made of a hard plastic. The Guedel and Berman are the two most frequently used types. The Guedel is tubular and has a hollow center. The Berman is solid and has channeled sides (Figure 3-4).

It is inserted into the oral cavity and displaces the tongue away from the posterior pharyngeal wall.

Even with this airway in place, it is necessary to maintain manual positioning of the airway by a head-tilt, chin-lift or jaw-thrust maneuver.

Indications for the Oropharyngeal Airway The oropharyngeal airway is used as an adjunct for airway control. The patient must be unresponsive and must not have a gag reflex. Insertion of the device in a patient with a gag reflex may stimulate gagging, vomiting, or laryngeal spasm, further complicating the airway. If the patient regains a gag reflex, it is necessary to remove the airway. The airway may be inserted following successful endotracheal intubation to serve as a bite block to prevent the patient from biting down on and possibly occluding the endotracheal tube.

Sizing the Oropharyngeal Airway Oropharyngeal airways come in a variety of infant, child, and adult sizes. The size is a measurement of the distance from the distal tip to the proximal flange. Determine the proper size by holding the airway next to the side of the patient's face and measuring the length of the airway from the corner of the mouth to the tragus of the ear or tip of the earlobe, or from the center of the mouth to the angle of the mandible (Table 3-1).

TABLE 3-1 RECOMMENDED SIZES OF OROPHARYNGEAL AIRWAYS		
	Length	Guedel Size
Large Adult	100 mm	5
Medium Adult	90 mm	4
Small Adult	80 mm	3

INSERTING AN OROPHARYNGEAL AIRWAY

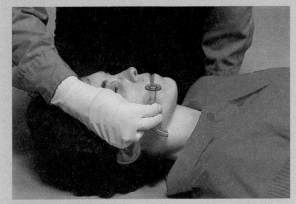

FIGURE 3-5a Measure to assure correct size.

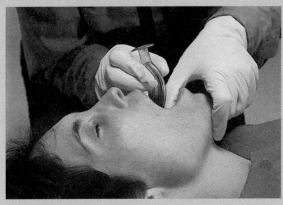

FIGURE 3-5b Insert with top pointing up toward roof of mouth.

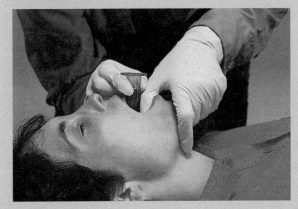

FIGURE 3-5c Advance while rotating 180°.

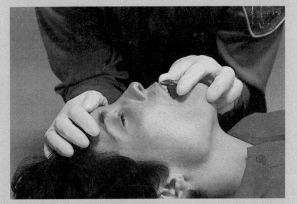

FIGURE 3-5d Continue until flange rests on the teeth.

Technique of Oropharyngeal Airway Insertion There are various methods of insertion. In the first method, insert the airway upside down with the distal tip facing the back of the hard palate. When the tip reaches the hard palate, rotate the airway to a ninety-degree position. As insertion continues, rotate the airway into the proper anatomical position until the flange of the proximal end of the airway is seated on the teeth (Figures 3-5a to 3-5d). Rotating the airway too early may actually push the tongue into the hypopharynx, worsening or causing an airway obstruction.

An alternative method is to insert the airway into the mouth at a ninety-degree angle, with the airway in a sideways position, then proceed with the insertion into the pharynx.

The preferred method of insertion, especially for infants and children, is with the use of a tongue blade (Figure 3-6). Insert the tip of the tongue blade into the mouth to the base of the tongue, then lift the tongue up and forward away from the posterior pharyngeal wall. Insert the airway in its correct anatomical position, past the tongue, into the airway. The airway is inserted properly when the tongue is displaced forward and the flange is seated on the teeth (Figure 3-7).

FIGURE 3-6 The preferred method of insertion, especially for infants and children, is with the use of a tongue blade.

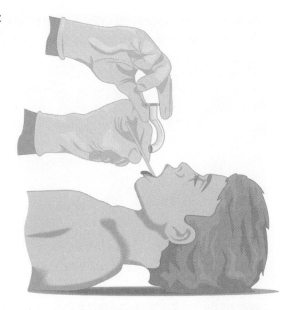

If the patient gags during insertion, immediately remove the airway and be prepared for vomiting. It may be necessary to see if the patient can tolerate a nasopharyngeal airway, if an adjunct is still desirable, or to reconsider the use of an adjunct. If the patient dislodges the airway with his tongue, remove it by gently pulling the airway out. Be prepared for vomiting.

Complications Associated with the Oropharyngeal Airway As already mentioned, insertion of the oropharyngeal airway in a conscious or responsive patient or one who has an intact gag reflex will likely cause vomiting. This will further complicate the airway and may lead to aspiration of gastric contents. Also, laryngeal spasm caused by insertion of the airway may result in airway obstruction at the level of the larynx. Positive pressure ventilation may be necessary to relieve the laryngospasm.

An improperly sized airway may result in one of two complications: If it is too long, it may push the epiglottis closed over the glottic opening of the larynx, causing a complete airway obstruction. Too short an airway may be easily misplaced and the distal opening of the airway obstructed by the tongue.

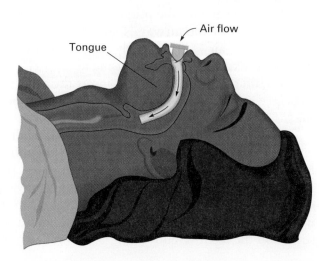

Air flow

Tongue

FIGURE 3-7 Oropharyngeal airway properly placed. The tongue is kept from falling back to occlude the patient's airway.

Complications may also arise from insertion. An improperly inserted airway can easily push the tongue back into the pharynx, causing or aggravating an airway obstruction.

Aggressive insertion, especially if using the technique in which the airway is inserted in its reverse position, may cause trauma to the upper airway and bleeding, particularly in children. To prevent any additional trauma, be sure that the lips and tongue are not between the teeth and the airway.

The lumen of the tube is not large enough to allow for suctioning. Suctioning must be performed around the tube.

Nasopharyngeal Airway

The nasopharyngeal airway, also known as the nasal airway, is a curved hollow tube constructed of soft plastic or rubber with a bevel at the distal end and a flange or flare at the proximal end (Figure 3-8). This airway is less likely to stimulate gagging and vomiting because the soft, pliable tube moves and flexes as the patient swallows, lessening the gag response. Therefore, it may be used in a less responsive patient who is spontaneously breathing but needs assistance in maintaining a patent airway. If a patient does not tolerate insertion of an oropharyngeal airway but needs an airway adjunct, insert the nasopharyngeal airway.

The tube is approximately 15 cm in length. When properly sized and inserted, the distal tip sits at the posterior pharynx while the proximal flare or flange is seated on the external nare. The hollow tube facilitates air flow from the proximal end, past the tongue, and into the hypopharynx.

The nasopharyngeal airway also requires that a manual airway maneuver, the head-tilt chin-lift or jaw-thrust maneuver, be maintained during its use.

Indications for the Nasopharyngeal Airway Insertion of the nasopharyngeal airway is indicated when the oropharyngeal airway is not able to be inserted due to trismus, mandibular trauma, mandibulo-maxillary wiring, or an intact gag reflex. This is the airway of choice for the spontaneously breathing, but less-responsive patient needing airway control.

Sizing the Nasopharyngeal Airway The size of the nasopharyngeal airway indicates the internal diameter (i.d.) in millimeters (mm). As the internal diameter increases, so does the length of the tube. To size the airway, place the proximal end of the tube at the tip of the nose and the distal end at the earlobe on the side of the face. The properly sized tube should extend from the tip of the nose to the earlobe. In addition, be sure not to select a tube with an external diameter that is greater than the internal diameter of the nare (Table 3-2).

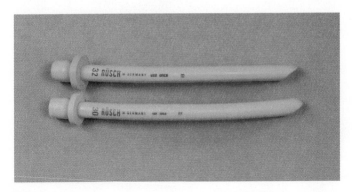

FIGURE 3-8 Nasopharyngeal airways.

TABLE 3-2 RECOMMENDED NASOPHARYNGEAL AIRWAY SIZES	
Large Adult	8.0 to 9.0 i.d.
Medium Adult	7.0 to 8.0 i.d.
Small Adult	6.0 to 7.0 i.d.

Technique of Nasopharyngeal Airway Insertion Make sure the nasopharyngeal airway is well lubricated with a water-soluble lubricant or an anesthetic jelly such as 2% lidocaine gel. This facilitates insertion and reduces the incidence of nasopharyngeal trauma and subsequent bleeding. Be sure to select the proper-sized airway prior to insertion. Advance the nasopharyngeal airway, with the distal beveled end toward the septum, posteriorly, aiming toward the back of the head (Figures 3-9a to 3-9c).

Attempting to advance the airway cephalically (upward) will only result in resistance. Gently guide the tube along the floor of the nostril

INSERTING A NASOPHARYNGEAL AIRWAY

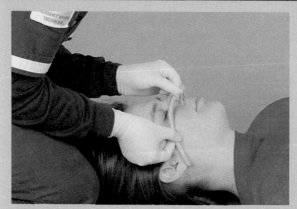

FIGURE 3-9a Measure the airway.

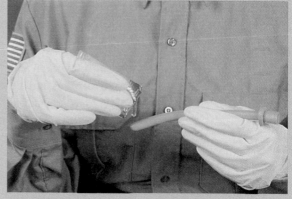

FIGURE 3-9b Lubricate it with water-soluble lubricant.

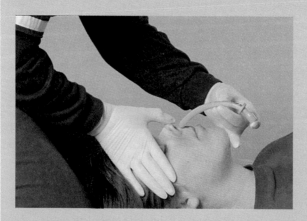

FIGURE 3-9c Insert with the bevel toward the septum or the base of the tonsil.

through the nasopharynx and into the posterior pharynx. In the spontaneously breathing patient, you should feel airflow at the proximal end of the tube. Immediately remove the tube if you feel no airflow in the spontaneously breathing patient.

If you meet resistance when inserting the airway, rotate the tube slightly while continuing. If you continue to meet resistance, you may have to remove the airway and insert it in the opposite nare. Significant trauma and bleeding may result if you force the airway into the nasopharynx.

Complications Associated with Use of the Nasopharyngeal Airway Several complications associated with the nasopharyngeal airway may arise during its use. An airway that has been improperly sized and is too long may be inadvertently inserted into the esophagus. This will result in gastric insufflation and subsequent gastric distention and hypoventilation during positive pressure ventilation. An airway that is too short may easily be occluded by the tongue in the posterior pharynx.

Insertion of the airway in the less responsive patient may cause laryngospasm. If the gag reflex is still intact and stimulated, vomiting may occur. This will further complicate airway management and may lead to aspiration of gastric contents.

Trauma to the nasal mucosa with bleeding may also result from insertion. Because the nasopharyngeal airway does not isolate the trachea, the blood may be aspirated into the trachea and lungs.

Advanced Airway Management Techniques

You may have to perform advanced airway management skills to establish, maintain, or protect the patient's airway. Also, when prolonged ventilation is necessary, you must consider advanced airway management to avoid some of the common complications associated with traditional airway management and ventilation techniques. Advanced airway management techniques are most commonly used:

- To protect the patient from aspiration of secretions, blood, vomitus, or other foreign substances
- To facilitate better oxygenation and ventilation when performed over a longer period of time
- When basic airway management techniques have failed or are inadequate
- To establish a limited drug route for the patient in cardiac arrest
- To create a means to perform tracheobronchial suctioning

Even though most advanced airways provide a more effective means of airway control and ventilation, you must usually initially establish an airway and ventilate the patient by using basic airway management techniques. However, there are some situations in which immediate intervention with advanced airway techniques is warranted, such as upper airway burns with laryngeal edema or massive bleeding into the upper airway.

The preferred method of advanced airway management is the insertion of an endotracheal tube. Other, less-desirable methods make use of the pharyngeo-tracheal lumen airway (PtL®), the esophageal-tracheal Combitube® (ETC), the esophageal obturator airway (EOA), or the esophageal gastric tube airway (EGTA).

Endotracheal Intubation

Endotracheal intubation is the preferred method of airway control in the patient with an altered mental status who lacks a gag or cough reflex, the non-breathing unresponsive patient, or the cardiac arrest patient. A properly placed endotracheal tube truly protects the airway by isolating the trachea and preventing aspiration of secretions, blood, vomitus or other foreign material into the lungs. In addition, the endotracheal tube limits the amount of dead air space during ventilation and ensures delivery of adequate tidal volumes.

When providing positive pressure ventilation to a patient who is not intubated, significant pressure must be generated to deliver the necessary tidal volume and subsequent lung inflation. During the process, high pharyngeal pressure may be created, thereby opening the esophagus and causing insufflation of large amounts of air into the stomach. This results in gastric distention, which may lead to regurgitation of gastric contents and potential aspiration. Also, the gastric distention may elevate the diaphragm and impede lung expansion during ventilation. This may reduce the tidal volume delivered and lead to hypoxia. To reduce the risk of these complications, the trachea should be intubated as soon as possible during resuscitation.

Placement of an endotracheal tube requires skill. A significant number of complications can occur from an improperly placed tube or poor technique of insertion. Therefore, only those health care providers who are well trained and perform or practice endotracheal intubation often should be intubating the patient.

Once an endotracheal tube is placed and confirmed, chest compressions and ventilations can be performed asynchronously. Ventilations should be done at 12–to–15 per minute while delivering a tidal volume of 10–to–15 ml/kg. At this rate and volume, with the addition of supplemental oxygen at as close to 100% as possible, adequate oxygenation should occur.

Advantages of Endotracheal Intubation

The following are advantages of intubation with an endotracheal tube:

- It isolates the trachea and prevents aspiration of foreign material.
- It permits tracheobronchial suctioning.
- It provides better oxygenation and more effective delivery of tidal volume and lung expansion.
- It provides a secondary route for administration of certain drugs.
- It prevents gastric insufflation and resultant gastric distention.
- It permits asynchronous chest compressions and ventilations, allowing faster compression rates.

Indications for Endotracheal Intubation

Not every patient requires endotracheal intubation. The following are indications for endotracheal intubation:

- Patient in cardiac arrest (intubate as soon as possible)
- Need for prolonged positive pressure ventilation
- Inadequate ventilation in the patient with no gag reflex
- Patient unable to protect his own airway due to altered mental status, coma, absent gag reflex, or cardiac arrest
- Inability to effectively ventilate the patient with other basic techniques

Evaluate the Patient

It is necessary to take a few seconds to minutes to evaluate the patient prior to intubation. This is done to identify a potentially difficult intubation due to the patient's anatomy or situations that may impede normal intubation procedures. The evaluation may aid you in selecting the most appropriate equipment and technique for intubation.

Information collected from a patient history could provide you with valuable indicators of possible difficult intubation. History of a previous surgery with difficult intubation is typically known by the family of the patient, which can predict difficult intubation in the present situation. Other indicators of potentially difficult intubation are:

- Oral surgery
- Neck surgery
- Temporal mandibular joint problems
- Rheumatoid arthritis
- Degenerative joint diseases
- Upper airway burns

Assess the oropharynx for potential signs of a difficult intubation. Measure the distance from the mandibular symphysis to the hyoid bone. If this distance is less than three fingerbreadths or 60 mm, a short, anterior larynx should be suspected. A straight blade is considered the preferred blade, rather than a curved, in this patient. Also inspect the oropharynx for dentures, loose teeth, caps, or plates which may become dislodged and possibly aspirated.

Inspect the neck for evidence of surgery, which may narrow and distort the airway anatomy and make visualization and tube insertion difficult. Thick and muscular necks typically have limited mobility, which may make alignment of the airway difficult. This would lead to problems in visualization.

Patients with spine and face trauma require in-line stabilization of the head and neck. Facial trauma also poses additional problems of bleeding in the airway, loss of bony structure, and distortion of anatomy for visualization and tube insertion. Bleeding in the airway may block visualization. Suction is required to clear the airway prior to the intubation technique. It may be necessary to continuously apply suction to the hypopharynx during the laryngoscopy.

Expect a large amount of secretions when intubating a near-drowning patient. A pulmonary edema patient may need to be intubated while in a seated position. This technique requires more skill than the conventional intubation.

Equipment Needed for Endotracheal Intubation

Several pieces of equipment are needed for endotracheal intubation. It is vital to check the equipment to ensure it is in proper working order prior to the procedure. The equipment needed for endotracheal intubation includes:

Body substance isolation equipment
Laryngoscope (includes handle and several blades)

Endotracheal tubes
Malleable stylet
Water-soluble lubricant
10-ml syringe
Device to secure the endotracheal tube
Suction unit
Stethoscope
Magill forceps (optional)
Confirmation device, such as a CO_2 monitor (optional)

Laryngoscope The laryngoscope consists of two parts, the handle and the blade. It is inserted into the hypopharynx where it is used to lift the epiglottis and view the glottic opening and the vocal cords. The procedure is termed *laryngoscopy*. Laryngoscopes may be reusable or disposable.

The laryngoscope blade is the component that is used to manipulate the tongue and epiglottis to expose and view the glottic opening and vocal cords. It is critical to be able to see this area in order to make sure that you are guiding the endotracheal tube between the vocal cords and into the trachea, and not misdirecting the tube into the esophagus. The laryngoscope handle holds batteries that provide energy for a light at the end of the blade that facilitates visualization. Fiber-optic handles contain the bulb within the handle. The light is transmitted by a fiber-optic strand to the end of the blade.

There are two types of laryngoscope blades: the curved blade (McIntosh) or the straight blade (Miller, Wisconsin, Flagg. (Figure 3-10). The name of each blade describes its shape. Both types of blades are designed to lift the epiglottis; however, each blade achieves this differently.

- **Straight Blade** The straight blade is a long, straight, hollow-channeled blade with a rounded distal end. It comes in a variety of sizes ranging from 0, the smallest, to 4, the largest. A 0 blade would be used in an infant, whereas, a 4 blade would be used to intubate a large adult. The straight blade is the preferred blade in infants and children. It is also the blade of choice in larger patients with short necks because the larynx is usually more anterior.

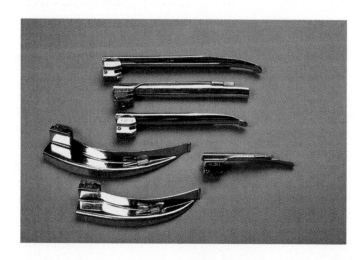

FIGURE 3-10 Straight and curved laryngoscope blades.

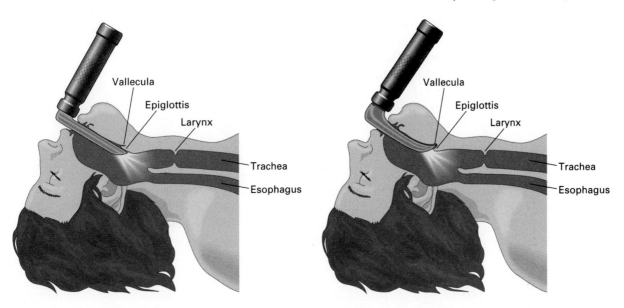

FIGURE 3-11 The straight blade is placed under the epiglottis and directly lifts the epiglottis upward to expose the vocal cords and glottic opening.

FIGURE 3-12 The curved blade is placed into the vallecula and indirectly lifts the epiglottis.

The straight blade is inserted into the hypopharynx and is used to directly lift the epiglottis (Figure 3-11). The blade is inserted in the right side of the mouth. With a sweeping motion to the midline, the blade moves the tongue to the left to provide for better visualization. The rounded distal end of the blade is inserted under the epiglottis. With an upward movement of the laryngoscope handle, the epiglottis is directly lifted upward, exposing the glottic opening and the vocal cords. The endotracheal tube is advanced along the right side of the blade. The hollow channel is a sight to allow for visualization of the tube passing through the vocal cords. Note that it is *not* a conduit for the tube insertion. This is a common mistake that ends in a torn or damaged endotracheal tube and the subsequent need to extubate and reintubate the patient.

- **Curved Blade** The curved blade has a round, beaded distal edge. The blade has a broad surface and a tall flange that is used to move and hold the tongue out of the way, allowing for better visualization of the airway anatomy during the intubation procedure. Like the straight blade, the curved blade comes in sizes ranging from 0 for infants to 4 for larger adults.

The distal, beaded end of the blade is inserted into the vallecula, the space located between the tongue and the epiglottis (Figure 3-12). With the edge of the blade resting on the glossoepiglottic ligament, upward and forward movement of the handle will put pressure on the ligament, causing the epiglottis to be indirectly lifted up off the glottic opening.

Assembly of the laryngoscope is a simple procedure. The indentation of the proximal end of the laryngoscope blade is designed to lock into the bar on the laryngoscope handle. The blade is lifted upward until at a right angle

FIGURE 3-13 A. Affix the laryngoscope blade to the handle. B. Lift the laryngoscope blade until the blade locks into place and the light at the end of the blade is lit.

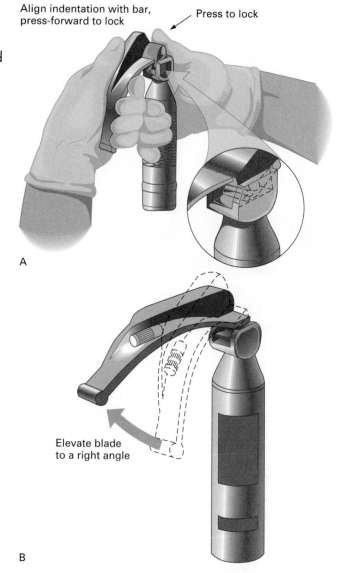

Align indentation with bar, press-forward to lock

Press to lock

A

Elevate blade to a right angle

B

to the handle. This will lock the blade into the handle, make electrical contact, and light the bulb at the distal end of the blade (Figure 3-13).

The light at the distal end of the laryngoscope should be white and bright. If the light is not lit or is poorly lit, check that the blade is properly locked in the handle. Also, check the bulb to be sure it is tightly screwed in. A loose bulb can be dislodged while intubating and aspirated down the trachea. An absent or poor light may indicate weak or dead batteries. Spare batteries and bulbs should be available.

Fiber-optic laryngoscope handles and blades are also available. The fiber-optic light source is located in the handle. The blade contains a fiber-optic strand, rather than a bulb, to provide illumination at the distal end of the blade. The light source is brighter than with the conventional bulb system.

Endotracheal Tube The endotracheal tube is a flexible, translucent tube made of polyvinyl chloride. It is open at both ends. The proximal end has a standard 15 mm connector that allows for attachment of a bag-valve or

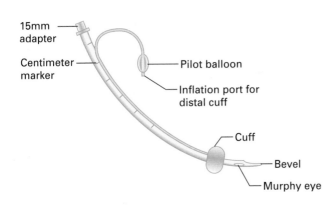

FIGURE 3-14 Endotracheal tube components.

15mm adapter

Centimeter marker

Pilot balloon

Inflation port for distal cuff

Cuff

Bevel

Murphy eye

other ventilation device. The distal end has a cuff that seals and isolates the trachea. An inflation tube extends from the cuff up the tube to a pilot balloon and a one-way inflation valve. A syringe is connected to the inflation valve to fill the distal cuff with air. The pilot balloon is designed to verify cuff inflation (Figure 3-14). Uncuffed endotracheal tubes are available and are used in children and infants, typically up until age eight.

The size noted on the outside of the tube is the internal diameter (i.d.). In general, an adult male will require an 8.0 to 8.5 mm i.d. tube, whereas an adult female will take a 7.0 to 8.0 mm i.d. tube. If you are uncertain as to what tube size to use, it is more prudent to use the smaller-sized tube to prevent damage to the glottic structures. In an emergency situation, both males and females can usually take a 7.5 mm i.d. tube. It is a good idea to have available, when intubating, one size larger and one size smaller than the selected tube size for the patient.

A Murphy eye (a small hole) is located at the distal end of the endotracheal tube opposite the side of the bevel. The eye reduces the chances of distal tube obstruction from the tracheal wall, blood clots, or secretions.

The length is measured in centimeters (cm) and is marked at several intervals along the tube. The average length of the tube for the adult is 33 cm. When properly placed, the front teeth of the patient will be at the 19–23 cm marking on the tube. These measurements are available to continually monitor for tube movement or displacement. The distal tip of the endotracheal tube sits midway between the carina and the vocal cords when properly placed. Once proper tube placement is confirmed, note the centimeter level marking on the tube at the front teeth. This will be used as one indicator of possible tube movement and dislodgement. The IT or Z79 markings indicate that the tube has met certain standards or tests.

Alternative types of endotracheal tubes are also available. An Endotrol tube contains a flexible stylet and trigger built into the side wall of the tube. When the trigger is pulled the stylet redirects the distal end of the tube upward. This facilitates placement of the tube in the patient with an anterior larynx. Also available is a tube with a built-in medication injection port and catheter for endotracheal medication administration.

Stylet The malleable stylet is a piece of pliable metal wire, typically coated in plastic, that is inserted into the endotracheal tube prior to insertion to alter its shape and provide stiffness (Figure 3-15). The stylet should be lubricated with a water-soluble jelly to facilitate easy removal. The stylet should

FIGURE 3-15 The stylet may be inserted to stiffen and shape the endotracheal tube.

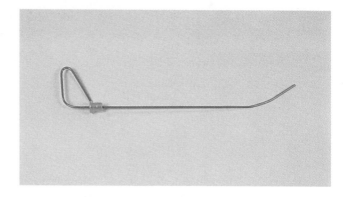

never project beyond the level of the Murphy eye and should always be recessed at least ½ inch from the distal end of the tube. Trauma to or perforation of the trachea may result from a stylet that is inserted beyond the distal end of the tube. Hold the tube securely while removing the stylet, so you do not accidentally dislodge the tube.

Other Equipment If time permits, water-soluble lubricant is applied to the distal end of the endotracheal tube to facilitate insertion into the trachea. In addition, the lubricant is applied to the stylet to allow for easier removal. Do not use petroleum-based products, since they can damage the endotracheal tube and irritate and inflame the mucosal lining of the airway.

A 10 ml syringe is used to inflate the distal cuff of the endotracheal tube. Test the cuff integrity with the syringe when checking the equipment prior to intubation. Once the air is inserted in the cuff, remove the syringe. If the syringe is left attached to the inflation port, the cuff may deflate.

Magill forceps are used to remove foreign material from the upper airway. Also, the forceps may be used to direct the tip of the endotracheal tube into the glottic opening.

Tape, intravenous tubing, or a commercially available securing device must be used to hold the tube in place once proper placement has been confirmed.

A suction unit must be available during endotracheal intubation to remove any fluid, vomitus, blood, or other material from the upper airway to prevent aspiration. A rigid catheter is used to suction the oropharynx, whereas, a soft suction catheter should be available to perform tracheobronchial suctioning.

A stethoscope must be at hand to listen for breath sounds at the lungs and epigastrium to help confirm correct placement of the endotracheal tube, or to help detect incorrect placement.

Sellick's Maneuver (Cricoid Pressure)
As explained earlier, a major complication associated with both basic and advanced airway management is the regurgitation and aspiration of gastric contents. When an endotracheal tube is not in place, high pharyngeal pressure is generated during positive pressure ventilation. This opens the esophagus and causes gastric insufflation. The resultant gastric distention may impede effective artificial ventilation or may lead to regurgitation of gastric contents with subsequent aspiration.

In an attempt to protect the airway, posterior pressure (Figure 3-16) is applied to the cricoid cartilage to seal off the esophagus when unprotected positive pressure ventilation is performed. This reduces the amount of air traveling down the esophagus to the stomach and blocks vomitus from being transmitted up the esophagus.

In addition, cricoid pressure is used to better visualize the glottic opening. By applying pressure on the anterior cricoid ring, displacing the larynx posteriorly, the glottis will be less anterior and the visual field used for endotracheal tube insertion is improved.

Technique of Oral Endotracheal Intubation

When properly placed in the trachea, the endotracheal tube is the ultimate airway. However, if the tube is misplaced in the esophagus, it will lead to rapid deterioration of the patient. If this mistake is not detected and corrected immediately, it can be fatal or result in irreversible brain damage from hypoxia.

The steps for endotracheal intubation (Figures 3-17a to 3-17g) are as follows:

1. *Take the necessary universal precautions against contact with body fluids.* In addition to gloves and eye protection, consider a surgical mask because of the potential for spattering of secretions during intubation.
2. *Clear the airway of any potential obstructions.* Establish the proper manual positioning of the airway, and insert an oropharyngeal or nasopharyngeal airway.
3. *Begin positive pressure ventilation to oxygenate the patient while the equipment is being prepared.*
4. *Assemble and check the equipment.* Select the proper laryngoscope blade according to patient size and personal preference. Assemble the laryngoscope blade and handle. If a conventional laryngoscope is used, check the

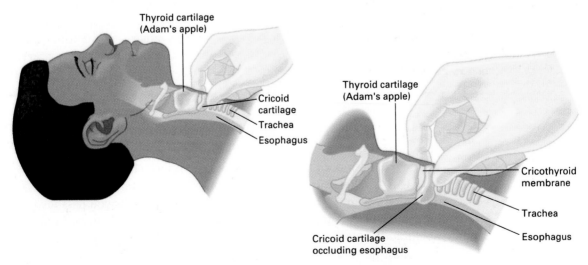

FIGURE 3-16 To perform Sellick's maneuver, locate the cricoid cartilage inferior to the thyroid cartilage. Apply firm posterior pressure with the thumb and index finger.

OROTRACHEAL INTUBATION

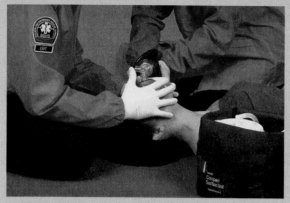

FIGURE 3-17a Prior to any intubation attempt, hyperoxygenate the patient at a rate of 24 ventilations per minute.

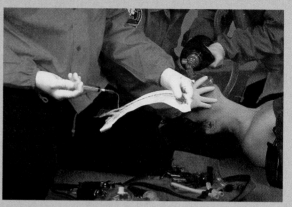

FIGURE 3-17b Assemble and test the equipment.

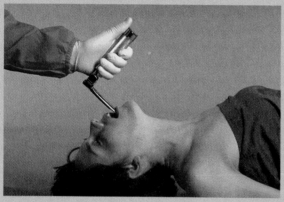

FIGURE 3-17c Insert the laryngoscope blade on the right and sweep the tongue to the left until the blade is midline. In the patient with no suspected spinal injury, point and direct the end of the handle at a 30- to 45-degree angle toward and above the patient's feet. This will place the patient's head and neck in the "sniffing position" to aid visualization of the glottic opening and vocal cords.

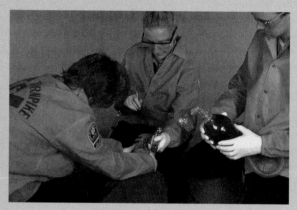

FIGURE 3-17d The trauma patient with suspected spinal injury must be intubated with in-line spinal stabilization maintained. The care provider intubating secures the patient's head with her thighs while a coworker holds the head from a position below the patient's neck.

light at the distal end of the blade. The light should be bright and secure. If the light is dim, you will have difficulty in visualizing the glottic opening and will be more likely to misplace the endotracheal tube in the esophagus. Oral endotracheal intubation is a completely "visual" technique, and it is imperative that you visualize the tube as you pass it through the vocal cords and into the larynx. Oral endotracheal intubation should not be performed blindly. Therefore, the light emitted from the blade must be very white and bright. Obtain another handle or change the batteries if necessary.

Select the proper-size endotracheal tube. Women usually require a 7.0 mm to 8.0 mm i.d. tube, whereas men usually take an 8.0 mm to 8.5 mm i.d.

OROTRACHEAL INTUBATION *(continued)*

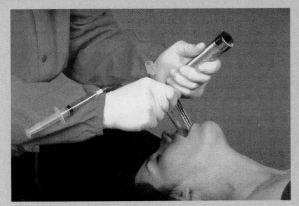

FIGURE 3-17e Visualize the vocal cords and insert the endotracheal tube. To visualize, lift the laryngoscope in the direction of the handle.

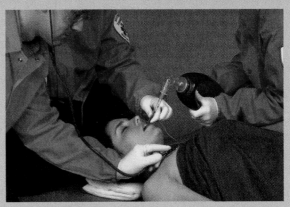

FIGURE 3-17f Confirm correct placement of the tube.

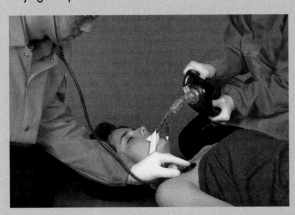

FIGURE 3-17g Secure the tube and reassess tube placement.

tube. In an emergency situation, a 7.5 mm i.d. tube is acceptable for use in both men and women.

Lubricate the stylet and insert it into the endotracheal tube. Be sure the stylet is recessed at least ½ inch (1.27 cm) from the distal end of the tube. The use of a stylet is based on your personal preference, the patient's anatomy, and any difficulty in passing the tube. The stylet merely conforms the tube to a desired configuration and facilitates insertion into the glottic opening and trachea. Shaping the tube and stylet into an open J, or "hockey-stick," configuration can facilitate the tube insertion.

Attach a 10 ml syringe to the inflation port, inject 10 ml of air, and check the distal cuff for leaks. The cuff and pilot balloon should remain inflated. Replace any defective tubes prior to intubation. Insertion of a tube with a defective cuff will not isolate the trachea, therefore leaving the airway unprotected and allowing for air leakage and potential subsequent aspiration.

Have a suction unit available. Check the suction unit to ensure it is working properly. Have both a rigid and soft suction catheter available.

If time permits, you can lubricate the endotracheal tube with a water-soluble lubricant to ease insertion of the tube.

5. *Open the patient's mouth and inspect for any potential obstructions. Suction any secretions, blood, or other substances from the oropharynx. Remove any loose dental appliances.*

6. *Position the patient's head to align the three axes of the mouth, pharynx, and trachea to achieve better visualization* (Figure 3-18a and Figure 3-18b). Place the head in a "sniffing" position. Accomplish this by extending the head and flexing the neck (extension at C_1 and C_2, flexion at C_5 and C_6). You can aid flexion of the neck by placing folded towels under the occiput. The neck is extended by the person performing the intubation. Do not allow the patient's head to hang over the end of the bed or table.

   If a cervical spine injury is suspected, you must place the patient's head and neck in a neutral in-line position. In this position, the nose is aligned with the umbilicus on a sagittal (vertical, midbody) plane, and the head and neck are maintained in a neutral position without any flexion or extension. To protect the patient's spine, open the airway with a jaw-thrust maneuver and perform laryngoscopy with a second person maintaining in-line stabilization. Apply cricoid pressure any time you are intubating a patient with a suspected cervical spine injury.

7. *Hyperoxygenate the patient at approximately 24 ventilations per minute for a 30-second period with a ventilation device delivering as close to 100% oxygen as possible.* This will raise the PaO_2 and reduce the effects of hypoxia associated with the absence of ventilation during the intubation procedure.

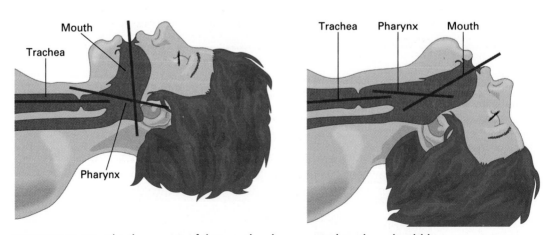

FIGURE 3-18 The three axes of the mouth, pharynx, and trachea should be aligned to achieve optimal visualization for endotracheal intubation.

At any time the intubation process reaches 30 seconds, stop the procedure and resume hyperventilation of the patient for at least 30 to 60 seconds before attempting intubation again.

8. *Open the mouth using the fingers of the right hand. If any secretions or other substance are again found inside the mouth, suction it out immediately.* Apply cricoid pressure until the endotracheal tube is successfully placed and the distal cuff is inflated.

9. *Insert the laryngoscope and visualize the vocal cords.* Hold the laryngoscope handle in your left hand. Insert the blade into the right side of mouth. Move the blade to the midline while advancing it to the base of the tongue. With the tip of the blade at the base of the tongue, lift the blade up and forward toward the patient's feet—in the direction that the handle is pointing. This should be a nice, fluid motion without prying or digging. Do not pull back on the handle or use the teeth as a fulcrum. This will potentially cause trauma to the lips, gums, or teeth. To avoid trauma to the lower lip, you can retract it with your right index finger during the laryngoscopy. In the patient without suspected spinal injury, point and direct the end of the handle at a 30- to 45-degree angle toward and above the patient's feet. This will place the patient's head and neck in the "sniffing position," which will allow for better visualization of the glottic opening and vocal cords.

   To visualize the vocal cords for tube insertion, you must use the laryngoscope blade to lift the epiglottis off the glottic opening. If you are using a straight blade, insert the tip under the epiglottis. With upward and forward movement on the laryngoscope handle, directly lift the epiglottis to expose the glottic opening. If you are using a curved blade, insert it into the vallecula, the space between the base of the tongue and the base of the epiglottis. Lift the handle to place pressure on the glossoepiglottic ligament, which will indirectly cause the epiglottis to be lifted away from the glottic opening.

   To aid in visualization, you may slightly elevate the patient's head. Also, cricoid pressure may be applied to slightly displace the laryngeal structures posteriorly, facilitating visualization. These measures should not be used, however, if a cervical spine injury is suspected.

   The identifiable structures that you should view during laryngoscopy are the epiglottis, the cuneiform, corniculate, and aretynoid cartilages, the glottic opening, and the vocal cords. If the straight laryngoscope blade is inserted too far, it may enter the esophagus, and no identifiable structures will be seen. Remember that the opening of the esophagus is more oval in shape and lacks cartilaginous structures, whereas the opening of the glottis is surrounded by cartilage and is round in shape. Pull back on the blade to remove it from the esophagus while watching for the glottic opening and vocal cords to come into view.

   If you do not see any identifiable structures, remove the blade and begin hyperventilation of the patient. Never exceed 30 seconds from the time artificial ventilation is stopped until it is resumed. Hyperventilate the patient for at least 30 to 60 seconds prior to any further attempt at intubation.

10. *With the vocal cords visualized, insert the endotracheal tube.* Insert the tube through the right side of the mouth. Watch the tube as it passes through the vocal cords. The proximal end of the cuff should be advanced ½ to 1

inch (1 to 2.5 cm) beyond the level of the vocal cords. This should place the tip of the endotracheal tube midway between the vocal cords and the carina. The tube marking in an average-sized adult will be between 19 and 23 cm at the level of the front teeth.

Hold the tube firmly in place and remove the stylet if you used it.

11. *Inflate the distal cuff with 8–to–10 ml of air.* Inject enough air to assure cuff inflation that is adequate to isolate the trachea. This may require 10–to–20 ml of air. Check the pilot balloon to ensure the cuff is still inflated. If the pilot balloon does not remain inflated, remove the endotracheal tube, hyperventilate the patient, and repeat the procedure using a new endotracheal tube. The cuff is used to isolate the trachea and prevent aspiration of foreign materials. It does not secure the tube in place. Be sure to hold the tube firmly until it is properly secured.

12. *Assess tube placement.* While simultaneously delivering the first ventilation, auscultate over the epigastrium while watching for chest rise and fall. If gurgling sounds are heard over the epigastrium, or the chest does not rise with the ventilation, assume the esophagus has been inadvertently intubated and immediately remove the tube. Immediately begin hyperventilation for approximately 30 to 60 seconds prior to another attempt. Be prepared to suction vomitus.

If the chest wall rises and no sounds are heard over the epigastrium, auscultate over the right and left lung fields, both apices and bases, with subsequent ventilation. If equal breath sounds are heard bilaterally, secure the device.

Right mainstem intubation may occur from insertion of the tube too far into the trachea. If diminished or no breath sounds are heard on the left but good breath sounds are heard on the right, deflate the cuff and pull back on the tube about 1 to 2 cm. Recheck breath sounds. Repeat this procedure until equal breath sounds are heard bilaterally. (A left mainstem intubation may also occur; however, because of the anatomy and angles of the right and left mainstem bronchi, it is much more likely that the right mainstem bronchus will be inadvertently intubated. The same procedure would be used to correct a left mainstem intubation.)

An end-tidal carbon-dioxide monitor may also be used to help confirm tube placement. Lack of CO_2 typically indicates an esophageal intubation in patients with spontaneous circulation. However, in pulseless patients or those with low pulmonary blood flow or large dead space, the amount of carbon dioxide may be negligible and not detected. Both electronic and less-expensive CO_2 detectors are available. Be familiar with the limitations of both devices. Esophageal detector devices are also available to assess for esophageal intubation.

These devices are only adjuncts to proper assessment of tube placement. A chest x-ray, if it is feasible to obtain one, can also be used to confirm tube placement. However, the best method to ensure proper tube placement is direct visualization. If in doubt, reconfirm the tube placement by performing a laryngoscopy and visualizing the tube between the vocal cords. If at any time you are in doubt that the tube is properly positioned, remove it and resume ventilation with a bag-valve mask or other acceptable ventilation device.

13. *Secure the tube with tape or a commercially available securing device.* IV tubing can be used as a temporary securing device, especially when sweat or vomit make taping impossible. Note the cm marker at the level of the front teeth. You may insert an oropharyngeal airway after the tube is secured to prevent the patient with spontaneous circulation and breathing from biting down and occluding the tube. Following any patient movement, you must reassess tube placement. Even when the tube is secured, it can become dislodged when the patient moves or is moved.

14. *Ventilate the patient with a tidal volume of 10–to–15 ml/kg.* You can adjust the volume up for larger patients and down for smaller patients. During respiratory or cardiac arrest, provide a 15 ml/kg tidal volume at a rate of 10 to 12 ventilations per minute (one every 5 to 6 seconds). Following successful resuscitation from cardiac arrest, initially increase the rate of ventilation to 12 to 15 ventilations per minute (one every 4 to 5 seconds). Deliver each ventilation slowly over a 2-second period. You must use a ventilation device that is capable of delivering close to 100% oxygen with each ventilation.

Complications Associated with Endotracheal Intubation Several complications are associated with the procedure of endotracheal intubation. These include the following:

- Trauma to the lips and tongue from compression between the teeth and the blade, causing lacerations
- Trauma to the teeth from the laryngoscope blade
- Bleeding, hematoma, or abscess formation associated with laceration of the pharyngeal or tracheal mucosa caused by the tip of the tube or an improperly placed stylet
- Rupture of the trachea
- Injury to the vocal cords and avulsion of an arytenoid cartilage
- Pharyngeal-esophageal perforation
- Intubation of the pyriform sinus
- Stimulation of the gag reflex with subsequent vomiting and aspiration of gastric contents
- Hypertension, tachycardia, and dysrhythmias from stimulation of the sympathetic nervous system in the patient with spontaneous circulation
- Right mainstem intubation—the most frequent complication, which can lead to hypoxia from underinflation of a lung
- Esophageal intubation, resulting in no ventilation or oxygenation
- Hypoxia resulting from prolonged interruptions in ventilation during attempts at intubation
- Airway obstruction associated with laryngospasm from stimulation of the epiglottis or larynx
- Accidental displacement of the tube during movement of the patient

To reduce the possibility of complications associated with endotracheal intubation, the following precautions must be observed:

- Only properly trained personnel should perform endotracheal intubation.
- Cardiac arrest patients should be intubated as quickly as possible to reduce the risk of gastric insufflation and aspiration of gastric contents.

- The intubation procedure must not exceed 30 seconds. (The 30-second time period is from cessation of ventilation to resumption of ventilation.) If the procedure is unsuccessful, the patient must be hyperventilated with a ventilation device connected to 100% supplemental oxygen. Hyperventilation must be provided for 30 to 60 seconds before intubation is reattempted.
- Apply cricoid pressure to reduce the incidence of gastric distention and aspiration of gastric contents into the lower airway. Once the patient is successfully intubated, there is no need to continue with cricoid pressure.
- A high-volume, low-pressure cuff is recommended for use during cardiac arrest management. The intracuff pressure should be adjusted to 25–to–35 cmH2O. An intracuff pressure of 25 cmH2O is the minimum required to isolate the trachea and prevent aspiration. An intracuff pressure greater than 40 cmH2O will reduce capillary blood flow to the mucosa and result in tissue ischemia or necrosis.
- Continually reassess and confirm endotracheal tube placement.

Special Considerations in the Patient with Severe Trauma   Patients who present with trauma to the face, neck, or head, or those with multiple injuries require special airway consideration due to the possibility of spinal cord or vertebral injury. If the mechanism of injury is consistent with a pattern that may cause spinal injury, take the necessary precautions against excessive manipulation of the head and neck while establishing an airway. During both manual and mechanical maneuvers to establish and maintain an airway, the head and neck must be maintained in a neutral in-line position until spinal injury can be ruled out.

When manually establishing an airway in the patient with suspected spinal injury, perform a jaw-thrust or a chin-lift maneuver without the head tilt. If the jaw thrust or chin lift alone does not clear the airway, slowly and carefully perform the head tilt until the airway is unobstructed. The goal is to keep the head in an in-line neutral position, with the nose in-line with the umbilicus and the head and neck not flexed or hyperextended. This position must be maintained until spinal injury is properly ruled out.

Blind nasal intubation may be performed in patients with suspected spinal injury since, unlike orotracheal intubation, nasal intubation does not require manipulation of the head and neck. Nasal intubation must be performed only by trained and experienced health care providers in spontaneously breathing patients. Spinal immobilization must be continuously maintained, since the technique may cause the patient to move his neck. This technique of intubation is relatively contraindicated in patients with suspected midfacial fractures and basilar skull fracture. In this case, orotracheal intubation should be performed while a second care provider maintains manual in-line stabilization of the head and neck. This procedure requires special training and skill.

If an endotracheal tube cannot be successfully placed, and if ventilation cannot be adequately achieved by other methods such as bag-valve-mask ventilation, a cricothyrotomy or tracheostomy may be necessary. Paralytic agents may aid in successful intubation when the patient presents with trismus and clenched jaws. Frequent suctioning may be necessary, as bleeding is associated with facial or airway trauma.

Alternative Orotracheal Intubation Techniques

There are several alternative techniques that can be used to insert an endotracheal tube orally. These methods do not use the conventional technique of insertion or the standard equipment. These techniques are not recommended in every situation nor for all patients needing endotracheal intubation.

Digital Intubation

In digital intubation you insert your fingers into the patient's hypopharynx and use them to lift the epiglottis and guide the endotracheal tube through the glottic opening. This is referred to as a "blind" technique because you do not use a laryngoscope and do not actually visualize the endotracheal tube passing through the vocal cords. (The word *digits* is another word for fingers or toes. The term *digital* means "with the fingers.") Digital intubation may be used in a patient who is in cardiac arrest or unresponsive and has no gag reflex.

The standard technique of using a laryngoscope is preferred because it allows you to visualize the endotracheal tube passing through the vocal cords. However, you may encounter situations where the patient's position or condition precludes effective use of a laryngoscope, for example in situations where visualization of the glottic opening is difficult because of bleeding in the airway.

Digital intubation may also be recommended in the patient with a possible cervical spine injury. Since this patient is immobilized and the head and neck cannot be manipulated, it is very difficult to achieve an axis that allows for proper visualization with a layrngoscope. Digital intubation can be performed without visualizing the vocal cords, so it eliminates the need to manipulate the head or neck.

Also, consider the patient who is entrapped in a vehicle and needs to be intubated. Extrication time may be lengthy and the airway problem may be severe. Proper positioning for intubation with a layrngoscope is virtually impossible to achieve, but digital intubation may be possible.

In addition, in the case of failure of the laryngoscope batteries or bulb when no spares are available or working properly, you may be able to insert an endotracheal tube using the digital technique.

Equipment Needed for Digital Intubation

The equipment needed to perform digital intubation includes:

- Appropriate size endotracheal tube
- Malleable stylet
- Water-soluble lubricant
- 10 cc syringe
- Bite block
- Device to secure the endotracheal tube

Digital Intubation Procedure

The procedure for digital intubation is listed below:

1. *Take the necessary body substance isolation precautions.* Gloves, eye wear, and a mask are recommended.

2. *Hyperventilate the patient for approximately 30 seconds prior to initiating the insertion technique.*

3. *Check and lubricate the endotracheal tube as you normally would.* Lubricate the tube with a water-soluble lubricant. Lubricate the stylet and insert it to form the tube into a J-shape.

4. *Assure correct positioning.* If spinal injury is suspected, have a trained rescuer or health care provider manually stabilize the patient's head and neck. Face the patient and kneel at his left shoulder.

5. *Instruct the person ventilating the patient to stop.* Quickly place a bite block between the patient's molars to prevent the patient from biting down on your fingers during the procedure.

6. *Insert the middle and index fingers of your left hand into the patient's mouth.* Advance your fingers down the midline while simultaneously lifting the tongue up and out of the way.

7. *Palpate the epiglottis with your middle finger. Press upward and move the epiglottis forward* (Figure 3-19a).

8. *Insert the endotracheal tube into the mouth with your opposite hand.* Advance the tube using your index finger to maintain the tip of the tube against the middle finger. The tip will be directed upward toward the epiglottis. Guide the tip of the tube into the glottic opening with the index and middle fingers (Figure 3-19b).

9. *Remove your fingers, hold the tube in place, and remove the stylet carefully.*

10. *Ventilate.* Inflate the cuff with 8 to 10 cc of air. Attach a bag-valve device to the tube and ventilate. Artificial ventilation must not be interrupted for greater than 30 seconds during the insertion.

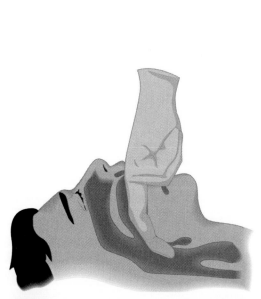

FIGURE 3-19a Insert your index and middle fingers into the patient's mouth. Elevate the epiglottis with your middle finger.

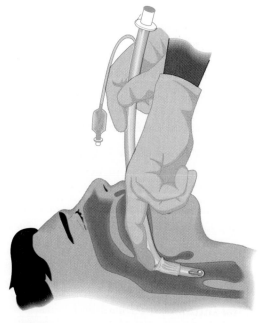

FIGURE 3-19b Guide the tube forward and into the glottic opening with your index and middle fingers.

11. *Confirm placement.* Auscultate over the epigastrium and watch for chest rise and fall while a ventilation is delivered. If no gurgling sounds are heard, auscultate over the right and left chest at the apex and bases of the lungs.

12. *If correct placement is not confirmed, remove or reposition the tube.* If gurgling sounds are heard over the epigastrium, cease ventilation through the tube and immediately remove it. Hyperventilate the patient with a bag-valve-mask device. If breath sounds are absent or diminished on the left but are good on the right, suspect a right mainstem intubation. Deflate the cuff and pull back on the tube until equal breath sounds are heard bilaterally and then re-inflate the cuff.

13. *If correct placement is confirmed, secure the tube.* If no sounds are heard over the epigastrium, breath sounds are heard equally bilaterally, and the chest rises and falls equally with each ventilation, secure the tube in place. Use tape or a commercial securing device.

14. *Resume hyperventilation of the patient for approximately 30 to 60 seconds. Then resume a normal ventilation rate.*

15. *Reassess tube position with each movement of the patient.*

Transillumination (Lighted Stylet) Intubation

Another alternative method of orotracheal intubation is transillumination, or the "lighted stylet" technique. In this technique, a special lighted stylet is inserted into the endotracheal tube which is then inserted through the mouth and hypopharynx and down into the trachea. If correctly placed in the trachea, the bright light can be seen through the soft tissues of the neck. If incorrectly placed in the esophagus, the light will be very dim or hard to see.

With the transillumination method, the intubator can confirm passage of the endotracheal tube through the glottic opening into the trachea without having to use a laryngoscope to directly visualize the glottic structures. This eliminates the need to manipulate the head or neck during intubation. For this reason, the transillumination technique can be an effective means of intubation in the trauma patient.

The transillumination stylet has a high intensity bulb at the distal end. Power for the device is supplied by a small battery housed at the proximal end and is controlled by an on-off switch. A major complication with this technique is the inability to effectively see the stylet light because of the ambient light. For this reason, transillumination is best performed in a darkened environment. In sunlight or a brightly lit room, shield the neck to be sure whether the stylet light is or is not shining through the neck.

Equipment Needed for Transillumination Intubation

The equipment needed to perform transillumination endotracheal intubation includes:

- Appropriate sized endotracheal tube
- Lighted stylet
- Water-soluble lubricant
- 10 cc syringe
- Scissors (to trim the tube)
- Securing device for the endotracheal tube

Procedure for Transillumination (Lighted Stylet) Intubation
The procedure for transillumination intubation is:

1. *Take the necessary body substance isolation precautions* including gloves, eye wear, and a mask.

2. *While maintaining ventilatory support, hyperventilate the patient for approximately 30 to 60 seconds prior to the attempt.*

3. *Assemble and check the equipment.* The endotracheal tube should be between 7.5 and 8.5 mm i.d., and will need to be cut to 25-27 cm in order to accommodate the stylet. Place the stylet into the tube and bend it just proximal to the cuff.

4. *Kneel on either side of the patient, facing the head.*

5. *Turn on the stylet light.*

6. *Insert the tube/stylet.* With your index and middle fingers inserted deeply into the patient's mouth and your thumb on the chin, lift the patient's tongue and jaw forward. Insert the tube/stylet combination into the mouth and advance it through the oropharynx and into the hypopharynx. Using a "hooking" motion, lift the epiglottis out of the way and advance the tube/stylet through the glottic opening into the larynx (Figure 3-20a).

7. *Confirm that the light is visible.* When you see a circle of light at the level of the larynx on the anterior neck, hold the stylet stationary (Figure 3-20b). Advance the tube off the stylet into the larynx approximately one-half to one inch. A diffuse, dim, or hard-to-see light indicates that the tube/stylet combination is in the esophagus. The tube should be immediately withdrawn and hyperventilation resumed. A bright light that appears laterally to the upper aspect of the thyroid cartilage (Adam's Apple) indicates that it is placed into the right or left pyriform fossa. Immediately withdraw the tube and resume hyperventilation. A second attempt can be tried after a few minutes. Artificial ventilation must not be interrupted for greater than thirty seconds when performing this technique.

8. *Hold the tube in place with one hand and remove the stylet.*

9. *Ventilate.* Inflate the cuff with 8-10 cc of air and attach the bag-valve device to the end of the tube.

10. *Confirm placement.* Auscultate for sounds over the epigastrium while inspecting for chest rise with the first ventilation. If gurgling is heard, immediately remove the tube and begin positive pressure ventilation with the bag-valve-mask device. If no sounds are heard, auscultate breath sound on both sides of the chest in the apical and basal zones of the lung. Breath sounds should be equal on each side. If breath sounds are diminished or absent on the left, suspect a right mainstem intubation. Deflate the cuff of the tube and pull back until breath sounds are heard equally bilaterally. Re-inflate the cuff. Observe for equal rise and fall of the patient's chest.

11. *Secure the tube* with tape or a commercial securing device that has been approved by medical direction.

12. *Reassess tube placement often, especially after each patient move.*

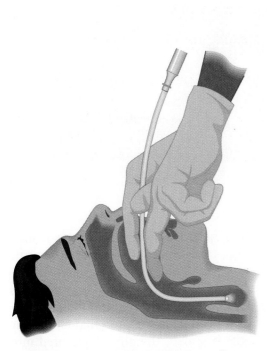

FIGURE 3-20a Lighted stylet (transillumination) endotracheal tube in position.

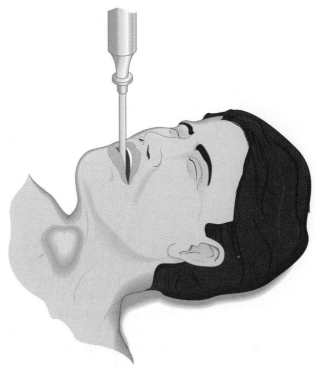

FIGURE 3-20b The properly positioned stylet should be visible at the front of the patient's neck.

Alternative Airway Adjuncts

A variety of alternative adjuncts for airway management are available. However, these adjuncts are not comparable with the endotracheal tube, which is the most effective airway. These alternative devices are designed to be inserted blindly; therefore, less skill is required for their use.

Esophageal Obturator Airway (EOA)

The esophageal obturator airway (EOA) was a widely used airway adjunct in the out-of-hospital setting (Figure 3-21). However, because of the complications associated with the device and the increase in training of prehospital providers in endotracheal intubation, its use has dropped drastically. According to the American Heart Association, the EOA is a Class IIb intervention, which is considered acceptable and possibly helpful. This device was recommended primarily in situations where the care provider was unable to successfully intubate the patient with an endotracheal tube, did not have the equipment to intubate the trachea, or was not permitted to perform endotracheal intubation.

The EOA is comprised of a mask and a cuffed esophageal tube with a sealed distal end. The tube connects with a clear face mask and has a series of openings at its proximal end several centimeters below the level of the mask. An inflation port is used to inflate the cuff with a syringe and a pilot balloon indicates the cuff volume.

FIGURE 3-21 The esophageal obturator airway (EOA).

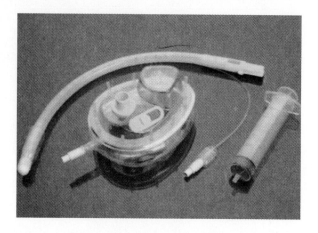

The tube is designed to be placed in the esophagus. The distal cuff seals the esophagus and does not allow any air to enter the stomach and prevents aspiration of gastric contents. The mask locks onto the tube and is used to form a seal around the patient's nose and mouth. The ventilation device is attached to the port on the top of the mask. During ventilation, the air is forced through the mask and out of the openings in the proximal end of the esophageal tube. Because the esophagus is sealed, the air is facilitated into the glottic opening and into the trachea. A good mask seal is imperative to effective ventilation.

Complications

Studies have shown that the risks of complications associated with insertion and ventilation with an EOA are higher than with endotracheal intubation. Also, clinical studies have indicated that ventilation and oxygenation with an EOA may be inferior to those with an endotracheal tube. Inadvertent placement of an EOA in the trachea is a fatal complication. Poor oxygenation and ventilation may result from operator misuse or fatigue. Also, the EOA does not protect the patient from aspiration of foreign substances found or originating in the mouth, nose, or pharynx. Other complications include the following:

- Esophageal rupture
- Laryngospasm
- Stimulation of vomiting during insertion
- Aspiration of gastric contents during insertion
- Soft tissue damage from the cuff pressure
- Inadequate mask seal
- Unrecognized tracheal intubation

Most of the complications are associated with operator misuse and not with the device itself. In order to reduce the incidence of these complications, the following recommendations should be adhered to:

- Only care providers specially trained and supervised should use the EOA.
- It should be used only in adults who are not breathing spontaneously and who have no gag reflex.
- Do not leave it in place for longer than 2 hours.

- Have suction available during insertion and removal.
- Do not use any force during the insertion.
- Remove the device only after endotracheal intubation or if the patient is alert enough to protect his own airway.

Contraindications
The EOA should not be inserted or used in the following conditions:

- The patient is alert, responsive, or has a gag reflex.
- The patient is less than 16 years of age.
- The patient has ingested a caustic substance (a strong acid or alkaline product such as lye) that may lead to esophageal rupture or perforation.
- The patient is less than 5 feet tall or greater than 7 feet tall. In a patient less than 5 feet tall, the esophageal tube may enter the stomach because of the short length of the esophagus. In the patient who is greater than 7 feet tall, the distal cuff of the esophageal tube will be at a level higher than the carina, the bifurcation of the trachea. Because the posterior tracheal wall is composed of soft fibroelastic tissue, it will become compressed from the volume in the distal esophageal cuff of the EOA once it is inflated. This may lead to obstruction of airflow through the trachea.
- The patient has significant bleeding in the oropharynx, nasopharynx, or pharynx. Remember, the cuff occludes the esophagus and does not isolate the trachea. Thus, aspiration of the blood may still occur.

Advantages
There are several advantages associated with the use of the EOA. They include the following:

- Insertion does not require visualization of the structures, and no additional equipment is required. Thus, it permits rapid, blind insertion.
- It prevents air from entering the stomach, thereby reducing the incidence of gastric distention.
- It prevents vomitus from traveling up the esophagus, therefore reducing the risk of aspiration of gastric contents.
- An endotracheal tube may still be inserted with the EOA in place.
- The head and neck of a suspected cervical-spine-injured patient may be maintained in a neutral in-line position during its insertion and use.

Disadvantages
Several disadvantages are associated with the device. They are as follows:

- A tight mask seal must be maintained the entire time the patient is being ventilated. Operator fatigue commonly leads to poor mask seal and ineffective ventilation.
- It may cause trauma to the esophagus or airway.
- It can be easily misplaced in the trachea, leading to asphyxia and possible tracheal damage.
- It cannot be left in place for prolonged periods of time.
- It does not isolate the trachea and prevent aspiration of contents from the upper airway.

- It cannot be used in patients less than 16 years of age, less than 5 feet tall, or greater than 7 feet tall.
- Tracheobronchial suctioning cannot be performed.
- It cannot be used to deliver drugs, as the endotracheal tube can.

Indications

Endotracheal intubation is the preferred method to secure and control the airway. The EOA should be considered if endotracheal intubation was unsuccessful after several attempts, the equipment is not available to perform endotracheal intubation, or the care provider is not trained or permitted to perform endotracheal intubation.

Technique

The EOA must be completely assembled prior to insertion. The mask seated on the face is the final indication that the tube has been inserted the proper depth. Insert the EOA following these steps (Figures 3-22a to 3-22c):

1. Hyperventilate the patient prior to insertion.
2. Assemble the mask and tube together and test the cuff for leaks. Deflate the cuff prior to insertion. Lubricate the tube with a water-soluble lubricant.
3. Place the patient's head midposition or slightly flexed. Grasp the tongue and mandible, displacing them upward and forward. Insert the EOA with the other hand, following the natural curvature of the posterior pharynx. Advance the tube until the mask is seated firmly on the patient's face. Do not force the tube if resistance is met. If this occurs, remove the tube, hyperventilate, and reattempt insertion. It may be necessary to reposition the tongue and jaw prior to reinsertion.
4. Deliver one or two ventilations while holding a tight seal with the mask. Auscultate over the epigastrium and watch for chest rise and fall. If the chest does not rise and fall or sounds are heard over the epigastrium with ventilation, immediately remove the tube and hyperventilate the patient. If the chest rises and falls and no sounds are heard over the epigastrium, inflate the distal cuff with 35 ml of air. After inflation of the cuff, reassess for chest rise and fall and epigastric sounds. If no sounds are heard in the epigastrium, resume ventilation and auscultate the chest for bilateral breath sounds in the midaxillary line. If gurgling sounds are heard in the epigastrium following inflation of the cuff, immediately remove the tube and resume ventilation.

The patient should be intubated with an endotracheal tube as soon as possible following insertion of the EOA. Be sure the airway is protected with an endotracheal tube or the patient is able to protect his own airway prior to removal of the EOA. With removal, be prepared for vomiting and possible aspiration.

Esophageal Gastric Tube Airway (EGTA)

The esophageal gastric tube airway (EGTA) is very similar to the EOA with some modifications. The EGTA's esophageal tube has an open distal end that allows for the insertion of a gastric tube into the stomach. The gastric tube is used to evacuate and decompress the stomach, reducing the incidence of aspiration of gastric contents. Also, impedance of ventilation from gastric distention is eliminated.

Alternative Airway Adjuncts

INSERTING THE ESOPHAGEAL OBTURATOR AIRWAY

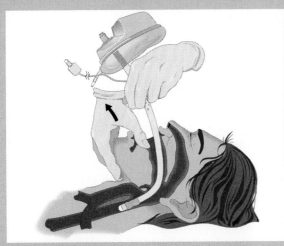

FIGURE 3-22a Insert the EOA completely assembled. Place the patient's head in a midposition or slightly flexed. Grasp the jaw and tongue. Lift up and forward.

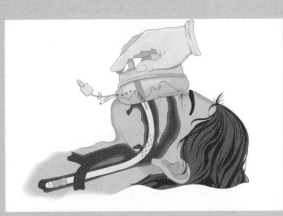

FIGURE 3-22b Advance the tube until the mask is seated snugly on the patient's face.

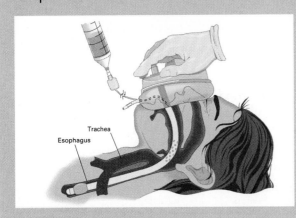

FIGURE 3-22c Deliver one or two ventilations. If the chest rises and falls and no sounds are heard over the epigastrium, inflate the distal cuff and reassess for chest rise and fall and epigastric sounds. If no sounds are heard, resume ventilation and auscultate the chest for bilateral breath sounds. If gurgling sounds are heard in the epigastrium following inflation of the cuff, immediately remove the tube and resume ventilation.

The EGTA, like the EOA, consists of a mask and esophageal tube. However, the mask has two ports: one for ventilation and the other for insertion of the gastric tube. Both are clearly marked. The complications, advantages, disadvantages, and insertion are the same as for the EOA.

Other Airway Adjuncts

Several other airway adjuncts are available that are similar to the EOA and EGTA. However, none of these devices is comparable to the endotracheal tube for airway control and ventilatory support. Two of the more common devices are the pharyngeo-tracheal lumen (PtL®) airway and the esophageal-tracheal Combitube® (ETC).

Pharyngeo-tracheal Lumen Airway (PtL®)

The pharyngeo-tracheal lumen (PtL®) airway is a dual-lumen device that is blindly inserted into the airway without the need for direct visualization. The PtL® is actually a tube within a tube, thus the dual lumen reference.

A long, clear endotracheal-type tube with a cuff at the distal end is located inside a shorter, wider tube that is designed to fit just proximal to the glottic opening. The shorter tube has a large balloon cuff that is used to seal the pharynx. The longer tube, which is designed to be inserted in either the trachea or esophagus, also has a distal cuff that is used to occlude the esophagus or isolate the trachea. An obturator is located within the long tube for cases of esophageal placement (Figure 3-23).

When the long, clear tube has been inserted into the trachea, the plastic obturator is removed and ventilation is performed through that tube. However, if the long tube is placed in the esophagus, the plastic obturator is left in place and the ventilation is performed through the green tube (Figure 3-24). The pharyngeal cuff seals the pharynx and allows for effective ventilation. The airway is secured in place with a strap that is fastened around the neck.

Two major advantages of the PtL® airway design are:

- The pharynx is sealed by the large balloon cuff located in the pharynx; therefore, a mask is not necessary for performing ventilation. This eliminates the complication of a poor mask seal during ventilation.
- The risk of inadvertent tracheal intubation is not considered a true complication since the tube is designed to be placed in either the trachea or esophagus.

Some studies have indicated that the seal with the pharyngeal balloon is still inadequate. In addition, difficulty in intubating with an endotracheal tube around the PtL® has been reported.

Esophageal Tracheal Combitube® (ETC)

The esophageal tracheal Combitube® (ETC) airway is a double-lumen airway that is structurally and functionally similar to the PtL® airway. Unlike

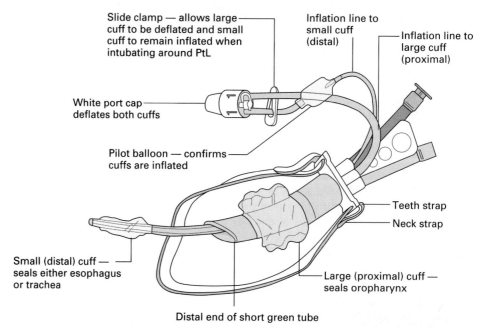

Slide clamp — allows large cuff to be deflated and small cuff to remain inflated when intubating around PtL

Inflation line to small cuff (distal)

Inflation line to large cuff (proximal)

White port cap deflates both cuffs

Pilot balloon — confirms cuffs are inflated

Teeth strap

Neck strap

Small (distal) cuff — seals either esophagus or trachea

Large (proximal) cuff — seals oropharynx

Distal end of short green tube

FIGURE 3-23 The pharyngeo-tracheal lumen (PtL®) airway.

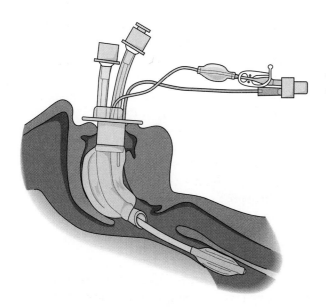

FIGURE 3-24 The PtL® airway in place. The longer tube is shown placed in the esophagus while ventilations delivered through the shorter tube are directed into the trachea.

the PtL®, the ETC lumens are not placed one inside the other. Instead, the lumens are situated side by side and separated by a partition wall within a larger tube (Figure 3-25).

The distal end of the ETC has a cuff that is used to seal either the esophagus or the trachea, depending on the placement. A proximal pharyngeal cuff, which is self-positioning and self-adjusting, is used to seal the pharynx, eliminating the need for a mask device. The #1 tube is slightly longer and delivers the ventilation through a series of holes located between the distal cuff and the pharyngeal cuff. The holes are located just proximal to the glottic opening when the tube is placed in the esophagus. The #2 tube is slightly shorter than the #1 tube and provides ventilation from the end of the tube below the distal cuff, similar to an endotracheal tube. The #2 tube is used to ventilate when the tube has been placed in the trachea. Based on

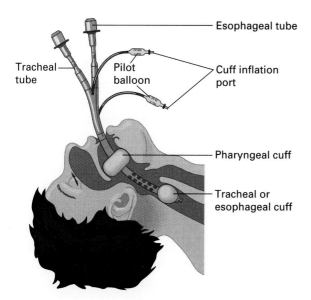

Esophageal tube

Tracheal tube

Pilot balloon

Cuff inflation port

Pharyngeal cuff

Tracheal or esophageal cuff

FIGURE 3-25 The esophageal tracheal Combitube® (ETC).

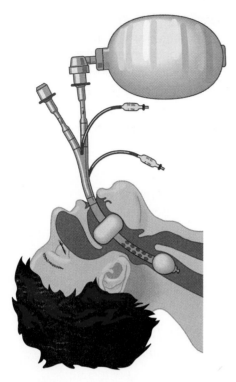

FIGURE 3-26a Esophageal placement of the Combitube® airway.

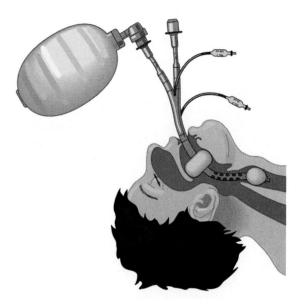

FIGURE 3-26b Tracheal placement of the Combitube® airway.

the tube design and operator use, it is more likely that the tube will be placed in the esophagus (Figures 3-26a and 3-26b).

The ETC carries the same advantages as the PtL®. However, the following are additional advantages of the ETC:

- There is no obturator in the distal lumen; therefore, immediate suctioning of gastric contents may be performed.
- A spontaneously breathing patient may breathe through the series of small holes in the opposite lumen.
- The pharyngeal cuff is self-positioning and self-adjusting, allowing for a better pharyngeal seal.

The complication rate with the use of the ETC has been low. Studies have shown that ventilation and oxygenation have been comparable to the endotracheal tube. However, experience with the device is limited. Both the PtL® and the ETC require the operator to make a proper assessment of the tube's placement, which requires some skill. Therefore, the endotracheal tube remains the airway device of choice.

Translaryngeal and Transtracheal Airways

In the event of an airway obstruction when it is not possible to establish an airway by using conventional manual or mechanical techniques, it may be necessary to puncture or incise the larynx or trachea to provide ventilation and oxygenation. These techniques are performed in the acute setting only after failure to gain control of the airway by endotracheal intubation and inability to ventilate using less invasive measures.

Transtracheal Catheter Ventilation

Transtracheal catheter ventilation, also known as needle cricothyrotomy or needle jet insufflation, is an emergency procedure for gaining rapid access to the airway in an acute obstruction that cannot be relieved by other methods. An over-the-needle catheter is inserted through the cricothyroid membrane in the lower larynx and angled downward into the trachea. Intermittent jet ventilation is provided through a valve system connected to a 100% oxygen source.

Equipment

Since this is performed only as an emergency procedure, it is important to have all the necessary equipment readily available. Unless a commercially made device is available, the following equipment is needed:

- A 12-14-gauge over-the-needle catheter (angiocath)
- A 5- or 10-ml syringe
- Pressure regulating valve and a pressure gauge
- High-pressure oxygen source (30–to–60 psi)
- High-pressure tubing to connect the pressure regulating valve to a hand operated release valve
- Relief valve connected by tubing to the catheter

Technique

The cricothyroid membrane forms the soft depression located just inferior to the thyroid cartilage (Adam's Apple) and superior to the cricoid cartilage, the large bulky circumferential ring that is the most inferior part of the larynx (Figure 3-27). A 5–to–10-ml syringe is attached to the back of the flashback chamber of the angiocath. Insert the angiocath at a 45-degree angle caudally (toward the feet) through the cricothyroid membrane (Figures 3-28a and 3-28b). Pull back on the syringe, creating a negative pressure during insertion. When air freely moves into the syringe, the angiocath is in the trachea. Stop the insertion to prevent inadvertent puncture and placement of the angiocath into the esophagus. Advance the catheter off of the stylet and

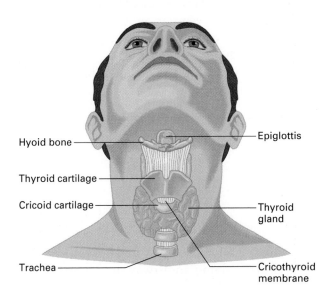

Hyoid bone —

Thyroid cartilage —

Cricoid cartilage —

Trachea —

— Epiglottis

Thyroid gland

Cricothyroid membrane

FIGURE 3-27 The cricothyroid membrane is inferior to the thyroid cartilage and superior to the cricoid cartilage (lower border of the larynx).

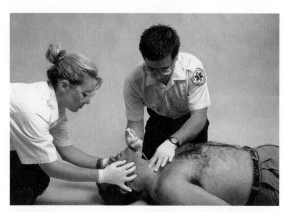

FIGURE 3-28a To perform a transtracheal catheter ventilation, insert the angiocath at a 45-degree angle caudally through the crico-thyroid membrane.

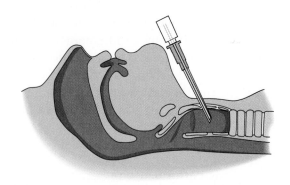

FIGURE 3-28b The angiocath properly placed through the cricothyroid membrane into the trachea.

into the trachea until the hub rests on the skin. The tubing is connected to the hub of the catheter while it is held in place. Open the release valve, allowing the oxygen under high pressure to flow through the catheter and inflate the lungs. Adjust the pressure so that the chest rises adequately with each insufflation. As soon as the chest rises during ventilation, stop the insufflation of oxygen. Exhalation occurs passively.

Generally, even with acute blockage of the airway, there is enough opening to permit passive exhalation through the pharynx. However, you must carefully monitor the chest during inhalation and exhalation. If the chest remains inflated after the exhalation period, a complete airway obstruction may be present proximal to the cricothyroid membrane, thus blocking passive exhalation. In this situation, a second catheter will need to be inserted next to the first to allow for adequate exhalation. If this procedure does not correct the exhalation problem, cricothyrotomy should be considered.

Complications

Several complications of transtracheal catheter ventilation may occur both from the insertion and from the technique of ventilation itself. A major disadvantage of using this device and technique is carbon dioxide retention and buildup from inadequate ventilation. Although transtracheal catheter ventilation provides oxygenation, adequate ventilation is not possible. The following are potential complications associated with the device:

- Barotrauma resulting in a pneumothorax from the high pressure and air entrapment
- Hemorrhage at the site of needle insertion
- Laceration of the thyroid gland
- Perforation of the esophagus
- Inability to suction secretions
- Subcutaneous or mediastinal emphysema

Employing this technique when other more suitable and less complicated methods of establishing and maintaining an airway are available is a major error. Transtracheal catheter ventilation should only be performed when all other conventional methods of airway control are not possible or not effective. This technique is used when an obstruction prevents successful intubation of the trachea. It is not intended to be employed as an alternative because of lack of skill of the health care provider to intubate the trachea successfully.

Cricothyrotomy

The cricothyrotomy is another technique that is used to establish an emergency airway in a patient when other methods are not possible or effective. An incision or puncture is made through the cricothyroid membrane and an endotracheal tube or other similar device is inserted into the trachea. Like transtracheal catheter ventilation, a cricothyrotomy provides a temporary avenue for ventilation and oxygenation. However, this technique provides a much better airway, ventilation, and oxygenation than the transtracheal catheter ventilation technique.

Indications

Indications for a cricothyrotomy include:

- Inability to intubate the trachea because of a complete airway obstruction that is not relieved by manual foreign body obstruction techniques or laryngoscopy
- Trauma to the face or upper airway, hemorrhage, or swelling that prevents endotracheal intubation or other airway techniques

Surgical Technique

The surgical technique uses conventional equipment that is readily available. There are commercially prepared devices specifically designed for cricothyrotomy that differ slightly from the surgical technique as described below:

1. Locate the cricothyroid membrane between the thyroid and cricoid cartilage.
2. Cleanse the site with alcohol or another antiseptic solution.
3. While stabilizing the larynx with your nondominant hand, make a horizontal incision with a scalpel into the cricothyroid membrane (Figure 3-29).
4. Insert the handle of the scalpel into the incision and rotate it 90 degrees.
5. Insert the largest possible endotracheal tube, usually a pediatric size (5.0 or 5.5 mm), into the opening. The tube only needs to be inserted a few centimeters until the cuff is completely in the trachea. The tip of the tube must be above the carina.
6. Inflate the cuff with 8–to–10 ml of air.
7. Attach a bag-valve-mask device to the 15/22 mm adapter on the tube and ventilate with the highest concentration of oxygen that can be provided.

Another suggested method requires the scalpel to be left in place. A curved hemostat is inserted in the opening in a closed position, rotated, and then opened widely to create a larger opening. Then the scalpel is removed. This provides a much larger opening that facilitates easier insertion of an endotracheal tube.

FIGURE 3-29 In the cricothyrotomy, a surgical incision or puncture is made into the cricothyroid membrane.

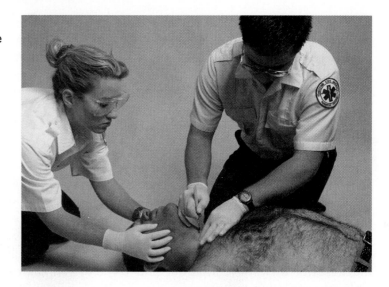

Complications

The following are complications associated with the cricothyrotomy technique:

- Damage to blood vessels, causing significant hemorrhage
- False passage
- Perforation of the esophagus
- Subcutaneous or mediastinal emphysema
- Tracheal stenosis

A contraindication to performing a cricothyrotomy is the ability to establish and maintain an airway using other possible techniques and devices. The risks of the procedure outweigh the potential benefits when other means are available.

Tracheostomy

Tracheostomy, which is a surgical opening directly into the trachea, is not a technique that should be performed in an emergency setting. It is better performed by a skilled care provider in the operating room under a controlled setting. The airway should first be secured by endotracheal intubation, transtracheal catheter ventilation, or cricothyrotomy prior to consideration of performing a tracheostomy.

Ventilation Techniques

Several techniques and devices are available to perform positive pressure ventilation when ventilatory support is necessary. These include mouth-to-mouth; mouth-to-nose; bag-valve-mask devices; flow restricted, oxygen-powered ventilation devices; and automatic transport ventilators.

Mouth-to-Mouth and Mouth-to-Nose Ventilation

This basic technique of ventilation uses the expired air of the care provider to provide positive pressure ventilation to the patient. Adequate tidal volumes of air can be delivered by this method. An average of 10–to–15 ml/kg of tidal volume is necessary to adequately inflate a person's lungs. The vital capacity of the average person is several liters more than that required to provide adequate lung inflation; therefore, this method provides sufficient tidal volumes during positive pressure ventilation.

Exhaled air contains approximately 17% oxygen. This is a limitation to effective oxygenation. The care provider can breathe oxygen from a simple face mask, nasal cannula, or other simple oxygen-delivery device to increase the percentage of delivered oxygen to the patient. This method may increase oxygen content delivered by almost 5%.

Cross contamination of infectious disease is also a concern. These techniques should be performed with a barrier device.

Mouth-to-Mask Ventilation

A mask, commonly referred to as a pocket mask, can be used to increase the effectiveness of ventilation by the care provider (Figure 3-30). The mask should:

- Be constructed of a transparent material to allow for detection of vomitus, secretions, or other substances in the mouth
- Be capable of fitting tightly to the face to provide a good mask seal
- Contain an oxygen inlet to increase the delivered oxygen to the patient
- Contain a one-way valve to reduce the risk of contamination by infectious secretions
- Be available in sizes for the adult, child, and infant

Advantages

Mouth-to-mask ventilation has the same advantage as mouth-to-mouth ventilation of providing more-than-adequate tidal volumes. This technique has actually been shown to be more effective in delivering adequate tidal volumes on mannikins than bag-valve-mask ventilation.

The other major advantages of mouth-to-mask ventilation are:

- Supplemental oxygen administration is possible.
- There is no direct contact with the patient's mouth or nose.
- Exhaled gases are diverted through a one-way valve.
- It provides effective tidal volumes.

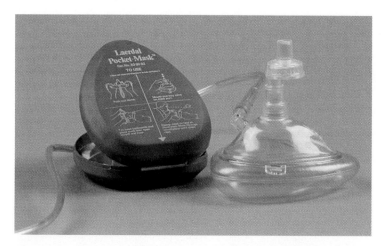

FIGURE 3-30 The pocket mask.

Technique

Connect a one-way valve to the ventilation port to eliminate exposure to the patient's exhaled gas. Connect oxygen tubing to the oxygen inlet valve and set it at 10–to–15 lpm. (At 10 lpm a concentration of inspired oxygen of 50% will be achieved, whereas at 15 lpm an 80% inspired oxygen concentration can be delivered.) To assure an open airway, you can use an oropharyngeal airway in conjunction with the appropriate manual airway maneuver, either a head-tilt, chin-lift or jaw-thrust maneuver. Fit the mask over the bridge of the nose and in the cleft of the chin. Place both hands over the mask with the thumb-sides of the hands placing pressure to the sides of the mask, creating an airtight seal. Use the index, middle, and ring fingers to bring the mandible upward toward the mask while maintaining the head tilt or jaw thrust. Blow into the ventilation port while watching for chest rise (Figure 3-31).

Deliver each breath over a 1½–to–2-second period for an adult and a 1–to–1½-second period for an infant or child. (Breaths delivered more quickly are likely to create high esophageal pressure and gastric insufflation with resultant gastric distention.) You can also apply cricoid pressure to reduce the incidence of gastric insufflation and distention.

Bag-Valve Devices

A bag-valve device can be used to provide positive pressure ventilation in conjunction with an endotracheal tube, with an alternative airway adjunct such as an EOA, PtL®, or ETC, or with a mask. The bag-valve device is comprised of a self-inflating bag, a nonrebreathing valve to vent all exhaled gases away from the bag, and a mask (Figure 3-32). Most bag-valve-mask devices have a volume of approximately 1600 ml. When used in conjunction with an endotracheal tube, the bag-valve device can usually deliver an adequate tidal volume of 10–to–15 ml/kg.

When performing ventilation with a bag-valve device connected to a mask, it is imperative that you establish and maintain a proper manual airway maneuver (head-tilt, chin-lift or jaw thrust). You can use an oropharyngeal airway to facilitate better airway control. Deliver each ventilation over a 1½–to–2-second period in the adult and 1–to–1½ seconds in the infant and child to reduce the likelihood of creating high esophageal pressure with resultant gastric insufflation and gastric distention. Cricoid pressure can also

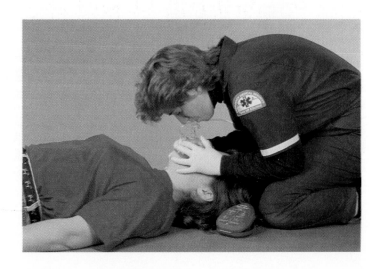

FIGURE 3-31 Mouth-to-mask ventilation.

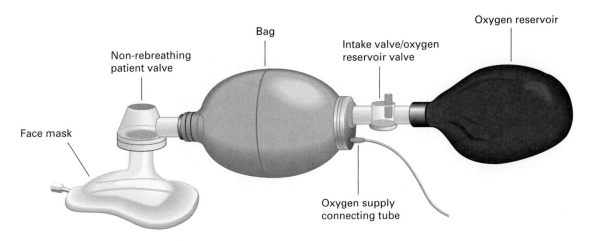

FIGURE 3-32 Bag-valve-mask device.

be used to reduce these complications. Oxygen should be attached to the bag-valve device and a reservoir used to maximize the concentration of delivered oxygen.

Desired Features

A bag-valve device that is acceptable for patient use should have the following standard features:

- A self-refilling bag that is either disposable or can be easily cleaned and sterilized
- A nonjam valve system that can accommodate at least 15 lpm oxygen inlet flow
- Standard 15/22 mm fittings to allow for connection with an endotracheal tube and other airway adjuncts
- Oxygen connection and a reservoir bag or tubing that facilitates the delivery of high concentrations of oxygen
- A nonrebreathing valve that does not allow any of the patient's exhaled gases to escape into the bag
- Manufacture of material that allows for proper function under all environmental conditions and temperature extremes
- Available in adult, child, and infant sizes

Advantages

Advantages to performing ventilation with a bag-valve device are as follows:

- It eliminates direct contact with the patient during ventilation.
- High concentrations of oxygen, up toward 98%, may be delivered to the patient during ventilations while using a reservoir tube or bag with high flow oxygen.
- The patient's exhaled gas is vented out of the bag so no rebreathing of oxygen-poor gas occurs.
- It can provide adequate ventilation when used with an endotracheal tube.
- The device is readily available and does not require an oxygen source to power it.
- It permits assessment of lung compliance during ventilation.

Disadvantages

The following are disadvantages of the bag-valve device ventilation:

- In adults, the bag-valve device may provide less tidal volume than mouth-to-mouth or mouth-to-mask ventilation.
- When used with a mask, one operator has difficulty in maintaining a tight mask seal and an adequate airway with one hand while squeezing the bag hard enough with the other hand to deliver an adequate tidal volume.
- The device is more effective when used with two experienced and well-trained care providers, one to hold the mask seal with two hands while the other squeezes the bag with two hands.
- Improperly over-squeezing the bag-valve device, or delivering the ventilations at too fast a rate, will increase the risk of gastric insufflation.

Technique

Position yourself at the top of the patient's head and establish an airway using the appropriate manual technique. If no cervical spinal injury is suspected, you can tilt the head back and place it on a towel or pillow to achieve a sniffing position. Insert an oropharyngeal airway if the patient has no gag reflex. Consider a nasopharyngeal airway in the patient who is not completely unresponsive but needs positive pressure ventilation. Fit the mask over the bridge of the nose and in the cleft of the chin (Figure 3-33). Hold the mask tightly against the face to form an airtight seal.

With the head in the proper position, squeeze the bag slowly to deliver an adequate tidal volume of 10–to–15 ml/kg. The volume should be delivered over 1½–to–2 seconds in the adult and 1–to–1½ seconds in the infant and child. If only one care provider is ventilating, he will squeeze the bag with one hand while holding a mask seal with the other (Figure 3-34a). This can be better accomplished by squeezing the bag slowly against his body to deliver a greater volume. One-person ventilation with a bag-valve-mask device often leads to early fatigue and inadequate ventilation. If two care providers are available, one will squeeze the bag with two hands to deliver an adequate tidal volume while the other holds the mask seal (Figure 3-34b). Observe the chest rise to determine if adequate volume is being delivered. A third care provider may apply cricoid pressure to reduce the incidence of gastric distention and aspiration.

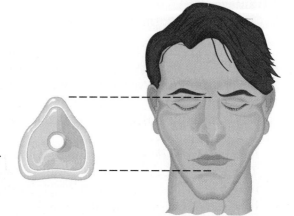

FIGURE 3-33 Always use the proper mask size. The mask should fit over the bridge of the nose and in the cleft of the chin.

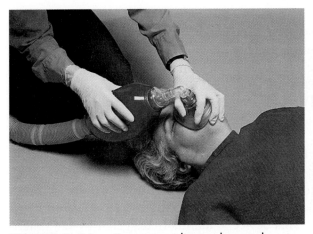

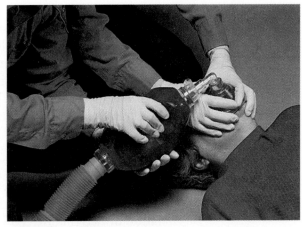

FIGURE 3-34a One-person bag-valve-mask method.

FIGURE 3-34b Two-person bag-valve-mask method.

If spinal injury is suspected, manual in-line stabilization of the patient's head must be established and maintained during ventilation, and cricoid pressure must be avoided (Figures 3-35a to 3-35c).

IN-LINE STABILIZATION DURING BAG-VALVE VENTILATION

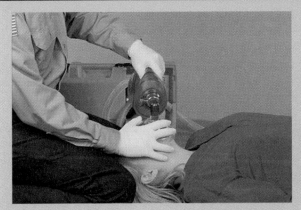

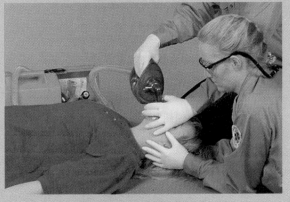

FIGURE 3-35a Technique for one-person in-line stabilization during bag-valve ventilation.

FIGURE 3-35b Technique for two-person in-line stabilization during bag-valve ventilation.

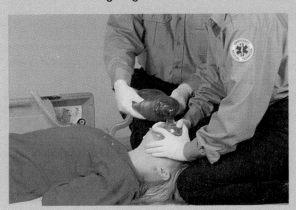

FIGURE 3-35c Alternative technique for two-person in-line stabilization during bag-valve ventilation

Complications

A major complication associated with bag-valve devices is the inability to provide adequate tidal volumes to patients who are not intubated. Operator fatigue occurs early in one-person bag-valve-mask ventilation, which may lead to inadequate mask seal and insufficient delivered volume. This leads to ventilatory insufficiency. The proper technique requires training, practice, and demonstrated proficiency.

Flow-Restricted, Oxygen-Powered, Manually Triggered Ventilation Device

Another method of providing positive pressure ventilation—to an adult patient only—is through the use of a flow-restricted, oxygen-powered ventilation device (Figure 3-36). This device is manually triggered by the practitioner to deliver the desired tidal volume. Since it is powered by an oxygen source, 100% oxygen is delivered with each ventilation. In the spontaneously breathing patient, the negative pressure generated with inspiration will automatically open the valve and allow the patient to breathe 100% oxygen. Oxygen flow ceases once inhalation ends. The device can be used in conjunction with an endotracheal tube, EOA, PtL®, ETC, mask, or other acceptable airway adjunct.

Features

The flow-restricted, oxygen-powered ventilation device should have the following features:

- A peak flow rate of less than 40 lpm of 100% oxygen
- An inspiratory-pressure-relief valve that opens at approximately 60 centimeters of water pressure and vents any remaining volume to the atmosphere or ceases gas flow
- An audible alarm that sounds whenever the relief-valve pressure is exceeded
- Adaptability to a variety of environmental conditions and extremes of temperature
- An activating trigger or on/off button positioned so the operator can keep both hands on the mask to hold a seal
- A standard 15/22 mm coupling to fit an endotracheal tube, mask, and other alternative airways

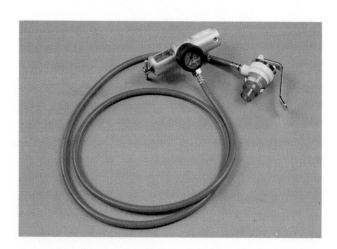

FIGURE 3-36 A flow-restricted, oxygen-powered ventilation device.

Technique
Follow the steps listed below when using a flow-restricted, oxygen-powered ventilation device:

1. Check the unit to ensure that it is functioning properly.

2. Open the airway using a manual maneuver.

3. Attach an adult mask to the ventilation port.

4. Position your hands over the mask and fit it to the patient's face, holding a tight seal with both hands.

5. Depress the button to activate the device and deliver the ventilation. As soon as the chest rises, release the button to deactivate the device and stop the airflow.

6. Exhalation occurs through the one-way valve and out to the atmosphere.

Complications
The flow-restricted, oxygen-powered ventilation device is designed to be used on adults only. Because of the high pressure and flow rates, it is not acceptable for infants or children. Also because of the high pressure and flow rates, gastric distention may easily occur. In addition, overinflation can lead to barotrauma, potentially resulting in a pneumothorax. High flow rates in intubated patients may lead to intrapulmonary shunting and maldistribution of ventilation. Because of the high rate of complications, only those specially trained should use the device for ventilation.

Automatic Transport Ventilator (ATV)

Another device used for positive pressure ventilation is the automatic transport ventilator, or ATV (Figure 3-37). Several different devices are currently available. They have been shown to be excellent at providing and maintaining a constant rate and tidal volume during ventilation and maintaining adequate oxygenation of arterial blood. In addition, most ATVs use oxygen as their power source, thereby providing 100% oxygen during ventilation.

Advantages
The ATV can deliver oxygen at lower inspiratory flow rates and for longer inspiratory times. Therefore, the device is less likely to cause gastric distention compared with other methods of positive pressure ventilation, including mouth-to-mask, bag-valve-mask, and flow-restricted, oxygen-powered

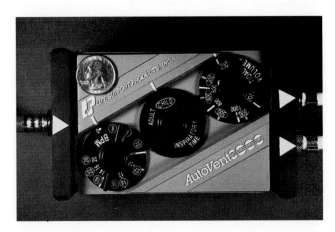

FIGURE 3-37 Automatic transport ventilator. (The coin shows relative size.)

ventilation devices. However, as with any other ventilation device, gastric distention can occur if the patient's head and neck are improperly positioned.

Advantages of the ATV are listed below:

- Oxygen can be delivered at lower inspiratory flow rates and for longer inspiratory times, thereby lessening the likelihood of gastric distention.
- The operator is free to use both hands to hold a mask seal or perform other responsibilities if the patient is intubated.
- The device can be set to deliver a specific tidal volume, respiratory rate, and minute volume.
- Alarms indicate low pressure in the oxygen tank as well as accidental disconnection from the ventilator.
- Cricoid pressure can be performed with one hand while the other holds the mask seal.

Disadvantages

There are a few disadvantages associated with the ATV:

- Because most ATVs are oxygen powered, a constant oxygen supply is needed to power the device. A bag-valve-mask device should always be readily available when using the ATV.
- The ATV cannot be used in children less than 5 years of age.
- When using the ATV, it is not possible to feel an increase in airway resistance or a decrease in lung compliance.

Features

The minimum desirable features of the ATV are as follows:

- A standard 15/22 mm adapter to fit an endotracheal tube, mask, or other airway adjunct
- A rugged design that is also lightweight (2–5 kg)
- Capable of operating under temperature extremes and under all environmental conditions
- A peak-inspiratory-pressure-limiting valve that is set at 60 cmH$_2$0 but can be increased to 80 cmH$_2$0
- An audible alarm that indicates high airway pressure or poor lung compliance when peak inspiratory limiting pressure is generated
- Minimal gas consumption so that the device can operate for a minimum of 45 minutes on an E cylinder
- Ability to deliver 100% oxygen with each ventilation
- Ability to deliver each ventilation over a 2-second period at a maximum flow rate of approximately 30 L/minute in the adult and 1 second duration in children with a maximum flow rate of 15 l/minute
- Ability to provide a rate of 10 ventilations/minute for an adult and 20 ventilations/minute for a child
- If it has a demand-valve feature, it should deliver an inspiratory flow rate of at least 100 L/minute and triggered at –2 cmH$_2$0 inspiratory pressure to reduce the work of breathing.

Technique

Check that the ATV is working properly and is attached to the endotracheal tube, mask, or airway adjunct. (These ventilators are most commonly used in intubated patients.) Set the tidal volume and ventilation rate if not already set on the unit. Turn the unit on and watch for adequate chest rise. Adjust the tidal-volume control to provide adequate ventilation. Continuously monitor the device to ensure adequate ventilation volumes and rate.

Suction

Oropharyngeal Suctioning

Two different types of suction catheters are available. A rigid catheter, commonly referred to as a Yankauer or tonsil tip catheter, is used to suction blood, secretions, or other foreign material from the mouth and oropharynx. A soft suction catheter is used to perform suctioning through an endotracheal tube to remove secretions from the tracheobronchial tree. The soft suction catheter is also used to clear secretions from the nasopharynx.

When suctioning the mouth or pharynx, high negative pressure is necessary. A suction pressure of greater than –120 mmHg should be used.

Tracheobronchial Suctioning

The soft suction catheter should have the following design features:

- Molded end and soft side holes to reduce mucosal trauma
- Available in various lengths to allow it to pass through the tip of the endotracheal tube
- Made of material that produces a minimal amount of friction during insertion through the endotracheal tube
- Sterile, disposable, and designed for one-time use

Technique

Follow these steps (Figures 3-38a to 3-38f) when performing tracheobronchial suctioning:

1. Check the equipment and make sure it is in proper working order. Place the patient on an ECG monitor if not already done.
2. Set the suction pressure at between –80 and –120 mmHg.
3. Hyperventilate the patient for 1 minute or preoxygenate the patient for 5 minutes.
4. Insert the catheter without suction pressure applied. This is accomplished by keeping your finger or thumb off of the suction port located proximally and on the side of the catheter.
5. Advance the catheter to the level of the carina.
6. Close the suction port and apply intermittent suction while spiraling and withdrawing the catheter.
7. Do not apply suction for greater than 15 seconds and continuously monitor the cardiac rhythm for indication of dysrhythmias. If bradycardia or other dysrhythmias are present, immediately stop the procedure and hyperventilate the patient.
8. Prior to repeating the procedure, hyperventilate the patient for approximately 30 seconds.

OROTRACHEAL SUCTIONING

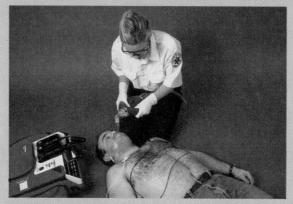

FIGURE 3-38a Hyperventilate the patient prior to suctioning.

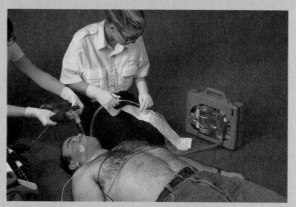

FIGURE 3-38b Meanwhile, check the suction equipment. Orotracheal suctioning is a sterile procedure, so be careful not to contaminate the suction catheter.

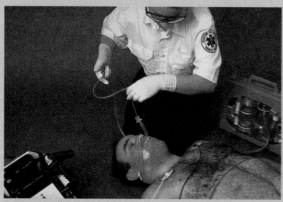

FIGURE 3-38c Insert the catheter without suction applied.

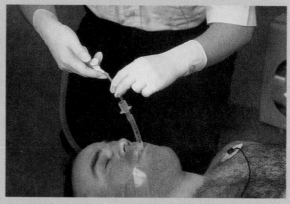

FIGURE 3-38d Advance the catheter.

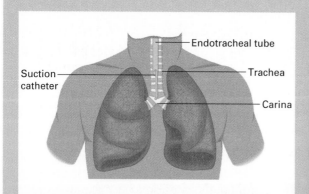

FIGURE 3-38e Continue to advance the catheter to the level of the carina.

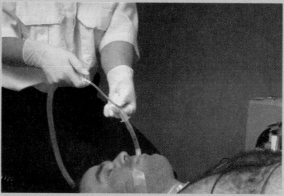

FIGURE 3-38f Apply suction by closing the suction port (covering the open part of the catheter). Apply intermittent suction while withdrawing the catheter.

Complications

The following are complications associated with tracheobronchial suctioning:

- Hypoxemia may occur secondary to a decrease in functional residual volume due to interruption of ventilation and the negative pressure of the suction itself. This is the most serious complication, and may lead to cardiac arrest.
- Stimulation of the airway may cause an increase in arterial pressure and tachycardia or increases in intracranial pressure.
- Cardiac dysrhythmias, particularly bradycardia, may occur due to a decrease in myocardial oxygen supply from hypoxemia or due to an increased myocardial demand from hypertension or tachycardia.
- Vagal stimulation may produce bradycardia and hypotension.
- An increase in intracranial pressure and decrease in cerebral blood flow may result from stimulation of coughing during suctioning.
- Mucosal damage may result in edema, ulceration, and tracheal infection from loss of integrity.

Oxygen Therapy

Any patient with an acute cardiac condition should receive supplemental oxygen, even in the absence of respiratory distress. A nasal cannula can be applied at 2 lpm for comfort. If the patient is exhibiting mild respiratory distress, the oxygen flow should be increased to 5–to–6 lpm. A high concentration of oxygen, preferably as close to 100% as possible with a nonrebreather mask, should be delivered to the patient with severe respiratory compromise or evidence of hypoxia. If positive pressure ventilation is being performed, supplemental oxygen should be attached to the ventilation device to deliver as high a concentration of oxygen as possible. Administration of 100% oxygen to any nonbreathing patient is advisable, likewise to any serious respiratory- or cardiac-compromised patient. Oxygen can then be titrated according to PaO_2, or oxygen saturation, values.

Equipment

Oxygen delivery equipment (Figure 3-39) normally consists of the following:

- An oxygen supply derived from a cylinder or wall unit
- Valve with a handle to open the cylinder
- Pressure gauge and flowmeter to regulate the oxygen flow
- Tubing to connect the delivery device to the regulator
- Humidifier to humidify the oxygen

Four common devices are used to deliver oxygen to a patient: nasal cannula, face mask, face mask with an oxygen reservoir, and Venturi mask. Each has advantages, disadvantages, and specific uses.

Nasal Cannula

The nasal cannula is considered a low-flow oxygen system (Figures 3-40a and 3-40b). The gas flow emitted from the nasal cannula is not enough to provide an adequate tidal volume; therefore, the gas is mixed with ambient air during inspiration. The amount of oxygen inspired is dependent on the liter flow as well as the tidal volume of the patient. As a general rule, for

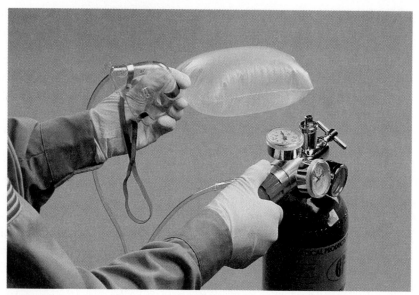

FIGURE 3-39 Oxygen delivery equipment.

every increase of 1 liter per minute, the inspired oxygen concentration will increase by 4%. Thus, at 1 lpm, the FiO_2 (concentration of inspired oxygen) will be approximately 25%, whereas at 6 lpm, the approximate FiO_2 will be 45%. However, the actual oxygen concentration range is said to be between 24% and 44%.

The patient must be breathing in an adequate tidal volume in order to use this device. The liter flow is restricted to no less than 1 lpm and no greater than 6 lpm. This device is best used in patients with minimal distress, when the desired FiO_2 to be delivered is low, or when the patient is unable to tolerate an oxygen face mask.

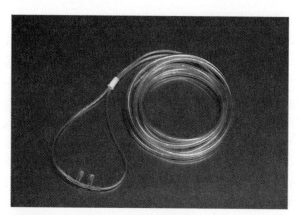

FIGURE 3-40a Nasal cannula.

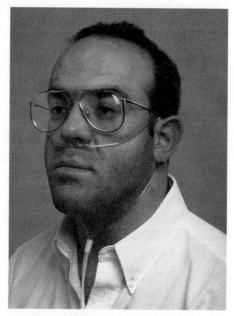

FIGURE 3-40b Nasal cannula applied to patient.

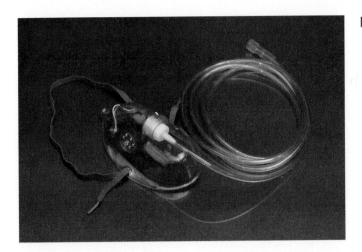

FIGURE 3-41 Simple face mask.

Face Mask

The simple face mask (Figure 3-41) is usually well tolerated by an adult patient. This device can deliver oxygen concentrations of between 40% and 60% at a recommended liter flow of 8–to–10 lpm. Like the nasal cannula, the simple face mask allows the patient to inspire ambient air, diluting the oxygen concentration. It is imperative that a minimum liter flow of 6 lpm be used to avoid accumulation of exhaled gas in the mask with subsequent rebreathing of that gas.

Face Mask with a Reservoir

This device, which consists of a face mask, nonrebreather valve, and reservoir, is commonly referred to as a nonrebreather mask (Figures 3-42a and 3-42b). A nonrebreather valve located between the mask and the reservoir bag prevents the patient's exhaled gas from entering the reservoir bag and diluting the oxygen concentration. Instead, the exhaled gas is diverted out of the mask through two side ports while the reservoir is filling with 100% oxygen. On the patient's next inspiration, the 100% oxygen that has collected in the reservoir is drawn up into the mask and breathed in. The side ports have rubber gaskets that occlude at least one port to reduce the amount of inspired ambient air. This provides the greatest concentration of oxygen.

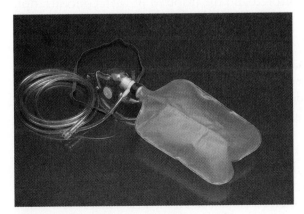

FIGURE 3-42a Nonrebreather mask.

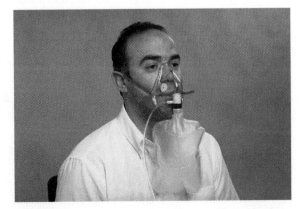

FIGURE 3-42b Nonrebreather mask applied to patient.

FIGURE 3-43 Venturi mask.

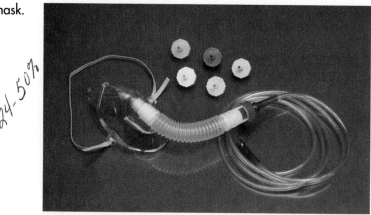

A constant flow of oxygen is required to keep the reservoir bag inflated. An oxygen flow of 6 lpm will provide an FiO$_2$ concentration of approximately 60%. With each liter/minute increase, a parallel increase of approximately 10% FiO$_2$ will occur. Thus, at 10 lpm the device may deliver up toward 100% oxygen.

This device is used on patients who are spontaneously breathing with an adequate tidal volume but who require high concentrations of oxygen. Carbon monoxide poisoning, head injuries, and near-drowning are just a few situations that may require high concentrations of oxygen delivered by a nonrebreather. It is important to monitor these patients closely for deterioration and respiratory insufficiency, vomiting, and airway occlusion.

Venturi Mask

The Venturi mask (Figure 3-43) is capable of delivering fixed concentrations of oxygen. This is accomplished by forcing the oxygen through an entrainment valve. The oxygen concentration is adjusted by changing the entrainment valve size and oxygen liter flow. Typical concentrations of 24%, 28%, 35%, and 40% are used.

A Venturi mask is commonly used in chronic obstructive pulmonary disease (COPD) patients who require low or restricted oxygen concentrations. In the acute setting however, if the COPD patient appears to be hypoxic, never withhold oxygen from him. The patient's oxygen saturation and ventilation efforts are monitored and the inspired oxygen concentration adjusted accordingly.

SUMMARY

Within this chapter we have reviewed techniques and equipment necessary to secure a patent airway, provide effective ventilatory support, and administer supplemental oxygen. It is imperative that the right techniques and equipment be used to ensure effective ventilation and oxygenation of the patient.

Dependent on the patient's condition, you may initially need to manage the airway with basic manual maneuvers and basic airway adjuncts, then move to more advanced techniques and equipment if necessary. In general, the endotracheal tube is the preferred advanced airway. As a last resort when endotracheal intubation cannot be performed, translaryngeal or transtracheal ventilation may need to be performed.

CASE STUDY FOLLOW-UP

Assessment

During your initial assessment of Mrs. Brookley, you find a 75-year-old female patient who is ashen gray and cyanotic and who has gasping respirations and vomitus streaming from her mouth. A carotid pulse is present, strong but irregular at a rate of 78/minute. You glance up at the cardiac monitor and note atrial fibrillation.

You instruct Mrs. Brookley's husband to leave the room as you call for additional help.

Treatment

You immediately attach a tonsil tip catheter to the suction tubing and set the wall suction at greater than −120 mmHg. You do a crossed-finger technique to open Mrs. Brookley's mouth and suction the vomitus from her oral cavity. Once the vomitus is clear, you perform a head-tilt, chin-lift maneuver to manually open her airway. You assess her chest for rise and fall and feel for air movement from her nose and mouth. Your patient has one gasping-type respiration. You immediately measure an oropharyngeal airway and begin to insert it into her oropharynx. She gags, so you immediately remove the airway. You quickly lubricate a nasopharyngeal airway and insert it into her right nare. She accepts the airway without incident.

With the head-tilt, chin-lift maintained, you place the mask of the bag-valve-mask device over Mrs. Brookley's face and form a tight seal. Two of your coworkers arrive. You instruct them to perform two-person bag-valve-mask ventilation. As they attempt ventilation, Mrs. Brookley begins to have projectile emesis. You turn her on her side and scoop out the vomitus with a finger sweep with a gloved hand. You then apply suction to remove the remainder of the vomitus from her airway, which now appears to be clear. Your coworkers resume ventilation and begin to hyperventilate at your command.

Because of the significant decrease in her mental status and the potential for a compromised airway, you elect to intubate Mrs. Brookley's trachea with an endotracheal tube to protect her airway. You select a 7.5 mm tube

based on the patient's size. You also choose a #3 straight blade and prepare your equipment. You lubricate a stylet, insert it into the endotracheal tube, and form the tube into a "hockey stick" shape. You lightly lubricate the tube with lidocaine jelly. You also assess the proper functioning of the laryngoscope.

You instruct your coworkers to stop ventilation. You insert the straight blade into the right side of Mrs. Brookley's mouth, sweeping her tongue to the left. You insert the blade to the base of the tongue, carefully noting the lack of a gag reflex, and then into the hypopharynx. As you lift the laryngoscope handle up and forward, you expose the glottic opening. You insert the endotracheal tube into the right side of her mouth and watch it disappear into the trachea past the cords. Once the proximal end of the cuff is about 1.5 cm beyond the level of the vocal cords, you stop the insertion and remove the laryngoscope handle and blade. You firmly hold the tube in place and remove the stylet while noting that the tube is at 23 cm at the level of her teeth. You inject 10 ml of air into the inflation port to inflate the distal cuff. The pilot balloon inflates, indicating that the cuff is inflated.

While holding the tube, your coworker attaches the bag-valve device to the tube and delivers a ventilation. You inspect Mrs. Brookley's chest for rise while auscultating over her epigastrium. Her chest wall rises with the ventilation and you hear no gurgling sounds over her epigastrium.

Having confirmed that the tube is not misplaced into the esophagus, you instruct your coworker to continue to ventilate while you auscultate at the second intercostal space midclavicular and fourth intercostal space midaxillary, comparing the breath sounds on the right and left. You hear good breath sounds on the right, but diminished sounds on the left. You suspect a right mainstem intubation, so you deflate the cuff and pull back on the tube about one centimeter to 22 cm at the level of the teeth. You reinflate the cuff and auscultate with each ventilation. The breath sounds are now equal and clear bilaterally.

(continued)

You reassess tube placement by watching for chest rise and fall, auscultating over the epigastrium for gurgling sounds, and listening for equal breath sounds. The chest continues to rise and fall, no gurgling sounds are heard, and equal breath sounds are heard with each ventilation.

You again note the tube is at 22 cm at the level of the teeth. You secure the tube with a commercial endotracheal tube holder.

The physician arrives and begins to assess Mrs. Brookley. He is impressed that she is already intubated and has a secure airway.

Select the appropriate device to ventilate the patient. The device must be capable of delivering an adequate tidal volume to ensure effective ventilatory volumes. In some cases, mouth-to-mask ventilation may be more effective in delivering a sufficient tidal volume than bag-valve-mask ventilation. An automatic transport ventilator has many advantages and should be considered in certain situations.

Supplemental oxygen administration is vital when providing positive pressure ventilation. In addition, you should administer oxygen to any patient suffering from respiratory or cardiovascular compromise.

Without a patent airway, and without adequate ventilation and oxygenation, all other therapies become futile. You must carefully assess the patient and approach airway and ventilatory support and oxygen therapy aggressively.

REVIEW QUESTIONS

1. Sonorous sounds heard upon inspiration indicate
    a. an increase in airway resistance in the bronchioles.
    b. a partial occlusion at the level of the pharynx.
    c. secretions or vomitus in the hypopharynx.
    d. laryngeal occlusion due to edema.

2. With the oropharyngeal airway in place
    a. it is not necessary to maintain a manual airway maneuver.
    b. tracheobronchial suctioning may be performed.
    c. a head-tilt, chin-lift or jaw-thrust maneuver must be maintained.
    d. stimulation of the gag reflex will not occur.

3. Which of the following is **not** an advantage of endotracheal intubation?
    a. It isolates the trachea, preventing aspiration of foreign material.
    b. It provides a route for administration of certain drugs.
    c. It permits asynchronous chest compressions and ventilation to be performed.
    d. It stimulates a sympathetic nervous system response.

4. The curved laryngoscope blade is designed to fit
    a. in the vallecula to indirectly lift the epiglottis.
    b. under the epiglottis to directly lift it up.
    c. in the glottic opening to expose the vocal cords.
    d. in the aryepiglottic fold to indirectly lift the epiglottis.

5. Which of the following endotracheal tube sizes would be most appropriate for both adult males and females in an emergency situation where immediate endotracheal intubation is necessary?
   a. 6.0 mm i.d.
   b. 7.0 mm i.d.
   c. 7.5 mm i.d.
   d. 8.0 mm i.d.

6. Insertion of the endotracheal tube in the glottic opening should be stopped when
   a. the proximal end of the cuff has passed 1 to 2.5 cm beyond the level of the vocal cords.
   b. resistance is met and the tip of the tube is suspected to be at the level of the carina.
   c. the 23 cm marker on the tube is at the level of the front teeth.
   d. the distal end of the cuff is at the level of the vocal cords.

7. Which of the following should be initially performed with the first ventilation following intubation to confirm endotracheal tube placement?
   a. Auscultate bilateral breath sounds.
   b. Assess chest rise and auscultate for epigastric sounds.
   c. Inspect for condensation in the endotracheal tube.
   d. Inspect the centimeter marker at the level of the teeth.

8. Which of the following should be done when performing orotracheal intubation in a patient with blunt trauma to the face?
   a. Only 5 ml of air should be used to inflate the cuff to reduce the cuff pressure.
   b. The patient should not be hyperventilated because of suspected intracranial hypertension.
   c. The head and neck must be maintained in a neutral in-line position.
   d. The distal end of the cuff should only be inserted to the level of the cords.

9. Which of the following is a contraindication to the use of the esophageal obturator airway?
   a. a patient who is greater than 7 feet tall
   b. a patient who is greater than 16 years of age
   c. an unresponsive patient with no gag reflex
   d. a narcotic drug overdose patient

10. The cricothyroid membrane is located
   a. inferior to the cricoid cartilage and superior to the thyroid cartilage.
   b. superior to the thyroid cartilage and inferior to the hyoid bone.
   c. inferior to the thyroid cartilage and superior to the cricoid cartilage.
   d. inferior to the cricoid and superior to the suprasternal notch.

11. The tidal volume that should be delivered to an adult patient when performing positive pressure ventilation is
   a. 5–to–10 ml/kg.
   b. 10–to–15 ml/kg.
   c. 15–to–20 ml/kg.
   d. 20–to–25 ml/kg.

12. Which of the following is a major complication associated with ventilation with a flow-restricted, oxygen-powered ventilation device?
    a. inability to deliver high concentrations of oxygen during ventilation
    b. delivery of inadequate tidal volume
    c. induction of barotrauma and a pneumothorax
    d. the device is restricted to use on pediatric patients only

13. Which of the following should **not** be done while performing tracheo-bronchial suctioning?
    a. Set the suction to greater than –120 mmHg.
    b. Hyperventilate the patient for one minute prior to applying suction.
    c. Insert the catheter without suction applied.
    d. Suction for less than 15 seconds at a time.

14. The most serious complication associated with tracheobronchial suctioning is
    a. stimulation of the cough and gag reflex.
    b. stimulation of the sympathetic nervous system with resultant tachycardia.
    c. mucosal damage and subsequent infection.
    d. hypoxemia secondary to a decrease in functional residual volume.

15. Which of the following is true regarding the simple face mask?
    a. An FiO_2 of 100% is possible with the mask.
    b. The liter flow should not be set at less then 6 lpm.
    c. Oxygen is collected in a reservoir bag prior to inhalation.
    d. The mask is well tolerated by pediatric patients.

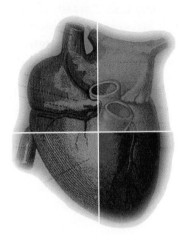

Gaining Intravenous Access

In an emergency situation with a patient experiencing severe cardiovascular instability, drug therapy is often used to help convert the abnormality. To obtain the desired effects, the drugs must reach the target cell or organ rapidly. To facilitate the quickest absorption, you will often deliver medications directly into the patient's venous circulation. You may also need to obtain samples of the patient's venous blood for analysis.

Both of these objectives—rapid delivery of medications and obtaining samples of venous blood—are accomplished by gaining intravenous (IV) access with a cannula, which may be a needle or a catheter. IV cannulation is generally a safe procedure, but there are risks, which can be reduced by following proper procedures.

The topics to be covered in this chapter are:

- IV Cannulas
- Peripheral IV Lines
- Techniques for Cannulating Peripheral Veins
- Complications

CASE STUDY

Bill, a 56-year-old male, begins having severe chest pain just after dinner. When the pain hasn't diminished after 20 minutes, his wife decides to drive him to the hospital where he is quickly moved into the emergency department. You are part of the Chest Pain Team that completes the assessment, starts Bill on oxygen, and places him on a cardiac monitor. Your team will be careful with injections and venipuncture, because you suspect that Bill might be a candidate for thrombolytic agents.

How should your team proceed to assess and manage this patient? What medications would be administered intravenously in this situation? This chapter will discuss the purposes of IV access in the emergency setting and describe the techniques of gaining IV access. Later we will return to the case to see how IV therapy is applied.

Introduction

In non-emergency situations, most medications are given orally, intramuscularly (I.M.), or subcutaneously (sq.). In emergencies, you must deliver medications so that they can enter the central circulation quickly. The most reliable way to administer medications in emergency situations and cardiac arrest is by injecting them directly into the venous circulation. This is accomplished by placing a catheter or needle directly into a vein.

Intravenous (IV) cannulation is performed for two main reasons:

1. To administer medications and fluids
2. To obtain venous blood samples

There are two general categories of IVs: central and peripheral. Peripheral IVs are relatively easy to locate, and can be accessed quickly, easily, and safely, even during CPR. Central veins, however, are more difficult to cannulate because they are deeper within the body. To become efficient in central line placement, a significant amount of practice and experience is necessary.

In this chapter we will take a very practical view of IV cannulation. You should review and understand the advantages and disadvantages of peripheral and central IVs (Tables 4-1 and 4-2). You should also be familiar with the technique of cannulating peripheral IVs and how to maximize the delivery of medication in cardiac arrest.

This chapter will not discuss the techniques of central vein cannulation. If you routinely perform central IV cannulation, it is unlikely that we could add to your knowledge about the skill in this chapter. It is not the intent of this chapter to teach the technique of central cannulation. Please read other texts available that cover intravenous techniques in greater detail and for an extensive review of central vein cannulation.

In some situations, either peripheral or central IV access will have been established in the patient before the cardiac emergency. In these cases, you

TABLE 4-1   ADVANTAGES AND DISADVANTAGES OF PERIPHERAL IVS

Peripheral Sites	Advantages	Disadvantages
Arm Leg External jugular vein	Relatively easy to master the technique Easy to locate Fast to cannulate Safe to perform Multiple practitioners can try at once Easily compressible to reduce bleeding from unsuccessful attempts Can usually be accomplished during CPR Low complication rate compared to central IVs	Collapse during shock or cardiac arrest Prolonged time for medication to reach the central circulation in cardiac arrest

should obviously use this access during the emergency care or resuscitation of the patient after confirming patency of the catheter.

In non-emergency situations, you usually can spend additional time to assure that you are paying strict attention to aseptic (sterile) technique. In an emergency you must gain IV access quickly, and occasionally you are not able to maintain the desired strict aseptic technique. In these cases, be sure that you remove the catheter as soon as possible after the emergency and replace it with an IV initiated under more aseptic conditions.

TABLE 4-2 ADVANTAGES AND DISADVANTAGES OF CENTRAL IVS

Central Sites	Advantages	Disadvantages
Femoral vein Internal jugular vein Subclavian vein	Do not collapse in shock Do not collapse during cardiac arrest Can be used to monitor central venous pressure Can be used for transvenous pacing The central veins accommodate large-bore catheters More rapid delivery of medication to the central circulation during cardiac arrest	Relatively difficult to master the technique Increased incidence of: Arterial puncture Pneumothorax Air embolism Catheter embolism Can usually not be accomplished during CPR Relatively contraindicated in patients who may receive thrombolytic agents

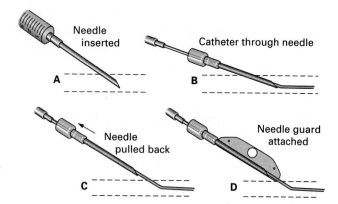

FIGURE 4-1 Insertion of catheter through needle.

Glucose-containing solutions, such as 5% dextrose in water, should be avoided. Some studies have shown worsened neurological outcomes following the use of dextrose in patients with intracranial pathology. The IV fluid of choice to keep the vein open in cardiac arrest is 0.9% sodium chloride (normal saline). The fluid should be adjusted to administer 10–20 cc/hr. Alternatively, you can also attach a saline lock to the IV cannula and eliminate the need for tubing and IV fluid.

IV Cannulas

There are different types of IV cannulas:

1. *Hollow needles.* These are commonly called butterfly needles and are occasionally used in pediatric patients. The problem with hollow needles is that the sharp, metal needle, when inserted in the vein, often damages the vessel.

2. *Catheters inserted through a needle.* These are used occasionally for central vein access, but are quite uncommon for peripheral access (Figure 4-1).

3. *Catheters inserted over a needle.* These are by far the most common IV catheters used for peripheral vein cannulation (Figure 4-2).

Peripheral IV Lines

If the emergency patient (or patient in cardiac arrest) has no venous access, you should consider peripheral IV cannulation as one of the first priorities of management. Peripheral veins used for venous access include the veins in

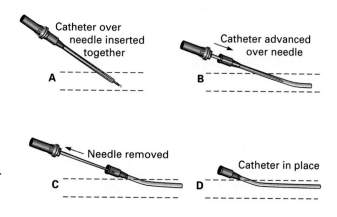

FIGURE 4-2 Insertion of catheter over needle.

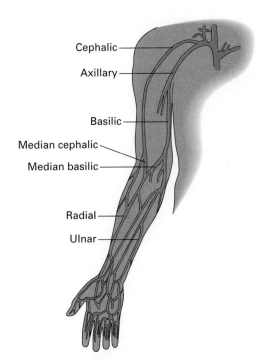

FIGURE 4-3 Veins of the hand and arm.

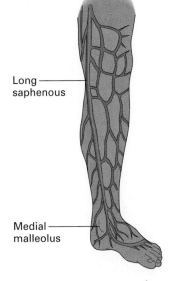

FIGURE 4-4 Long saphenous vein of the leg.

the arm, the leg, and the external jugular vein (Figures 4-3, 4-4, and 4-5). These veins lie superficially and are easy to see and palpate. Although a relatively easy skill, cannulating peripheral veins requires practice.

In cardiac arrest, venous blood flow is severely compromised. As a result, medications administered peripherally have significant delays in reaching the central circulation. To increase the effectiveness in cardiac arrest, you should raise the extremity and follow each medication administration with a 20–50 cc flush of saline. When selecting a site for cannulation, the closer to the central circulation you can cannulate a vein the better. Try to use the large antecubital or external jugular veins in cardiac arrest (Figures 4-6 and 4-7).

In non-arrest situations, the veins in the dorsum of the hand, the wrist, and the forearm are the preferred IV sites (Figure 4-8). As a last resort, you can use the long saphenous vein in the leg, but a higher rate of thrombophlebitis and other complications is associated with IVs started in the lower extremities.

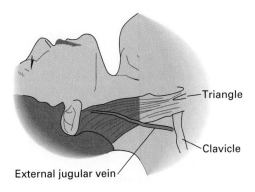

FIGURE 4-5 External jugular vein.

FIGURE 4-6 Antecubital venipuncture.

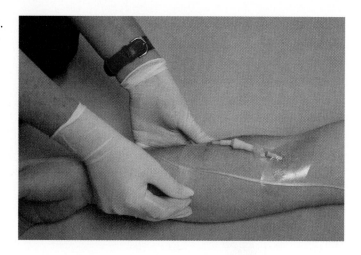

Techniques for Cannulating Peripheral Veins

Cannulating an Arm or Leg Vein

The vast majority of IVs are started in the upper extremities. The veins are superficial and easily located on the back of the hand, the forearm, and the antecubital fossa. In cardiac arrest, the preferred sites are the antecubital and external jugular vein. Below are the steps of cannulating a superficial arm or leg vein.

1. Apply a venous tourniquet proximally to the site of the attempt. The purposes of the constricting band are to impede venous return and to engorge the veins. Engorgement makes the distal veins easier to locate.

2. Locate the vein and cleanse the skin with alcohol or a similar antiseptic.

3. Hold the skin taut.

4. With the needle bevel-up, puncture the skin.

5. Enter the vein either from the side or from above. You will feel a "pop" as you enter the vein, and you will see a flash of blood returning through the flash-back chamber

6. Advance the needle slightly to be sure that the catheter is completely within the lumen (interior) of the vein.

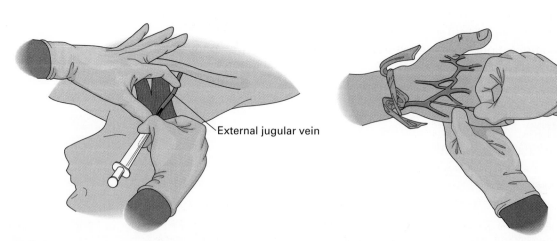

External jugular vein

FIGURE 4-7 External jugular venipuncture.

FIGURE 4-8 Dorsal hand venipuncture.

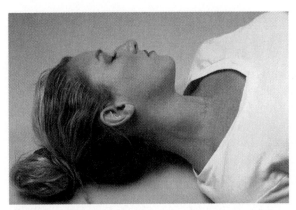

FIGURE 4-9a Location of the external jugular vein.

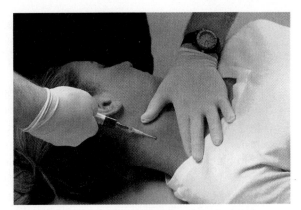

FIGURE 4-9b Cannulation of the external jugular vein.

7. Advance the catheter over the needle and into the vein. Remove the tourniquet.

8. Completely remove the needle stylet, attach the tubing to the catheter, and slowly start the flow of fluids.

9. Cover the injection site with sterile dressing material and tape the catheter in place.

10. Watch for complications. (See "Complications" below.)

Cannulating an External Jugular Vein

The external jugular vein is considered a peripheral vein because it lies superficially in the neck (Figure 4-9a). However, it is very close to the central circulation and has significant advantages over other peripheral IVs. Below is the technique for cannulating the external jugular vein (Figure 4-9b).

1. Place the patient in a Trendelenburg position (supine, feet slightly elevated) and turn the patient's head to the side.

2. Cleanse the injection site.

3. Attach a 10 cc syringe filled with a few cc's of saline to the angiocath.

4. Occlude the venous return by placing one finger on the external jugular vein just above the clavicle.

5. Puncture the vein midway between the angle of the jaw and your finger.

6. Enter the vein while withdrawing the plunger of the syringe. Stop when blood flows briskly into the syringe.

7. Advance the catheter into the vein and remove the needle stylet.

8. Attach the tubing to the catheter, start the flow of fluid, and secure the catheter.

9. Watch for complications.

Complications

IV cannulation is not without some risks. The complications can be divided into local and systemic complications. Local complications of IV cannulation include hematoma formation, cellulitis, thrombosis, and phlebitis. Systemic complications are sepsis, pulmonary embolism, and air or catheter

CASE STUDY FOLLOW-UP

Assessment

Bill, a 56-year-old male who is suffering from chest pain, has been brought to the emergency department. As part of the Chest Pain Team, you quickly insert an over-the-needle catheter into a vein in his right forearm. You take blood samples from the IV site and then attach the IV line to the catheter hub. You start an IV of normal saline running at 20 cc/hr. Then, as the staff is preparing to do a 12-lead ECG, Bill suddenly slumps over, unconscious. The monitor shows ventricular fibrillation.

Treatment

The team performs the defibrillation sequence, which is unsuccessful in converting the rhythm. You administer a 1 mg bolus of 1:10,000 epinephrine through the IV. Since the IV is in Bill's antecubital fossa, you raise his arm and open the line to let about 20 cc of fluid flush the medication into the vein. The fourth defibrillation is successful, and you administer a bolus of 1 mg/kg of lidocaine followed by an infusion of lidocaine into the primary line.

Bill leaves the hospital four days later, starts a cardiac rehabilitation program, and recovers fully.

emboli. The probability of any of these complications can be reduced by following proper technique, as described above.

For patients who are potential candidates for thrombolysis, special care must be taken to avoid unnecessary bleeding. Sites of I.M. injections, blood draw, IV cannulation, and unsuccessful IV attempts can result in bleeding or significant hematomas after thrombolytics are administered, since thrombolytics act to dissolve clots and will therefore increase the risk of or aggravate bleeding or hematomas. In this situation be especially diligent in attempting to establish a patent IV on the first attempt. Candidates for thrombolytic therapy are NOT the patients to practice IVs on. Let the most experienced practitioner start the IV. Finally, watch for bleeding or hematomas at any injection site and control the bleeding with direct pressure if necessary. A pressure dressing should be applied to a site of potential bleeding in any patient who is a candidate for thrombolytic therapy.

SUMMARY

Access to the venous circulation is a critical part of emergency management. Typically, the initial IV access is accomplished by cannulating a peripheral vein in the arm. If the patient is in cardiac arrest, select an IV site as close as possible to the central circulation. Preferably, place a large-bore catheter in the antecubital fossa and elevate the arm, or place the catheter in the external jugular vein. Following any drug administration, flush the line with at least 20 cc of saline to speed circulation to the cells.

In non-arrest situations, the veins in the dorsum of the hand, the wrist, and the forearm are the preferred IV sites. As a last resort, you can use the long saphenous vein in the leg.

In an emergency you must gain IV access quickly and may not be able to follow strict aseptic (sterile) technique. In these cases, remove the catheter as soon as possible after the emergency and replace it with an IV initiated with a strict aseptic technique.

REVIEW QUESTIONS

1. Which of the following types of catheters is most commonly used for peripheral venous cannulation?
    a. catheter over the needle
    b. catheter through the needle
    c. hollow needle
    d. intraosseous catheter

2. What is the preferred solution to be used to keep the vein open during cardiac arrest?
    a. 5% dextrose in water
    b. 5% dextrose in lactated Ringer's
    c. normal saline
    d. sterile water

3. Which of the following is **not** an advantage of peripheral IV cannulation (as compared to central IV cannulation)?
    a. It is easier to locate a larger number of suitable veins with peripheral cannulation.
    b. Delivery of medication to the central circulation is more rapid with peripheral cannulation.
    c. Peripheral cannulation is a relatively easy skill to master.
    d. Peripheral cannulation can be accomplished without interruption of CPR.

4. In cardiac arrest, which of the following would be the preferred site for peripheral IV cannulation?
    a. saphenous vein
    b. dorsum of the hand
    c. subclavian vein
    d. antecubital fossa

5. List two strategies for improving the delivery of medications to the central circulation in cardiac arrest.

    a. _____

    b. _____

6. What precaution should be taken when performing IV cannulation in a patient who is a possible candidate for thrombolysis?

    _____

Chapter**Five**

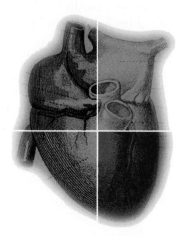

Dysrhythmia Recognition

When treating a patient with an apparent cardiac problem, it is important to determine whether a mechanical or electrical dysfunction exists. Electrical activity and conduction malfunctions cause changes in the myocardial rhythm. An electrocardiogram can reveal the abnormal rhythm and provide information about the location and nature of the malfunction. This information is critical to treatment decisions you will make. Improper rhythm identification will almost certainly lead to improper management. So the ability to read and interpret an ECG is an essential skill in advanced cardiac life support.

The topics to be covered in this chapter are:

- Basic Electrophysiology
- The Electrocardiogram
- Monitoring Systems
- Analyzing the ECG
- The Normal ECG and Sinus Rhythms
- Abnormal ECGs

CASE STUDY

You are a paramedic called to the house of Alma Brown, a 48-year-old woman who called 911 for a "fluttering sensation" in her chest. Upon your arrival, you find a conscious, alert female who is in no particular distress and who denies chest pain and shortness of breath but says that she feels like her heart is racing. This has happened a few times before, Mrs. Brown tells you, but it always ended within 2 or 3 minutes. She called for help when the sensation did not stop after 20 minutes.

The cardiac monitor shows the following:

What additional assessment steps would you take to differentiate the origin of the dysrhythmia? What parameters would you use to determine the appropriate treatment? This chapter will discuss electrocardiograms and analysis of a variety of normal and abnormal cardiac rhythms. Later we will return to the case to see how these skills are applied.

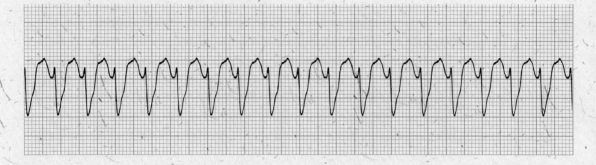

Introduction

One of the critical aspects of assessing the status of a cardiac patient is determining the mechanical and electrical status of the heart. The patient's pulse and blood pressure are simple measures of myocardial function. Advanced diagnostics, such as the echocardiogram, give you information about heart wall movement. To assess the electrical activity of the heart, you need to know how to interpret the electrocardiogram (EKG or ECG). Analyzing the ECG is one of the most important skills of advanced cardiac life support.

It is worth emphasizing early that the ECG provides information only about the electrical activity of the heart, not about the mechanical function. It is possible for the ECG to be perfectly normal in the absence of mechanical contraction. Always remember the popular phrase: "Treat the patient, not the monitor."

Basic Electrophysiology

Electrophysiology is often presented as complex, abstract, and frustrating. Many beginning students become so intimidated by the physiology that they never learn how to interpret ECGs. The intent of this chapter is to limit the amount of technical information to what you will need to identify the basic, life-threatening cardiac rhythms used in ACLS. Once you have mastered basic rhythm recognition, we encourage you to tackle electrophysiology, which will increase your understanding of cardiology and ACLS. Electrophysiology becomes less overwhelming once you have a grasp of the basics.

The heart is an unique organ. It is made up of muscle tissue that has the property of automaticity. Automaticity is the ability of the heart, or any of its individual muscle cells, to contract on its own—without any nervous system control. In fact, if you quickly remove the heart from the body, place it in a saline bath, and provide it with oxygen and glucose, the heart will continue to beat for quite some time. If you cut it into tiny pieces and separate them, each chunk of heart muscle will beat separately! This is an amazing physiological phenomenon and makes the heart dramatically different from any other organ in the body.

To contract, a myocardial cell must be depolarized. Depolarization is a process where a shift in the electrical properties of the cell occurs from the movement of electrically charged molecules across the cell's membrane. When the electrical properties of the cell change, the cell is capable of contracting.

Some areas of the heart have evolved to perform special functions. The three specialized types of myocardial cells are:

- Pacemaker cells
- Conduction cells
- Working cells

Pacemakers

For the heart to pump blood and generate a pulse, the myocardial working cells must contract in a coordinated fashion. The coordination is provided by pacemaker cells, which control the heart's rate and rhythm by depolarizing at regular intervals. Through influence from the autonomic (sympathetic and parasympathetic) nervous system, the impulse emmission rate of the pacemakers can be altered.

The primary pacemaker of the healthy heart is the sinoatrial (SA) node. It is a bundle of cardiac tissue that is located on the inner wall of the heart, near the junction of the right atrium and the vena cava. Without nervous control, the SA node will normally depolarize 60–100 times per minute. If the body demands changes in cardiac output, the autonomic nervous system can increase (as a sympathetic action) or decrease (as a parasympathetic action) the rate at which the SA node emits impulses.

If the SA node fails to emit an impulse, there are some backup functions that assure that the heart will continue to beat. If the SA node fails, the atrioventricular (AV) node at the junction of the atria and ventricles will take over as a pacemaker and will depolarize at a rate of 40–60 times per minute. If both the SA and AV nodes fail, the Purkinje fibers of the ventricles will depolarize at a rate of less than 40 times per minute.

The Cardiac Conduction System

The impulse from the pacemakers travels through the heart in a couple of ways. There are internodal pathways that connect the SA node to the AV node. In normal conduction, the AV node is the only electrical connection between the atria and the ventricles; therefore, any stimulation for the ventricles to contract that originates above the ventricles must pass through the

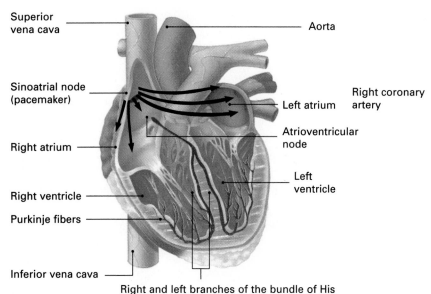

Superior vena cava

Aorta

FIGURE 5-1 The cardiac conduction system.

Sinoatrial node (pacemaker)

Right coronary artery

Left atrium

Atrioventricular node

Right atrium

Left ventricle

Right ventricle

Purkinje fibers

Inferior vena cava

Right and left branches of the bundle of His

AV node. Below the AV node the impulse for contraction travels through the bundle of His, the bundle branches, and the Purkinje fibers.

The overall cardiac conduction pathway in the normal heart (Figure 5-1), therefore, is:

$$\text{SA node} \longrightarrow \text{internodal pathways} \longrightarrow \text{AV node} \longrightarrow \text{bundle of His}$$
$$\longrightarrow \text{bundle branches} \longrightarrow \text{Purkinje fibers}$$

Myocardial Working Cells

The actual contraction of the heart occurs when electrical depolarization is coupled with physical contraction. It is important to remember that the physical contraction is what generates blood flow—not the electrical activity. However, the physical contraction requires organized electrical activity.

The physical contraction of the heart is created by the myocardial working cells. These muscle cells are bundled into an interconnecting weave of muscle fibers. Contraction of these fibers causes a rapid decrease in the internal size of the atria and ventricles, which in turn ejects the blood from the chambers.

The Electrocardiogram

The body is a giant conductor of the electrical impulse transmission that occurs within the heart. These events can be detected by two electrodes, one positive and one negative, placed on the skin. Typically, the signal is amplified and then displayed on an oscilloscope or printed on graph paper. Theoretically, electrodes can be placed anywhere on the body, but this causes subtle differences in the relative size of each wave. For convenience and standardization, there are some conventional electrode placements that you should remember. Figure 5-2 shows the location of the positive, negative, and ground leads; for the placements known as Lead I, Lead II, Lead III, and Lead MCL$_1$. These placements conventionally display a clearer tracing of the ECG.

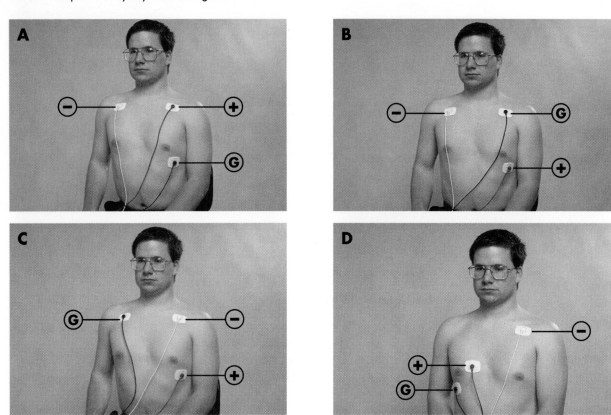

FIGURE 5-2   ECG placements: (A) Lead I, (B) Lead II, (C) Lead III, and (D) Lead MCL$_1$.

The electrical events of the heart rhythm produce waves that have been labeled alphabetically P through T. In some cases, a U wave is present, the significance of which is unknown. You should become familiar with these components of the normal ECG, as shown in Figure 5-3.

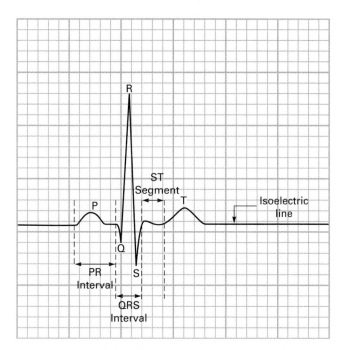

FIGURE 5-3   The electrocardiogram (ECG).

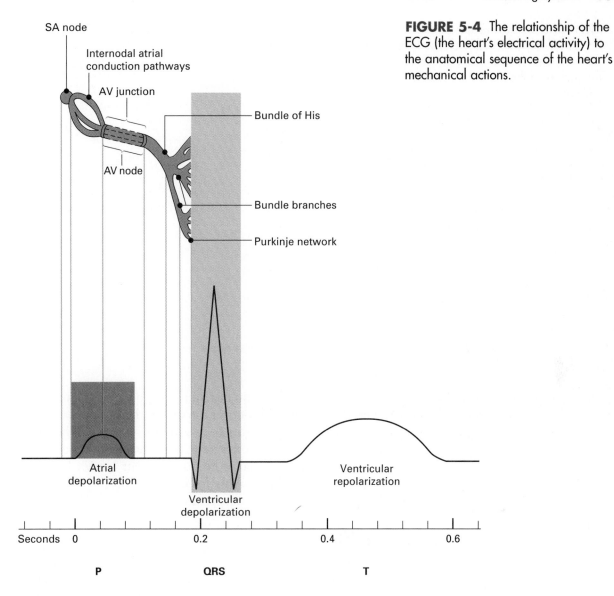

FIGURE 5-4 The relationship of the ECG (the heart's electrical activity) to the anatomical sequence of the heart's mechanical actions.

Each wave represents the summation of the depolarization or repolarization of a mass of heart tissue. Atrial depolarization produces the P wave. Ventricular depolarization produces the QRS complex, and ventricular repolarization produces the T wave. Atrial repolarization is buried in the QRS complex (Figure 5-4).

Occasionally, there are variations in how the waves look and even if they are present. In fact, these alterations are how you will be able to recognize dysrhythmias. If you keep this in mind, dysrhythmia recognition becomes much easier.

Monitoring Systems

There are many different cardiac monitors on the market. There are many features, with various configurations of switches and buttons, but basically all cardiac monitors are the same. They generally consist of a screen (or oscilloscope) and usually have a printer that provides you with an opportunity to print a hard copy of the patient's cardiac rhythm.

FIGURE 5-5 ECG graph paper. The horizontal axis represents elapsed time in seconds. The vertical axis represents the magnitude of the electrical impulse in millivolts.

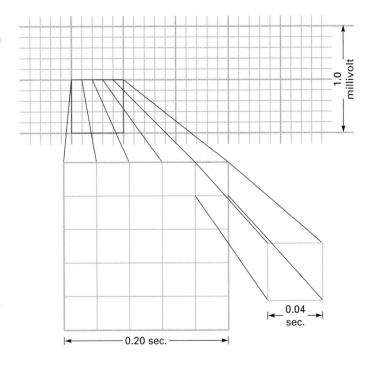

Cardiac monitors print the ECG on a strip of graph paper (Figure 5-5). Since the paper exits the machine at a constant speed, the horizontal boxes represent time. (Each large box represents 0.20 seconds; each small box represents 0.04 seconds.) The vertical boxes represent the magnitude of the electrical impulse in millivolts. (Two large boxes represent 1 mV.) It is very important to remember the time increments for each box on the ECG, since they will be used extensively in ECG interpretation.

Analyzing the ECG

Now that you know how to identify each wave of the ECG, analyzing the cardiac rhythm simply becomes a matter of looking at a number of parameters and applying a couple of rules. We will use the "red flag" method of ECG interpretation. The "red flag" method looks at five parameters in each ECG and, by understanding what they mean, you will easily be able to interpret the ECG. The five parameters (Table 5-1) are:

- Rate
- Regularity
- QRS width
- P waves
- P-R interval

Rate

As we mentioned earlier, the SA node normally depolarizes 60–100 times a minute. This represents the normal range of heart rate. Any rate that is faster than 100 beats per minute is called *tachycardia* and any rate slower than 60 beats per minute is *bradycardia*. We assess the rate by looking at the number of QRS complexes.

TABLE 5-1 FIVE PARAMETERS OF ECG ANALYSIS
Analyze
Rate What is the rate? (Normally 60–100 per minute)
Regularity Is the rhythm regular? (Normally a variance of less than 0.04 seconds)
QRS Complex Do all of the QRS complexes look alike? (Normally yes) What is the width of the QRS complex? (Normally less than 0.12 seconds)
P Waves Is there a P wave before every QRS complex? (Normally yes) Is there a QRS complex after every P wave? (Normally yes)
P-R Interval What is the P-R interval? (Normally less than 0.20 seconds) Is the P-R interval constant? (Normally yes)

There are two ways to determine the heart rate by looking at the ECG. The easiest way is to count the number of QRS complexes that occur in 6 seconds and multiply that number by 10. For your convenience, ECG paper is often marked in 3- or 6-second increments (Figure 5-6). This method is best used to count irregular rhythms.

The second way to determine the heart rate is to look for a QRS complex that falls on one of the heavy lines on the strip. You then count how many large boxes are between this and the next QRS complex. Then divide that number into 300—because 300 large boxes represent 60 seconds, or 1

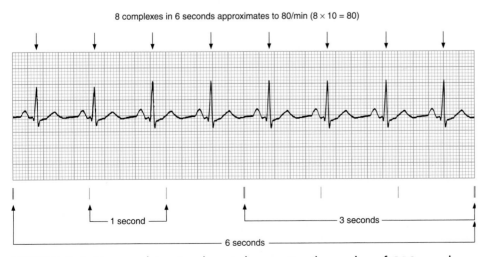

8 complexes in 6 seconds approximates to 80/min (8 × 10 = 80)

1 second
3 seconds
6 seconds

FIGURE 5-6 You can determine the rate by counting the number of QRS complexes in 6 seconds and multiplying by 10.

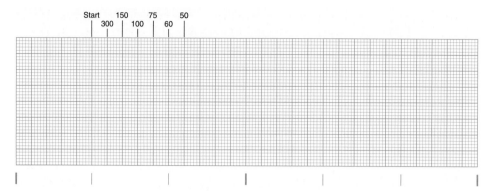

FIGURE 5-7 You can determine rate, or the regularity of rhythm, by counting the number of boxes between QRS complexes.

minute. Therefore, if the next QRS fell exactly three heavy lines away, the rate would be 100 beats per minute (300÷3=100) (Figure 5-7).

Usually, you are not lucky enough to have the subsequent QRS fall directly on a heavy line, so this technique is often used just to estimate the heart rate. Study Figure 5-8. Can you see why the rate is estimated to be 70 on this strip?

Regularity

The next variable to analyze is the regularity of the rhythm. The normal heart rhythm is highly regular. A variance of more than 0.04 seconds, or 1 small box, between the complexes is considered abnormal. This is best analyzed using calipers. Simply measure the distance between two QRS complexes and then check the distances between others to determine if they are within 0.04 seconds of each other.

The QRS Complex

After evaluating the rate and the regularity of the rhythm, next analyze the QRS complexes. Remember that the QRS complex represents ventricular depolarization. Specifically, you are examining the QRS complexes to see if they have the same morphology (look the same) and if they are the same width. If all QRS complexes look alike, they are all following the same conduction pathways below the AV node.

The width of the QRS complex has special significance. If the QRS complex is narrow, defined as less than 0.12 seconds (3 small boxes), the wave of depolarization has followed the normal conduction pathways below the AV node. In other words, the impulse did NOT originate in the ventricles. The rhythm is therefore referred to as *supraventricular*, i.e., "above the ventricles."

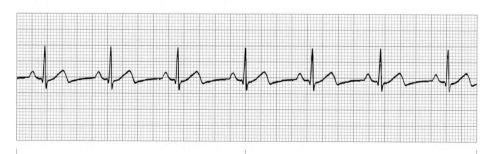

FIGURE 5-8 An ECG strip with a heart rate estimated at 70.

If the QRS complex is wide, the opposite is not necessarily true. If the QRS complex is greater than 0.12 seconds (3 small boxes), there are three common causes:

- The impulse may have originated in the ventricles.
- The impulse may have originated above the ventricles but circumvented the normal conduction pathway through the AV node. This is known as *aberrant conduction*.
- The impulse may have originated above the ventricles and traveled through the AV node but experienced a delay in one side of the ventricular conduction system. This is called a bundle branch block. Bundle branch blocks represent another type of aberrant conduction.

KEY POINT: Narrow QRS complexes are always of a supraventricular origin, whereas wide QRS complexes may have either a ventricular origin or a supraventricular origin with aberrant conduction.

The P Waves

Remember that the P wave represents atrial depolarization. There are two questions to ask about the P waves:

- Is there a P wave before every QRS complex?
- Is there a QRS complex after every P wave?

The P-R Interval

The normal delay of conduction that occurs at the AV node is less than 0.20 seconds (1 big box or 5 small boxes). You need to know two things about the P-R interval to correctly interpret the ECG:

- Is the P-R interval less than 0.20 seconds?
- Is the P-R interval constant?

The Normal ECG and Sinus Rhythms

Now that you know the five parameters for analyzing any ECG (rate, regularity, QRS complex, P waves, and P-R interval), interpreting and understanding cardiac rhythms simply becomes a matter of answering each question and applying a few rules. We call this the "red flag" method, because by knowing which of the five variables falls out of the normal range (raises a "red flag"), you can interpret any rhythm.

A WORD OF CAUTION: After you have analyzed many ECGs, you will have a tendency to "cut to the chase" and attempt to interpret the rhythm without going through each step of analysis. Although this will often result in a correct interpretation, you will sometimes miss important findings. We suggest that you use this sequential method of ECG analysis until you have gained much more experience in ECG interpretation.

Normal Sinus Rhythm

Very simply, any rhythm where all of the variables fall within the normal limits is called normal sinus rhythm (NSR). There can be significant variations on how some of the waves look, but if the answer to every question falls within normal limits, the rhythm is normal (Table 5-2 and Figure 5-9).

TABLE 5-2 NORMAL SINUS RHYTHM

Analyze	ECG
Rate	60–100 per minute
Regularity	Variance of less than 0.04 seconds

QRS Complex
    Do all of the QRS complexes look alike?
    What is the width of the QRS complex?
	
	Yes
	Less than 0.12 seconds

P Waves
    Is there a P wave before every QRS complex?
    Is there a QRS after every P wave?
	
	Yes
	Yes

P-R Interval
    What is the P-R interval?
    Is the P-R interval constant?
	
	Less than 0.20 seconds
	Yes

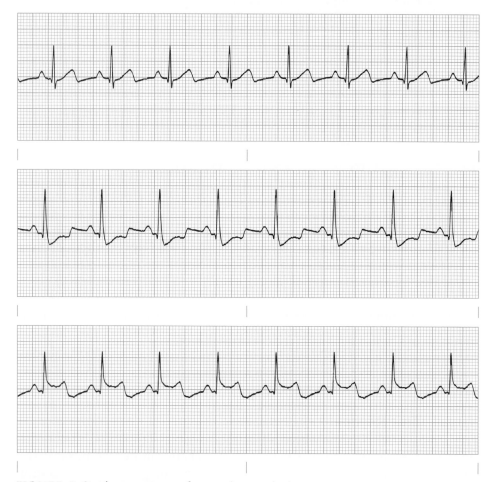

FIGURE 5-9 Three variants of normal sinus rhythm.

Sinus Tachycardia

Sinus tachycardia is a common variant of NSR where the only "red flag" is that the rate is over 100 (Table 5-3 and Figure 5-10). Every beat is stimulated by an impulse from the SA node. This is a common dysrhythmia caused by exercise, stress, fever, fear, or shock.

TABLE 5-3 SINUS TACHYCARDIA	
Analyze	**ECG**
Rate	**Greater than 100 per minute**
Regularity	Variance of less than 0.04 seconds
QRS Complex Do all of the QRS complexes look alike? What is the width of the QRS complex?	 Yes Less than 0.12 seconds
P Waves Is there a P wave before every QRS complex? Is there a QRS after every P wave?	 Yes Yes
P-R Interval What is the P-R interval? Is the P-R interval constant?	 Less than 0.20 seconds Yes

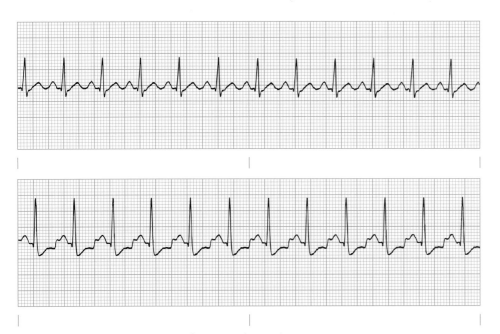

FIGURE 5-10 Two variants of sinus tachycardia.

Sinus Bradycardia

Sinus bradycardia is characterized by all of the variables falling within normal limits, except a rate that is less than 60 beats per minute (Table 5-4 and Figure 5-11). This is very common in well-conditioned athletes, but in an emergency it may be caused by a myocardial infarction or excessive parasympathetic stimulation.

TABLE 5-4 SINUS BRADYCARDIA	
Analyze	ECG
Rate	**Less than 60 per minute**
Regularity	Variance of less than 0.04 seconds

QRS Complex
    Do all of the QRS complexes look alike?
    What is the width of the QRS complex?
	Yes
	Less than 0.12 seconds

P Waves
    Is there a P wave before every QRS complex?
    Is there a QRS after every P wave?
	Yes
	Yes

P-R Interval
    What is the P-R interval?
    Is the P-R interval constant?
	Less than 0.20 seconds
	Yes

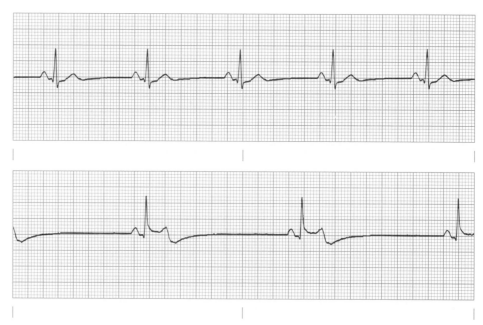

FIGURE 5-11 Two variants of sinus bradycardia.

Sinus Dysrhythmia

Sinus dysrhythmia is characterized by all variables being within normal limits except the regularity (Table 5-5 and Figure 5-12). Variation in the regularity is common and is normal in some people. It is thought that this results from the changes in venous return associated with breathing.

TABLE 5-5 SINUS DYSRHYTHMIA	
Analyze	**ECG**
Rate	60–100 per minute
Regularity	**Variance of more than 0.04 seconds** 🚩
QRS Complex 　Do all of the QRS complexes look alike? 　What is the width of the QRS complex?	 Yes Less than 0.12 seconds
P Waves 　Is there a P wave before every QRS complex? 　Is there a QRS after every P wave?	 Yes Yes
P-R Interval 　What is the P-R interval? 　Is the P-R interval constant?	 Less than 0.20 seconds Yes

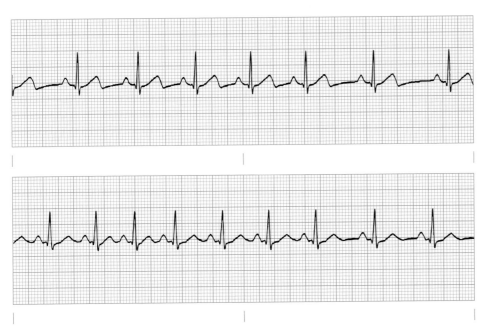

FIGURE 5-12 Two variants of sinus dysrhythmia.

Abnormal ECG's

There are some very confusing terms that are used when discussing ECGs. Technically, a dysrhythmia is an abnormality in the rhythm and arrhythmia is the absence of rhythm. In practice, the terms are used interchangeably.

There are only a few causes of abnormal ECGs and they are very easy to remember. If you think of cardiac dysrhythmias in terms of their causes, the interpretation becomes logical. Most textbooks teach dysrhythmia interpretation anatomically, i.e., atrial, junctional, and ventricular dysrhythmias. Although this is a convenient way to group dysrhythmias, it does not help to understand the causes of the rhythm disturbances.

In the "red flag" method of ECG interpretation, we evaluate each rhythm strip using the five criteria discussed. The answers to the questions direct us toward the correct interpretation. If you remember the questions, a little about the causes of the dysrhythmias, and a few rules, the pattern of abnormal findings leads you to the correct interpretation.

A brief word of caution: For clarity, we will only consider one dysrhythmia at a time in this chapter. In real life, patients can exhibit multiple dysrhythmias at the same time. When you are first learning, it is much easier to consider "textbook" ECG strips, which illustrate the concepts of dysrhythmia interpretation.

Fibrillatory Dysrhythmias

As we mentioned earlier, each cardiac muscle cell has the ability to initiate contraction on its own. Normally, this does not happen; instead, the heart produces a coordinated sequence of muscle cell contractions, which is required to pump blood. Unfortunately, there are some cases where the muscle cells of the heart lose their coordination and do not respond to the impulses from the heart's pacemakers. When this happens, the cells contract on their own and there is no coordination to the myocardial rhythm. This phenomenon is referred to as *fibrillation*. Effectively, no blood is pumped by fibrillating myocardial tissue, and no pulse is generated.

There are two fibrillatory dysrhythmias that you must know: atrial fibrillation and ventricular fibrillation.

Atrial fibrillation

When the tissue of the atria fibrillates, the atria do not contract. The patient will continue to have a pulse since the ventricles are still pumping, but the effectiveness of the myocardial contraction is decreased since the atria are not effectively filling the ventricles with blood. There are two primary ways to identify atrial fibrillation. First, there are no P waves, since there is no coordinated atrial contraction. The millions of individual atrial cells depolarizing at random causes the baseline to be wavy with fibrillatory waves (fib-waves).

The second identifying characteristic of atrial fibrillation is its irregularity (Figure 5-13). The ventricles will contract when enough fibrillatory impulses combine to send a signal through the AV node and down the conduction system. This does not occur at regular intervals and therefore causes an irregular ventricular response, represented on the ECG as a variance in the R-to-R interval of greater than 0.04 seconds (Table 5-6).

CLINICAL TIP: If you see a rhythm with no regularity whatsoever (that is irregularly irregular), think atrial fibrillation.

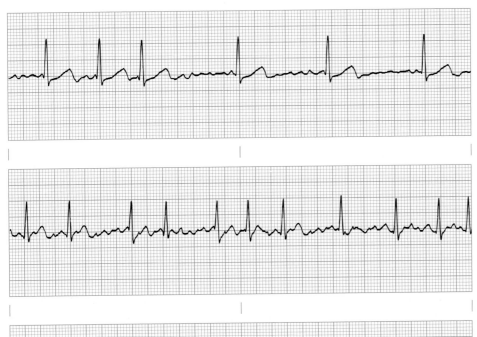

FIGURE 5-13 Three variants of atrial fibrillation.

TABLE 5-6 ATRIAL FIBRILLATION	
Analyze	**ECG**
Rate	Ventricular rate varies but is usually faster in the unmedicated patient.
Regularity	**Variance of more than 0.04 seconds, irregularly irregular** ⚑

QRS Complex
   Do all of the QRS complexes look alike?
   What is the width of the QRS complex?
	Yes
	Less than 0.12 seconds

P Waves
   Is there a P wave before every QRS complex?
   Is there a QRS after every P wave?
	There are no discernible P waves. ⚑
	The wavy baselines are called fibrillatory waves (f-waves).

P-R Interval
   What is the P-R interval?
   Is the P-R interval constant?
	NA (not applicable)
	NA

Ventricular Fibrillation

When the ventricular muscle tissue fibrillates, the ventricles cannot contract, resulting in no cardiac output and no pulse. Ventricular fibrillation is a cardiac arrest rhythm, but one that may be survivable with rapid defibrillation. It is also one of the easiest rhythms to identify, characterized by large fibrillatory waves and no discernible P waves, QRS complexes, or T waves (Table 5-7 and Figure 5-14).

TABLE 5-7 VENTRICULAR FIBRILLATION

Analyze	ECG
Rate	None 🚩
Regularity	NA 🚩
QRS Complex	Only fibrillatory waves are present. 🚩
Do all of the QRS complexes look alike?	NA
What is the width of the QRS complex?	NA
P Waves	Obliterated by the fibrillatory waves 🚩
Is there a P wave before every QRS complex?	NA
Is there a QRS after every P wave?	NA
P-R Interval	
What is the P-R interval?	NA 🚩
Is the P-R interval constant?	NA

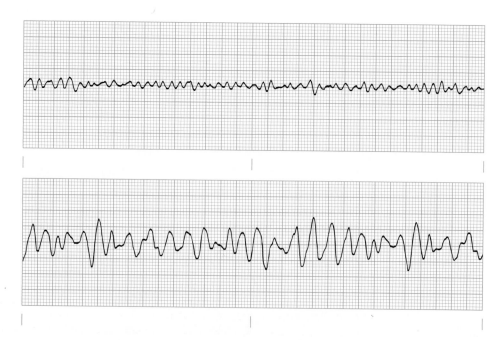

FIGURE 5-14 Two variants of ventricular fibrillation.

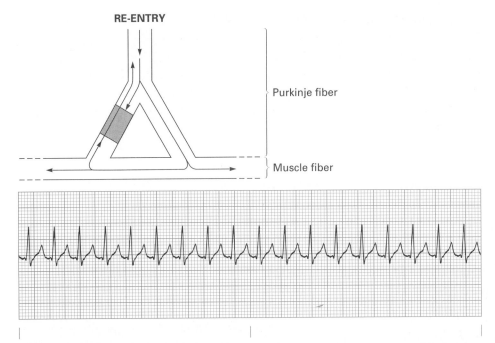

FIGURE 5-15 Reentry is a phenomenon usually created by a one-way block that causes a wave of depolarization to be rapidly propagated in a circular motion. Above: schematic drawing. Below: ECG tracing.

Reentry dysrhythmias

The reentry phenomenon is very complex, but basically it represents a "short circuit" of the conduction system. This short circuit may be caused by local damage (infarct or ischemia) or a congenital defect. Typically, reentry involves a situation in which a portion of the conduction system will allow an impulse to travel in only one direction. When this occurs, a vicious cycle of very fast depolarization ensues as the impulse moves in a circle throughout the heart tissue (Figure 5-15). The characteristics of reentry dysrhythmias are that they are fast and they are comparatively easy to convert, either electrically or pharmacologically.

Atrial Flutter

Atrial flutter is a reentry dysrhythmia in which the reentry circuit is propagated through the atria. Atrial flutter is characterized by a baseline that looks like the top of a picket fence, commonly referred to as "picket-fence" or "saw-tooth" waves. These are flutter waves (abbreviated F-waves) and represent the rapid circle of depolarization of the atria (Table 5-8 and Figure 5-16).

Paroxysmal Supraventricular Tachycardia

Supraventricular tachycardia is a catch-all term that technically applies to any tachycardia rhythm that originates above the ventricles (Table 5-9 and Figure 5-17). There are quite a few causes of supraventricular tachycardia. By convention, if you are able to identify where the tachycardia is originating, you should be as specific as possible.

You will recall that sinus tachycardia has a P wave which is evident. When the rate of sinus tachycardia gets above 160-170 beats per minute,

TABLE 5-8 ATRIAL FLUTTER

Analyze	ECG
Rate	Can be any rate, depending on the ventricular response and presence of AV block.
Regularity	Variance of less than 0.04 seconds
QRS Complex Do all of the QRS complexes look alike? What is the width of the QRS complex?	 Yes Less than 0.12 seconds
P Waves Is there a P wave before every QRS complex? Is there a QRS after every P wave?	**Flutter waves; no P waves discernible.** ⚑ **NA** **NA**
P-R Interval What is the P-R interval? Is the P-R interval constant?	 NA NA

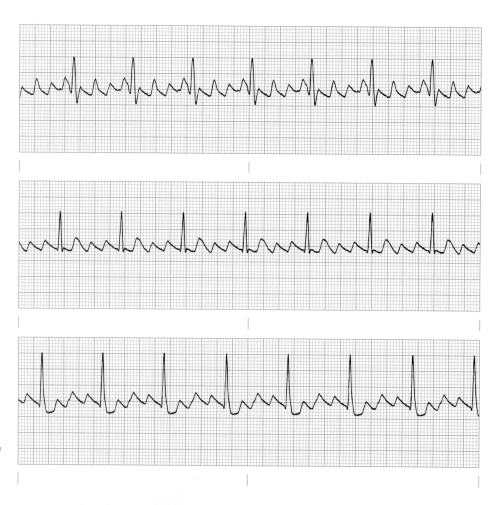

FIGURE 5-16 Three variants of atrial flutter.

TABLE 5-9 PAROXYSMAL SUPRAVENTRICULAR TACHYCARDIA

Analyze	ECG
Rate	140–220 per minute ⚑
Regularity	Variance of less than 0.04 seconds

QRS Complex
  Do all of the QRS complexes look alike?
  What is the width of the QRS complex?
	
	Yes
	Less than 0.12 seconds

P Waves
  Is there a P wave before every QRS complex?
  Is there a QRS after every P wave?
	No P waves are identifiable. ⚑
	NA
	NA

P-R Interval
  What is the P-R interval?
  Is the P-R interval constant?
	
	NA
	NA

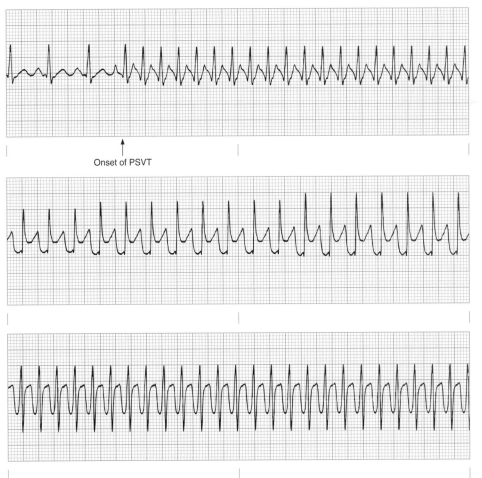

Onset of PSVT

FIGURE 5-17 Three variants of paroxysmal supraventricular tachycardia (PSVT).

the P wave gets buried in the previous T wave. Once this happens, it is impossible to tell if the tachycardia is created by rapid firing of the sinus node or by a reentry phenomenon. For narrow complex tachycardia from 150-200, it is important to look at the patient history to determine the electrophysiological cause of the dysrhythmia.

Shock, fear, fever, stress, or exercise usually indicates a sinus mechanism caused by sympathetic stimulation. Sudden onset and termination of tachycardia tend to be reentry in nature. A "run" of tachycardia that starts and stops abruptly is called paroxysmal, and is almost always a reentry mechanism. It is unusual for the SA node to discharge more than 200 beats per minute, so once the rate gets above 200, the dysrhythmia is probably caused by reentry.

Ventricular Tachycardia

Ventricular tachycardia (VT or V-tach) is a reentry phenomenon occurring in the ventricles. Like other reentry dysrhythmias, it is regular and fast. Since the rhythm does not follow the normal conduction pathways of the heart, the QRS complexes are wide (Table 5-10 and Figure 5-18). Mechanically, V-tach may cause the ventricles to contract, but if it occurs in patients with underlying cardiovascular disease, it is not well tolerated and may lead to ventricular fibrillation or pulselessness.

In some cases, it may be difficult to distinguish supraventricular tachycardia with aberrant conduction from ventricular tachycardia. If uncertain, it is best to assume that the rhythm is V-tach.

CLINICAL TIP: In an emergency, consider any wide complex tachycardia to be ventricular tachycardia until proven otherwise.

The Absence of Rhythm: Asystole

Probably the easiest rhythm to interpret is asystole. Asystole is the absence of any ventricular contraction or QRS complexes. Occasionally, you may see isolated P waves or slow, wide QRS complexes that are generally called "agonal" (Table 5-11 and Figure 5-19).

The Blocks

The atria and ventricles are isolated from each other electrically except for the atrioventricular (AV) node. The AV node, therefore, acts as a "gate" that any supraventricular signal must pass through if it is going to cause the ventricles to contract. Usually it takes less than 0.20 seconds for an impulse to pass through this gate. All of the blocks are caused by a delay at the AV junction. We will use the "gate" analogy to explain each of the blocks.

There are four AV blocks. It is easiest to consider the two ends of the spectrum, and then the intermediate situation. Therefore, we will start with a look at first and third degree blocks and then discuss the two types of second degree block.

First Degree AV Block

First degree AV block represents a slight closing of the "gate." In first degree AV block, the signal is delayed at the AV node, but all of the impulses get through. This is represented on the ECG as a constant P-R interval of greater than 0.20 seconds (Table 5-12 and Figure 5-20).

TABLE 5-10 VENTRICULAR TACHYCARDIA

Analyze	ECG
Rate	**Greater than 100 per minute** 🚩
Regularity	Variance of less than 0.04 seconds

QRS Complex
  Do all of the QRS complexes look alike?
  What is the width of the QRS complex?
	
	Yes
	Greater than 0.12 seconds 🚩

P Waves
  Is there a P wave before every QRS complex?
  Is there a QRS after every P wave?
	There are no P waves 🚩
	NA
	NA

P-R Interval
  What is the P-R interval?
  Is the P-R interval constant?
	
	NA
	NA

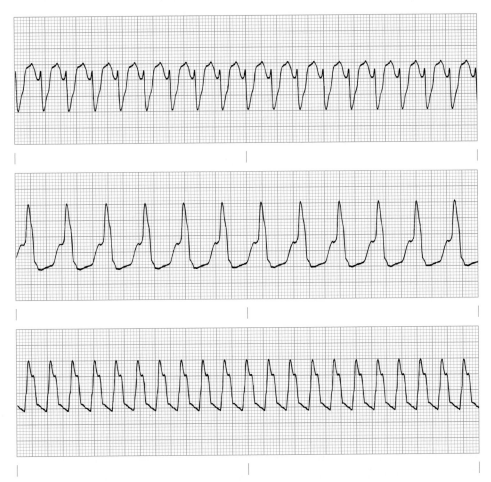

FIGURE 5-18 Three variants of ventricular tachycardia (V-tach).

TABLE 5-11 ASYSTOLE

Analyze	ECG
Rate	None 🚩
Regularity	NA 🚩
QRS Complex Do all of the QRS complexes look alike? What is the width of the QRS complex?	NA 🚩
P Waves Is there a P wave before every QRS complex? Is there a QRS after every P wave?	NA 🚩
P-R Interval What is the P-R interval? Is the P-R interval constant?	NA 🚩

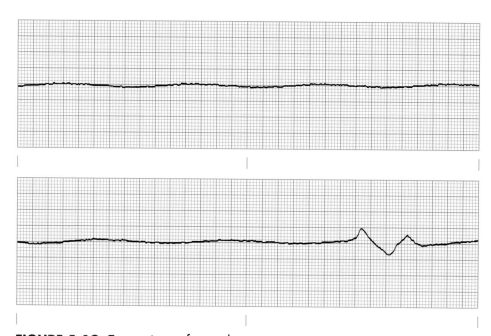

FIGURE 5-19 Two variants of asystole.

Third Degree AV Block

Third degree AV block is also called complete heart block. As the name implies, the "gate" is completely closed. There is no electrical connection between the atria and the ventricles; therefore, the atria and ventricles contract totally independently of each other. On the ECG, this is identified by a lack of relationship between the P waves and the QRS complexes (Table 5-13 and Figure 5-21). The P waves and QRS complexes have their own independent regular rates.

TABLE 5-12 FIRST DEGREE AV BLOCK

Analyze	ECG
Rate	60–100 per minute
Regularity	Variance of less than 0.04 seconds
QRS Complex Do all of the QRS complexes look alike? What is the width of the QRS complex?	 Yes Less than 0.12 seconds
P Waves Is there a P wave before every QRS complex? Is there a QRS after every P wave?	 Yes Yes
P-R Interval What is the P-R interval? Is the P-R interval constant?	 **Greater than 0.20 seconds** ⚑ **Yes**

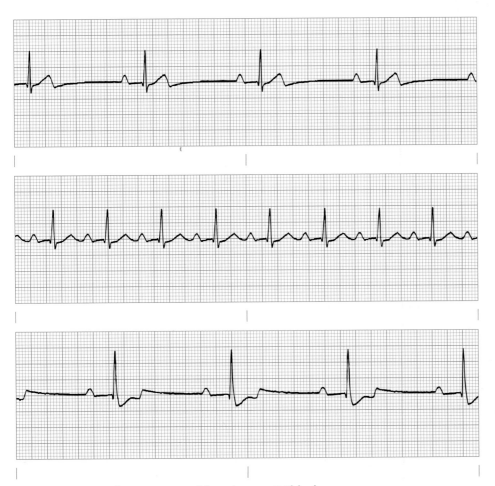

FIGURE 5-20 Three variants of first degree AV block.

TABLE 5-13 THIRD DEGREE AV BLOCK

Analyze	ECG
Rate	Less than 60 per minute
Regularity	Variance of less than 0.04 seconds

QRS Complex
  Do all of the QRS complexes look alike?
  What is the width of the QRS complex?
	Yes
	May be narrow or wide, depending on the location of the escape rhythm

P Waves
  Is there a P wave before every QRS complex?
  Is there a QRS after every P wave?
	There is no relationship between the P waves and the QRS complex. ⚑

P-R Interval
  What is the P-R interval?
  Is the P-R interval constant?
	Variable ⚑
	Variable

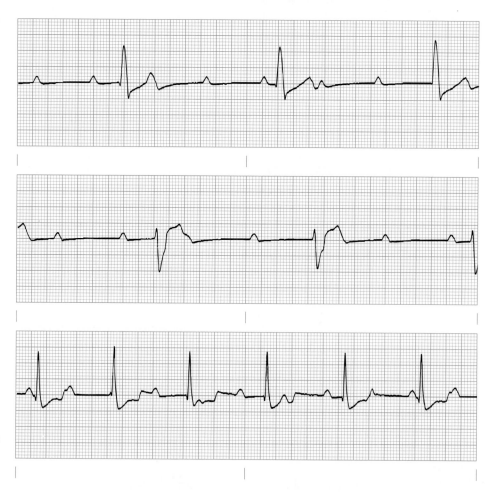

FIGURE 5-21 Three variants of third degree AV Block.

Second Degree AV Block

Second degree AV blocks represent some intermittent closing to the AV "gate." Since the gate does not remain closed, some of the beats get through and others do not. In second degree AV blocks, there are always more P waves than QRS complexes since some of the P waves are prevented from causing ventricular contraction by a gate that is opening and closing.

- **Type I.** Second degree AV block, Type I (which is also called second degree, Mobitz I or Wenckebach) is identified by a progressive prolongation of the P-R interval until one beat fails to get through, and then the pattern repeats itself (Table 5-14 and Figure 5-22).
- **Type II.** Second degree AV block, Type II (also called second degree, Mobitz II) is the intermittent closing of the "gate" at regular intervals. This leads to a pattern of grouped beats (P waves followed by QRS complexes) with pauses (P waves with no QRS complexes) (Table 5-15 and Figure 5-23). Typically, you can see the pattern developing if you look at a long-enough strip. Often, second degree blocks are referred to by the ratio of P waves to QRS complexes. When compared to Mobitz I second degree block, the interval between P wave and QRS complex does not lengthen in Mobitz II. It is also important to remember with this type of block that the intervals of the *transmitted* P waves are constant.

Ectopic Beats

An ectopic beat occurs when a site *other than the primary pacemaker of the heart* depolarizes. Remember that myocardial cells have the property of automaticity, which may cause depolarization if the conditions are right. This can cause depolarization of the surrounding muscle tissue. If the ectopic beat originates above the ventricles, the impulse can follow the normal ventricular conduction system and result in the depolarization of the ventricles. If the ectopic focus is located in the ventricles, it will most likely depolarize just the ventricles and typically does not follow the normal conduction of the heart. If the ectopic beat comes earlier than the next-expected beat, based on the underlying rhythm, the ectopic beat is called "premature." If it comes after a pause in the underlying rhythm, it is referred to as an "escape" beat.

In the past, premature beats were thought to indicate increased cardiac irritability. Especially in the case of premature ventricular contractions, increased ectopic beats were thought to be a warning of sudden cardiac arrest from ventricular fibrillation and were typically treated aggressively. Routine treatment of PVCs has not been supported by scientific studies, but you should still consider the presence of ectopic beats in the setting of a suspected myocardial infarction significant.

The process for determining where ectopic beats are coming from is slightly different than interpreting the rhythm. Technically, ectopic beats are not dysrhythmias. All rhythms with premature beats are irregular, but the underlying rhythm that is interrupted by the premature beat may be regular.

TABLE 5-14 SECOND DEGREE AV BLOCK, TYPE I

Analyze	ECG
Rate	60–100 per minute
Regularity	**Missed beats, regularly irregular** 🚩
QRS Complex Do all of the QRS complexes look alike? What is the width of the QRS complex?	Yes Less than 0.12 seconds
P Waves Is there a P wave before every QRS complex? Is there a QRS after every P wave?	Yes No 🚩
P-R Interval What is the P-R interval? Is the P-R interval constant?	**The P-R interval is variable and progressively lengthens until a QRS is dropped. Then the pattern repeats.** 🚩

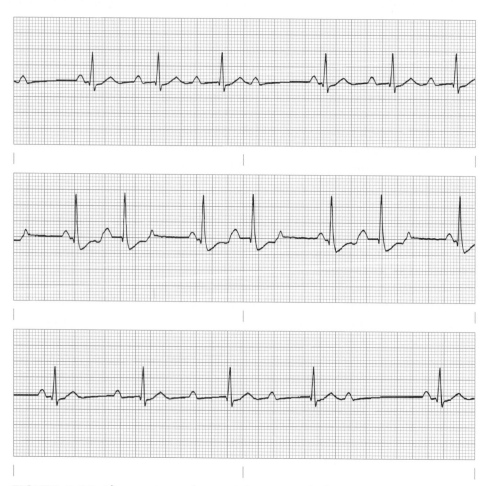

FIGURE 5-22 Three variants of second degree AV Block, Type I.

TABLE 5-15   SECOND DEGREE AV BLOCK, TYPE II

Analyze	ECG
Rate	60–100 per minute
Regularity	**Dropped QRS complexes result in an irregular rhythm.**
QRS Complex Do all of the QRS complexes look alike? What is the width of the QRS complex?	Yes Less than 0.12 seconds
P Waves Is there a P wave before every QRS complex? Is there a QRS after every P wave?	Yes No
P-R Interval What is the P-R interval? Is the P-R interval constant?	**Non-conducted P waves are not followed by QRS complexes. Conducted P waves have a constant P-R interval, typically less than 0.20 seconds.**

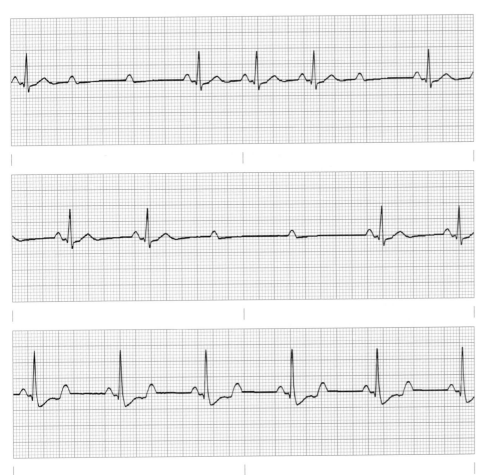

FIGURE 5-23 Three variants of second degree AV Block, Type II.

You should think of the possibility of ectopic beats in the following two situations:

- When all of the beats do not look the same
- When there is some regularity to the rhythm, but none of the blocks seem to fit.

Once you suspect the presence of ectopic beats, you should do the following:

1. *Identify the underlying rhythm.* If the ectopic beats look different, this is very easy. Unfortunately, this is not always the case and you should look at the patterns of the rhythm.
2. *Determine where the ectopic beats are originating.* There are three possibilities: the atria, the AV node, or the ventricles. Determining the origin of the ectopic beat is accomplished by looking at the P wave, QRS complex, and the interruption of the underlying rhythm that is caused by the ectopic beat, as explained below.

Premature Atrial and Premature Junctional Contractions

Premature atrial contractions (PACs) are caused by an ectopic focus located somewhere in the atrial tissue. Premature junctional contractions (PJCs) are caused by the AV node firing prematurely. The difference between PACs and PJCs is minor and, in the setting of a cardiac emergency, considered to be clinically insignificant. We will therefore discuss PACs and PJCs together.

The PAC may have a P wave if the ectopic beat is high enough in the atria, but it will usually look somewhat different from the P wave of the underlying rhythm. If the premature beat originates lower in the atria, or in the AV junction, the P wave may be absent or upside down. The QRS complexes of PACs and PJCs are usually narrow, since the ectopic beats follow the normal ventricular conduction pathway (Figure 5-24).

The SA node is reset by a premature atrial contraction and by most premature junctional complexes. Therefore the R-to-R interval for the beat immediately following the ectopic beat is usually the same as the R-to-R intervals of the underlying rhythm. If you measure the distance from the R wave of the last beat of the intrinsic rhythm to the R wave of the next beat after the ectopic beat, it is less than 2 R, the distance of two R-R intervals. This is called a non-compensatory pause (Table 5-16).

Premature Ventricular Contractions

Premature ventricular contractions (PVCs) are caused by an ectopic focus in the ventricles. Since the ectopic beat originates in the ventricles, there is no P wave. The ectopic beat does not follow the normal ventricular conduction pathway, and therefore the morphology of the PVC is always wide (Figure 5-25).

CLINICAL TIP: Not all wide premature beats are PVCs!

It is important not to make the mistake of assuming that all wide premature beats are PVCs. The underlying rhythm's QRS complexes can be narrow, and a PAC or PJC can be wide. Be sure to look at all the variables.

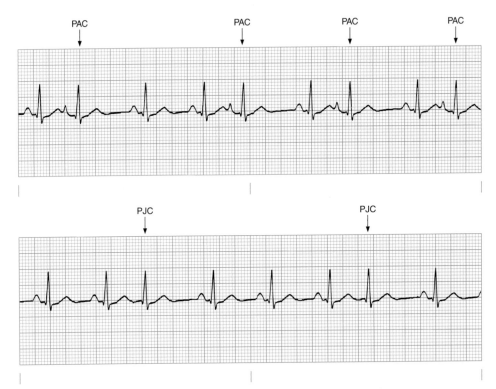

FIGURE 5-24 (Top) premature atrial contraction (PAC); (Bottom) premature junctional contraction (PJC).

Since the PVC originates in the ventricles, the SA node is not affected by the ectopic beat. The SA node continues to fire uninterrupted and is not reset by a PVC. For that reason, the distance from the R wave of the beat

TABLE 5-16 PACs AND PJCs	
Analyze	**ECG**
P wave of the ectopic beat	Usually looks different from the P waves of the underlying rhythm. May be upright if the ectopic foci are high in the atria. The P wave may be absent or upside down if it is low in the atria or in the AV junction.
QRS complex of the ectopic beat	Usually narrow. It is possible that the QRS is wide, even if the QRS of the underlying rhythm is narrow.
Interruption of the underlying rhythm that is caused by the ectopic beat	Non-compensatory pause

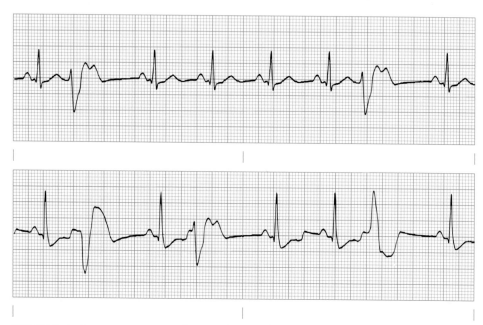

FIGURE 5-25 Two variants of normal sinus rhythm with PVCs.

immediately preceding a PVC to the R wave of the beat following the PVC will be 2R of the underlying beat. This is called a compensatory pause (Table 5-17 and Figure 5-26).

TABLE 5-17 PVCs	
Analyze	**ECG**
P wave of the ectopic beat	Usually none
QRS complex of the ectopic beat	Always wide
Interruption of the underlying rhythm that is caused by the ectopic beat	Compensatory pause

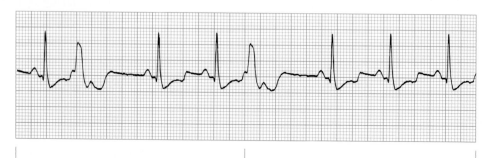

FIGURE 5-26 A compensatory pause following a PVC.

There are several types of PVCs with which you should become familiar.

- **Unifocal.** All of the PVCs look the same and probably come from one ectopic focus (Figure 5-27).

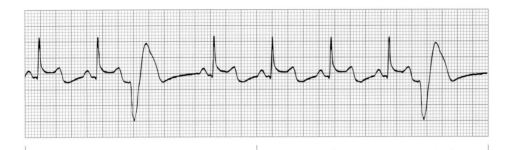

FIGURE 5-27 Normal sinus rhythm with unifocal PVCs.

- **Multifocal.** The PVCs look different from each other and likely come from more than one ectopic foci (Figure 5-28).

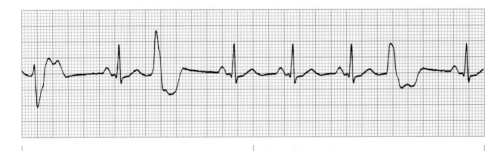

FIGURE 5-28 Normal sinus rhythm with multifocal PVCs.

- **Salvos or couplets.** Two or three PVCs in a row (Figure 5-29).

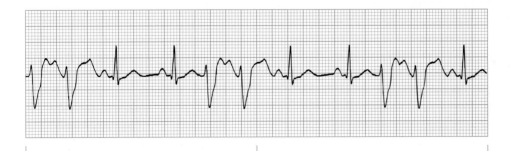

FIGURE 5-29 Normal sinus rhythm with PVC couplets.

- **Bigeminy.** A PVC every other beat (Figure 5-30)

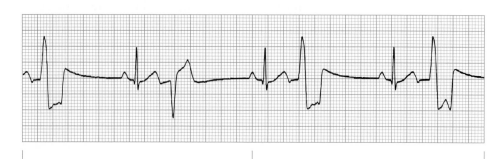

FIGURE 5-30 PVCs bigeminy.

- **Trigeminy.** A PVC every third beat (Figure 5-31).

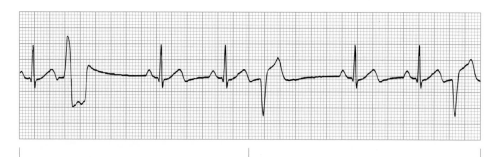

FIGURE 5-31 PVCs trigeminy.

CASE STUDY FOLLOW-UP

Assessment

Mrs. Brown is alert and oriented, she denies chest pain or shortness of breath, her pulse is 180, respirations 20 and unlabored, blood pressure 124/78. You remember that the majority of wide complex tachycardias are ventricular tachycardia. Often, you can get additional clues from the patient's history, but in this case it does not help, since she has not had the problem previously diagnosed. In this case, Mrs. Brown is stable and you are unsure of the origination of the dysrhythmia. This could be either ventricular tachycardia or a supraventricular tachycardia with aberrant conduction.

Treatment

You choose to administer lidocaine. The rhythm does not convert, and en route to the hospital, Mrs. Brown begins to complain of lightheadedness and dizziness. Reassessment reveals a pulse of 180, respirations of 22 and unlabored, and a blood pressure of 98/64. She is pale and diaphoretic.

Mrs. Brown is now unstable. You decide to abandon the pharmacological approach. You administer an intravenous sedative and cardiovert her at 100 joules. The rhythm converts to NSR and her blood pressure returns to 114/78.

Electrophysiology studies indicate that the rhythm was indeed ventricular tachycardia. Mrs. Brown is now taking Quinidine and doing fine.

SUMMARY

The recognition of dysrhythmias is one of the most important aspects of ACLS and a necessary component of the patient assessment for any cardiac patient. Many clinicians become intimidated by the electrophysiology of the heart and fail to learn a systematic method of evaluating ECGs. By using the "red flag" method and applying a few rules and an understanding of the etiology of dysrhythmias, dysrhythmia recognition becomes much easier.

REVIEW QUESTIONS

1. Myocardial cells possess the unique property of
    a. depolarization.
    b. repolarization.
    c. contractility.
    d. automaticity.

2. Which of the following is **not** one of the three specialized types of myocardial cells?
    a. pacemaker
    b. conduction
    c. depolarizing
    d. working

3. What is the purpose of pacemaker cells?
    a. to contract when a wave of depolarization reaches them
    b. to depolarize at regular intervals
    c. to repolarize contracted muscle tissue
    d. to delay the conduction from the atria to the ventricles

4. The main pacemaker of the healthy heart is the
    a. SA node.
    b. atrium.
    c. AV node.
    d. ventricle.

5. The AV node depolarizes spontaneously at what rate?
    a. greater than 100 times per minute
    b. 60–100 times per minute
    c. 40–60 times per minute
    d. less than 40 times per minute

6. The cells responsible for mechanical contraction of the heart are
    a. pacemaker cells.
    b. conduction cells.
    c. myocardial working cells.
    d. all of the heart cells.

7. What mechanical event corresponds to the QRS complex in the normal heart?
    a. atrial contraction
    b. the delay between atrial and ventricular contraction
    c. ventricular contraction
    d. reentry

8. A variance of greater than .04 second in the R-R interval is called
    a. irregularity.
    b. automaticity.
    c. ectopy.
    d. dysrhythmia.

9. Which of the following is a cause of wide QRS complexes?
    a. hypothermia
    b. bundle branch block
    c. hypernatremia
    d. acute myocardial infarction

10. What do we know for sure about a narrow QRS complex?
    a. It cannot have been generated by the SA node.
    b. The impulse was delayed at the AV node.
    c. It must have originated above the ventricles.
    d. It must have followed the internodal pathways.

11. What is the maximum normal P-R interval?
    a. .04 seconds
    b. .12 seconds
    c. .20 seconds
    d. .50 seconds

12. What is/are the "red flag(s)" in sinus tachycardia?
    a. rate
    b. regularity
    c. QRS complex
    d. P wave
    e. P-R interval
    f. If more than one "red flag," fill in the letters of the correct responses:
    _____

13. What is/are the "red flag(s)" in sinus dysrhythmia?
    a. rate
    b. regularity
    c. QRS complex
    d. P wave
    e. P-R interval
    f. If more than one "red flag," fill in the letters of the correct responses:
    _____

14. What dysrhythmia is **irregularly** irregular?
    a. second degree, Type I heart block
    b. third degree heart block
    c. sinus rhythm with PVCs
    d. atrial fibrillation

15. What is/are the "red flag(s)" in atrial fibrillation?
    a. rate
    b. regularity
    c. QRS complex
    d. P wave
    e. P-R interval
    f. If more than one "red flag," fill in the letters of the correct responses:
    _____

16. Which of the following is **not** a reentry dysrhythmia?
    a. atrial fibrillation
    b. supraventricular tachycardia
    c. atrial flutter
    d. ventricular tachycardia

17. What is/are the "red flag(s)" in atrial flutter?
    a. rate
    b. regularity
    c. QRS complex

    d. P wave

    e. P-R interval

    f. If more than one "red flag," fill in the letters of the correct responses:

    _____

18. What is/are the "red flag(s)" in supraventricular tachycardia?

    a. rate

    b. regularity

    c. QRS complex

    d. P wave

    e. P-R interval

    f. If more than one "red flag," fill in the letters of the correct responses:

    _____

19. What is/are the "red flag(s)" in ventricular tachycardia?

    a. rate

    b. regularity

    c. QRS complex

    d. P wave

    e. P-R interval

    f. If more than one "red flag," fill in the letters of the correct responses:

    _____

20. What is/are the "red flag(s)" in first degree AV block?

    a. rate

    b. regularity

    c. QRS complex

    d. P wave

    e. P-R interval

    f. If more than one "red flag," fill in the letters of the correct responses:

    _____

21. What is/are the "red flag(s)" in third degree AV block?

    a. rate

    b. regularity

    c. QRS complex

    d. P wave

    e. P-R interval

    f. If more than one "red flag," fill in the letters of the correct responses:

    _____

22. All PVCs are _____, but not all PACs and PJCs are _____.

    a. narrow, narrow

    b. wide, wide

    c. wide, narrow

    d. narrow, wide

23. Most PVCs have a _____, and most PACs have a _____ pause.

    a. compensatory, compensatory

    b. non-compensatory, non-compensatory

    c. compensatory, non-compensatory

    d. non-compensatory, compensatory

24. What is the name for PVCs that occur "every third beat"?
    a. trigeminy   c. multifocal
    b. bigeminy   d. salvos

25. Identify the following rhythm.

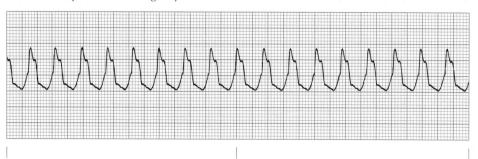

_____

26. Identify the following rhythm.

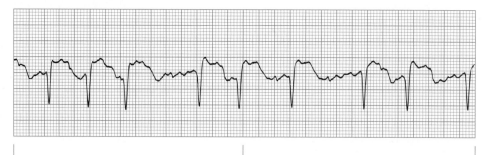

_____

27. Identify the following rhythm.

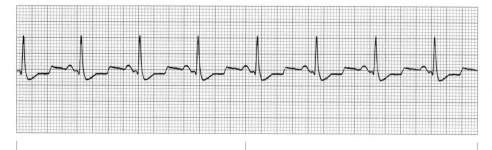

_____

28. Identify the following rhythm.

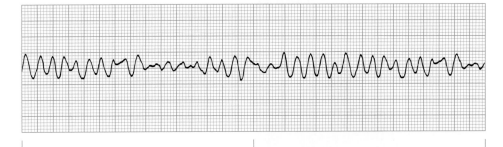

_____

29. Identify the following rhythm.

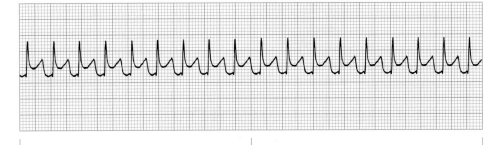

_____

30. Identify the following rhythm.

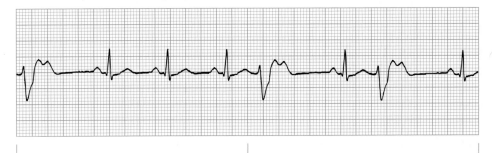

_____

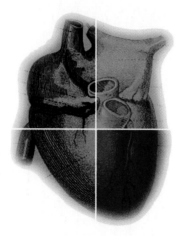

Electrical Therapy

Occasionally you will encounter a patient whose cardiac problem is likely to deteriorate before drug treatment would have time to be effective. In other cases, the patient may be suffering from a dysrhythmia that is unresponsive to any currently known drug therapy. In these situations, a form of emergency electrical therapy may be the most appropriate intervention.

Topics to be covered in this chapter are:

- Defibrillation
- Automated External Defibrillation
- Emergency Synchronized Cardioversion
- Special Situations Involving Electrical Therapy
- Emergency Cardiac Pacing

CASE STUDY

You are working the midnight shift at a small community hospital. The night has been quiet, and you have been catching up on some light reading between the sparse patients. As you near the end of your shift, the triage nurse calls you to assist her with a patient experiencing chest pain who arrived by private vehicle. You quickly walk to the triage desk, and there you see an anxious middle-aged man sitting in a wheelchair, his left hand clenched over his sternum.

As you escort him into the emergency department, the patient—Mr. Griffiths—tells you that the chest pain started about 4 hours ago when it woke him from his sleep. He adds that, shortly thereafter, he started having trouble breathing and became "sweaty." As a fellow health care provider starts removing his shirt, you rapidly obtain a set of vitals which reveal a blood pressure of 102/62, a heart rate of 220 and regular, and a respiratory rate of 36 with slight retractions. With an anxious look and a scared voice, Mr. Griffiths asks you, "Am . . .I . . .going to be O.K.?"

How would you proceed to assess and care for this patient? This chapter will describe the assessment and necessary treatment of a patient with a cardiac emergency that requires the use of electrical therapy. Later, we will return to the case and apply the procedures learned.

Introduction

During the course of emergency cardiac care, the health care provider may encounter a patient for whom traditional treatment with pharmacology may be ineffective or require more time to exert a desired physiologic action than is available. As well, there are certain cardiac dysrhythmias that are unresponsive to any type of drug therapy. It is in these specific instances that the most appropriate choice of therapeutic intervention may well be electrical therapy.

Electrical therapy can be used to terminate specific cardiac dysrhythmias. Depending on the type of dysrhythmia, you may need to apply defibrillation, synchronized cardioversion, or transcutaneous pacing. While all of these interventions require the administration of electricity to the patient's body, their delivery methods and indications differ significantly.

In this chapter, each method of administering electrical therapy will be discussed with its rationale, indications, and procedures. We will also discuss the automated external defibrillator, a device designed to reduce the incidence of out-of-hospital deaths from sudden cardiac arrest.

Defibrillation

The therapeutic benefit of electrical defibrillation (also known as asynchronous cardioversion) is its ability to terminate a fibrillating heart by passing a current of electricity through it.

As a reminder, ventricular fibrillation is a life-threatening dysrhythmia in which a grave disruption in the normal conduction system has occurred. Multiple cells within the heart are discharging and repolarizing independently of other cardiac cells. Since there is no organized depolarization wave spreading through the myocardium to cause muscle contraction, there can be no cardiac output. Ventricular fibrillation is a self-propagating and self-defeating dysrhythmia, as the varying degrees of depolarization prohibit organized repolarization. Thus, ventricular fibrillation will eventually degrade into asystole as the heart becomes damaged from ensuing acidosis and hypoxia. Without correction, the heart's ability to propagate any impulse will eventually cease.

There are two theories about how defibrillation works. By passing a large amount of electrical current through the heart over a brief period of time, the first theory maintains, a "critical mass" of ventricular cells are depolarized as a unit, thereby allowing repolarization to occur more uniformly—after which, it is hoped, when a normal pacemaker in the heart provides its electrical impulse, the impulse can now travel down a repolarized (and ready) conduction system.

The second theory views the multiple depolarizations as mini "wave fronts" passing through the heart in search of repolarized tissue. In this second theory, the act of passing a large current of energy through the heart will depolarize all primed (repolarized) muscle tissue, subsequently leaving nowhere for the "wave front" to spread next, eliminating the fibrillation.

Regardless of the exact mechanism of defibrillation, however, the fact remains that if ventricular fibrillation is left untreated, the patient will die. It is important to understand that electrical defibrillation is currently the most effective method of terminating ventricular fibrillation. CPR does not terminate fibrillation, nor do intravenous drugs, intubation, or IV fluids. While these may make a more favorable environment in which to achieve successful defibrillation, a fibrillating heart must receive early electrical therapy. Pulseless ventricular tachycardia (VT, or V-tach) will rapidly degrade into ventricular fibrillation (VF, or V-fib), so either of these rhythms should receive immediate defibrillation.

Importance of Defibrillation

A significant portion of all heart-related deaths can be classified as *sudden cardiac death*, which is defined as cardiac arrest occurring within hours of the onset of signs and symptoms of a cardiac problem. The most frequent rhythm underlying sudden cardiac death is ventricular fibrillation. So if health care providers want to make a significant impact in reducing the number of sudden cardiac deaths, one way to achieve this is by providing rapid defibrillation.

Defibrillation is inextricably time dependent. For example, the likelihood of successfully resuscitating a person in ventricular fibrillation is highest (greater than 90%) if defibrillation is delivered within the first minute of cardiac arrest. However, after only 9 minutes of cardiac arrest, a successful resuscitation occurs in less than 1 out of every 10 attempts. While CPR is effective and necessary in a cardiac arrest situation, studies indicate that the main benefit of CPR is not in converting ventricular fibrillation but rather in maintaining coronary and cerebral blood flow until a defibrillator is available.

Components of a Defibrillator

The defibrillation unit may be a stationary device requiring an external power source, a portable device that can be carried to the patient's side, or an integral part of a cardiac monitor.

Irrespective of type, all defibrillation machines share common components. A direct-current defibrillator has a variable transformer that will generate a high-voltage charge, which is stored in an electrical capacitor to be delivered to the patient at the desired time. To complete the circuit, the defibrillator is equipped with connections from the energy capacitor to the patient via defibrillation electrodes (paddles or pads) that are placed in contact with the patient's thorax.

Defibrillators manufactured today have numerous energy-level settings which the health care provider selects before charging the capacitor and delivering the energy. The specific amount of energy is selected based upon patient needs and is measured in *joules*, or watt-seconds.

What is a watt-second? How much energy is that? Try to picture the following analogy between a defibrillator and a light bulb. A common energy level used in defibrillation is 360 watt-seconds. Now picture putting four fingers into four empty light sockets specifically designed only for 90-watt light bulbs. Now, if someone turns on the light switch to these sockets for one full second and then shuts it back off, the amount of energy you just received (i.e., were shocked by) totals 360 watt-seconds (four 90-watt light sockets turned on for one second equals 360 watt-seconds). This is certainly not an experiment the authors recommend that you try at home! It is intended solely to help illustrate the amount of energy you are delivering when you defibrillate your patient.

Transthoracic Resistance to Energy Flow

Electricity, as is well known, will travel along the pathway of least resistance. This is why electrical cables and high tension wires are constructed of the materials they are—because these materials conduct electricity well. However, the materials that conduct electricity best are not found within the human body. In fact, the chest can offer a high resistance to electrical flow (termed *transthoracic resistance*) during defibrillation attempts.

Because it is typically not possible to defibrillate the heart directly during emergency cardiac care (unless the thorax has been previously opened), the energy must pass through the chest wall and associated structures before it reaches the heart. Since a portion of the energy delivered is used up in overcoming the high transthoracic resistance of the chest, the amount of current available for defibrillation, once the current reaches the heart, is less than that initially delivered through the paddles. The concern is that, if transthoracic resistance (the resistance to current flow) is not lowered during the defibrillation process, a subtherapeutic amount of energy may reach the heart and be unable to defibrillate a "critical mass" of the myocardium.

Many factors determine the amount of transthoracic resistance to current flow. These include electrode size, electrode position, electrode-skin interface material, phase of ventilation, size of the patient, electrode contact pressure, successive defibrillations, and energy level selection (Table 6-1).

The following sections outline these factors and describe methods to decrease the resistance to current flow.

Electrode Size

The size of the electrode applied to the patient's chest can decrease resistance if the proper size is used. For an adult, the defibrillation electrode should be

TABLE 6-1 METHODS OF REDUCING TRANSTHORACIC RESISTANCE DURING DEFIBRILLATION

Electrode Size	8.5–12 cm adult 8 cm child 4.5 cm infant
Electrode Position	anterior-apex placement anterior-posterior placement
Electrode Interface	electrode gel pads electrode paste
Phase of Ventilation	end expiration
Electrode Contact	25 pounds (11 kg) of muscular pressure on paddles
Time Interval of Previous Countershocks	deliver shocks in rapid succession
Energy Level	start 200 J, then 200-300 J, 360 J from then on

8.5 to 12 cm in diameter. Infant paddles, when needed, typically clip onto the adult paddle and have a smaller surface area that a child under 1 year of age can accommodate. Infant defibrillation paddles are typically 4.5 cm, and a child's size would be about 8 cm. The most important aspect to choosing electrode size is to use the size that can comfortably and appropriately fit on the patient's chest and that does not allow for large gaps under the paddle.

Electrode Position
Placement of the defibrillation electrodes in one of two recommended positions will assure that the maximum amount of electricity will flow through the myocardium. The anterior-apex placement will put the negative electrode to the right of the sternum, just beneath the clavicle. The positive electrode will then be placed to the left of the nipple of the left thorax, positioned midaxillary (left apex). The anterior-posterior placement will find the anterior (negative) electrode over the left precordium, with the posterior (positive) electrode in the infrascapular space of the left scapula. Either method is equally effective in enhancing the amount of energy reaching the heart. The anterior-apex placement is more commonly used because it is the easier of the two to use during a cardiac arrest (Figure 6-1).

The health care provider may also encounter situations where the patient has had a permanent pacemaker or defibrillator surgically implanted in the thorax. The presence of such a device does not, however, preclude defibrillation when necessary. In these and other situations where other medical devices are in close proximity to your defibrillation landmarks, common sense dictates repositioning your electrodes slightly to avoid defibrillating directly over top of one of these devices. If necessary, change the position of the monitor electrodes to gain additional space.

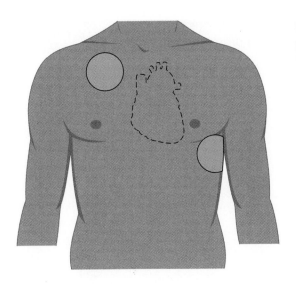

FIGURE 6-1 The anterior-apex position for placement of defibrillation electrodes.

Electrode-Skin Interface

Some type of commercially available gel pad or electrode gel is necessary to eliminate the resistance between the bare chest and the dry metal electrode. You must ensure that there are adequate amounts of conductive medium after repeated defibrillations. It is also important to ensure that there is no contact between the mediums of each paddle, which would make the electricity flow across the chest rather than through it. Arcing between paddles is also a potentially dangerous complication of improperly performed defibrillations.

Phase of Ventilation

The phases of ventilation will change the distance between the electrodes and the heart as the size of the thorax increases and decreases with inspiration and expiration. Delivering the defibrillation during the end-expiratory phase will eliminate resistance caused by an expanded thorax. This will not be a factor in the cardiac arrest patient, who has no spontaneous respiration.

Electrode Contact Pressure

Contact pressure is also an important aspect to successfully defibrillating a patient. By applying about 25 pounds of muscular pressure, you will ensure good contact of the paddle to the conductive medium against the chest. This will also help eliminate the chance for arcing of the electricity.

How much is 25 pounds of muscular pressure? Try placing a standard bathroom scale on the floor and applying pressure to it until you achieve 25 pounds on the display. Practice exerting *only* the muscular strength of your arms and *not* using the weight of your body. If you slip while leaning over a patient, you run the risk of shocking yourself, a bystander, or another care provider near the patient.

Time Interval of Previous Countershocks

Transiently, the degree of transthoracic resistance will decrease with successive countershocks as long as they are administered rapidly. (The terms *countershock* and *shock* are used interchangeably.) After the first defibrillation, the body becomes "polarized," and subsequent discharges flow against reduced resistance. This allows more electricity to be delivered to the heart.

STEPS OF DEFIBRILLATION

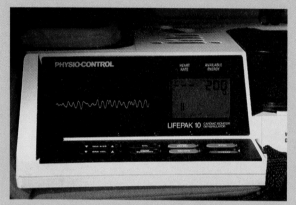

FIGURE 6-2 a Identify ventricular fibrillation on the cardiac monitor.

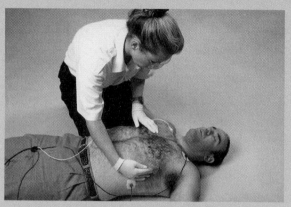

FIGURE 6-2 b Charge the defibrillation paddles.

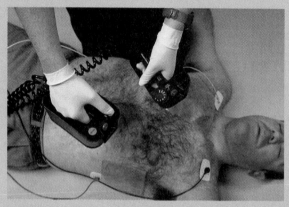

FIGURE 6-2 c Apply electrode gel to the paddles or place commercial defibrillation pads on the patient's exposed thorax.

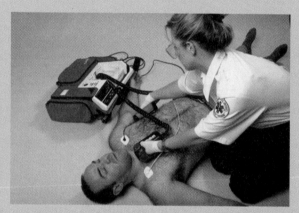

FIGURE 6-2 d Reconfirm the rhythm on the cardiac monitor.

Selected Energy Level

Naturally, the higher the amount of energy selected, the more energy that will be delivered to the heart. However, anytime you defibrillate someone you run the risk of causing myocardial damage. Therefore, you start with an energy level that is likely to convert the rhythm from fibrillation but is not so high that it will cause unnecessary damage. A setting of 200 joules is appropriate for the initial defibrillation attempt in a patient with pulseless VF or VT. The second countershock can be 200-300 joules (remember that the chest resistance drops with the first shock), the third and highest energy level is 360 joules. Successive defibrillations for persistent VF or pulseless VT are delivered at 360 joules. And if the VF/VT recurs after previously being successfully converted, select the energy level that was previously successful.

Procedure for Defibrillation

Once the decision for defibrillating the patient is made, follow these steps to perform defibrillation (Figures 6-2 a to 6-2 g).

STEPS OF DEFIBRILLATION *(continued)*

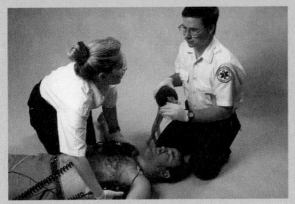

FIGURE 6-2 e Verbally and visually clear everybody from the patient (including yourself).

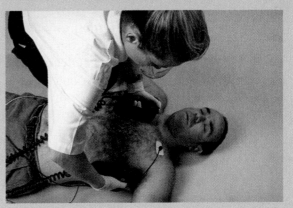

FIGURE 6-2 f Deliver a defibrillatory shock by depressing both buttons simultaneously.

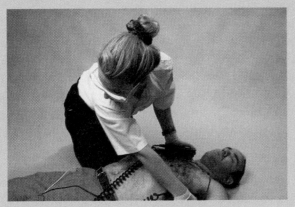

FIGURE 6-2 g Reconfirm the rhythm on the cardiac monitor.

1. Confirm ventricular fibrillation or pulseless ventricular tachycardia on the cardiac monitor.
2. Place the patient in a safe environment if initially in contact with some electrically conductive material (e.g., metal, water).
3. Apply electrode gel to the paddles, or place commercial defibrillation pads on the patient's exposed thorax.
4. Turn on and charge the defibrillator to 200 J for the first shock.
5. Ensure that the electrodes are appropriately placed on the patient's thorax with proper pressure.
6. ENSURE THAT NO ONE ELSE IS IN CONTACT WITH THE PATIENT. Verbally and visually clear everybody prior to any defibrillation attempt (including yourself).
7. Deliver a defibrillatory shock by depressing both red buttons simultaneously (depressing only one will result in no shock being delivered).
8. Reconfirm the rhythm on the monitor screen; if still VF/VT, recharge and repeat steps 5–7, using higher energy levels.

See Figure 10-2 in Chapter 10, the Ventricular Fibrillation/Pulseless Ventricular Tachycardia (VF/VT) algorithm.

Defibrillation and Asystolic Hearts

When you recognize asystole on the heart monitor, you should confirm it in two different leads, since fine ventricular fibrillation may "hide" or be "masked" in one lead but not another. And if asystole does in fact turn out to be fine VF in another lead, you should manage the rhythm as VF and carry out defibrillation attempts as previously discussed.

However, if asystole is truly asystole in multiple leads, defibrillation attempts are not warranted. Randomly shocking an asystolic heart under the premise that "no harm can be done" is inaccurate. The defibrillation attempt actually induces a profound increase in vagal tone, which can inhibit the natural pacemakers of the heart to an extent that any chance for recovery is eliminated.

Current-Based Defibrillation: "Smart Defibrillators"

Presently under investigation is an alternative approach to defibrillation called current-based defibrillation. With current-based defibrillation, you can select the desired electrical current to be delivered to the heart (in amperes), rather than the customary energy level delivered from the defibrillator (in joules). Then, the defibrillator determines the degree of resistance offered by this specific patient's thorax by passing a small amount of energy through it from electrode to electrode. Once it has determined the amount of energy required to overcome the resistance, the defibrillator adjusts the current flow to allow the exact energy selected to be delivered to the heart. This technology will be beneficial to patients with varying degrees of resistance due to differences in the size and/or integrity of the thorax.

Automated External Defibrillation

Defibrillation was once a skill reserved specifically for those health care providers capable of identifying the appropriate rhythms by reading and interpreting ECGs and trained in the use of manual defibrillation. However, the success of conversion from ventricular fibrillation is directly related to the speed with which defibrillation is provided. Unfortunately, there has often been a delay in getting a team trained in ECG interpretation and manual defibrillation to the patient's side.

Fortunately, with advances in medical technology, devices were invented that could distinguish between rhythms that are or are not ventricular fibrillation. After this, it was easy to create the computer programming that could deliver sequential countershocks independent of human interpretation. Thus, the device known as the automated external defibrillator (AED) was created. Because the AED is so simple to operate, laypersons and first responders can now be trained to provide early defibrillation to cardiac arrest patients, making possible a reduction in out-of-hospital cardiac arrests.

Components of an Automated External Defibrillator

There is striking similarity between an AED and a standard manual defibrillator. With both, a power source charges the capacitors to a specified amount of energy. They both have cables that attach to electrodes that are in contact with the patient's chest in order to deliver the defibrillation. (The AED also interprets the ECG through the electrodes attached to the chest.) The main difference between the two is how the rhythm is detected.

While the manual defibrillator requires a person to interpret the rhythm on the monitor, the AED has an internal rhythm analysis system capable of identifying VF, or VT above a preset rate. Its rhythm analysis system does not determine every dysrhythmia known; rather it looks simply for the presence of VF/VT. If the criteria it analyzes (amplitude, frequency, and slope of the ECG) fit the requirement for VF/VT, a shock is recommended. If the criteria for defibrillation are not met, no shock is advised.

Types of AEDs

There are basically two types of AEDs. Their main difference is based on the degree to which there is human input to the delivery of defibrillation shocks. The first type is known as "fully" automated. A fully automated AED will analyze the rhythm, charge the capacitors, and automatically discharge if VT/VF is present. It will deliver a shock independent of human involvement.

The second type, known as a "semi" automated AED, relies more heavily on human involvement in the administration of the defibrillatory shocks. In this type, the provider must activate the "analyze" button for the unit to interpret the rhythm. Then, if the unit identifies VF/VT, it will emit an audible tone or voice synthesizer, alerting the care provider to depress the "discharge" or "shock" button after verifying the rhythm and charging the capacitors to the appropriate level. This allows the care provider to visually and verbally clear the patient prior to the shock. While the fully automated type of AED is easier for the layperson to use, the semi-automated type of AED perceptively provides a greater amount of safety since it never enters the analysis or discharge mode without the operator's direction.

Fortunately, both units have been proven safe and effective to use by a wide variety of laypersons and health care professionals.

Procedure for Defibrillation with an AED

There are numerous AEDs from various manufacturers with a multitude of different options available on each model. For example, a basic unit may just have an audible tone and lights to alert the operator to defibrillate. Other models may have paper strip recorders, an oscilloscope for rhythm interpretation, tape back-up of the cardiac arrest events, voice synthesizer, and more. It is your responsibility to become familiar with the operational steps of the AED used in your service or unit.

Although they vary, the basic steps for use of all AEDs (Figures 6-3a to 6-3f) are:

1. Initiate and maintain CPR until the defibrillator is available.
2. Apply the device to the patient once confirmed to be pulseless.
3. Turn the main power switch on.
4. Apply the self-adhesive monitoring/defibrillation electrodes to the thorax in the standard "anterior-apex" or "anterior-posterior" location.
5. Clear the patient for "hands-off" analysis of the patient's rhythm.

USING A SEMI-AUTOMATED AED

Ideally, at least two practitioners should be present when defibrillation is to be performed with a semi-automated AED—one to operate the AED, the other to perform CPR.

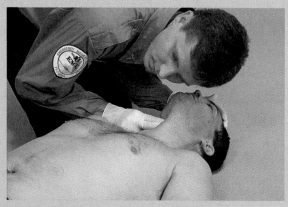

FIGURE 6-3a Conduct primary survey and verify absence of pulse and breathing.

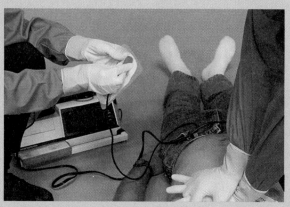

FIGURE 6-3b One practitioner should initiate CPR while the other prepares the AED.

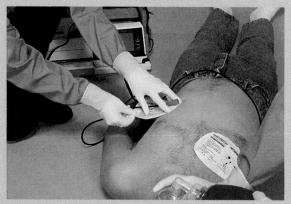

FIGURE 6-3c Place the defibrillator electrodes on the patient's chest.

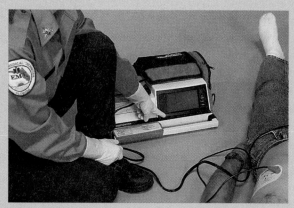

FIGURE 6-3d Turn on the defibrillator and begin narrative.

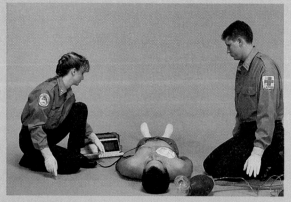

FIGURE 6-3e Stop CPR and get completely clear of the patient as the AED analyzes the rhythm.

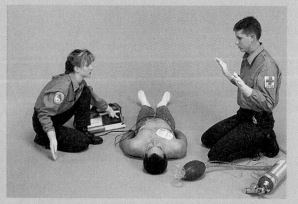

FIGURE 6-3f If a shock is advised, clear all people from the patient and deliver the shock.

6. Initiate analysis of the rhythm.

7. Be sure everyone is clear of the patient and deliver the defibrillation shock, if advised.

Refer to Figure 6-4 for the AED treatment algorithm.

The sequence of defibrillation for an AED is also slightly different than when using a manual defibrillator. With AEDs, after the first stack of three shocks is delivered (200 J, 200–300 J, 360 J), pulselessness should be reconfirmed and CPR instituted for 1 minute. After one minute of CPR, the patient is reanalyzed, and if VF/VT is persisting, another stack of three shocks is delivered (200 J, 200–300 J, 360 J—although the energy levels can be programmed differently). So the overall sequence when using an AED is a stack of three shocks followed by 1 minute of CPR, then another stack of three shocks followed by 1 minute of CPR.

This sequence will continue until the "no shock indicated" message is received.

Coordination of ACLS with AEDs

With the widespread acceptance and use of AEDs by laypersons and initial care providers (e.g., police, fire personnel, EMT-Bs, LPNs), the likelihood of responding to a patient in cardiac arrest with an AED attached is rapidly increasing. To promote a smooth transition from initial care using an AED to the provision of ACLS, the following guidelines are recommended:

- The ACLS provider with the greatest amount of emergency cardiac care education always assumes responsibility as team leader.
- The ACLS providers should ask for a brief summary of the arrest situation and any defibrillations that have been delivered by AED. If the personnel are still completing their stacked countershocks using the AED, the ACLS providers should allow them to proceed with their protocol.
- As long as the AED has a monitoring screen that will allow the ACLS providers to interpret the underlying rhythm, leave the AED device on and use it to deliver any additional defibrillations as appropriate. The personnel familiar with the AED should be allowed to operate the device. However, if the unit has no monitoring screen, the AED should be rapidly removed and replaced with a conventional monitor/defibrillator.
- Factor any defibrillations administered by the AED into your algorithm for the treatment of VF/VT. In other words, if the last defibrillation delivered was at 360 J, any subsequent defibrillations by the ACLS provider should be at 360 J rather than starting back at 200 J. The same applies for the first three stacked defibrillations in the ventricular fibrillation algorithm. There is no need to repeat the stack of three defibrillations (200 J, 200–300 J, 360 J) if they were already delivered using the AED.
- During transport with an AED in place, special considerations must be made. While it is not inherently dangerous to transport a patient attached to an AED, it is required to bring the vehicle to a complete stop before reanalyzing the rhythm. Some services also recommend turning the engine off prior to reanalyzing the rhythm. This is to avoid any rhythm disturbance caused by the moving vehicle. En route, be sure to maintain CPR, airway management, and drug therapy as appropriate.

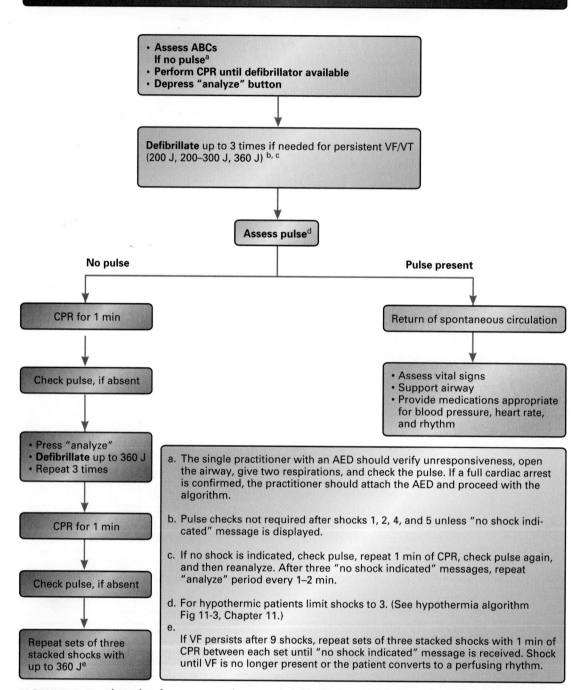

ALGORITHM: AUTOMATED EXTERNAL DEFIBRILLATION (AED)

- Assess ABCs
  If no pulse[a]
- Perform CPR until defibrillator available
- Depress "analyze" button

Defibrillate up to 3 times if needed for persistent VF/VT
(200 J, 200–300 J, 360 J) [b, c]

Assess pulse[d]

No pulse

CPR for 1 min

Check pulse, if absent

- Press "analyze"
- **Defibrillate** up to 360 J
- Repeat 3 times

CPR for 1 min

Check pulse, if absent

Repeat sets of three stacked shocks with up to 360 J[e]

Pulse present

Return of spontaneous circulation

- Assess vital signs
- Support airway
- Provide medications appropriate for blood pressure, heart rate, and rhythm

a. The single practitioner with an AED should verify unresponsiveness, open the airway, give two respirations, and check the pulse. If a full cardiac arrest is confirmed, the practitioner should attach the AED and proceed with the algorithm.

b. Pulse checks not required after shocks 1, 2, 4, and 5 unless "no shock indicated" message is displayed.

c. If no shock is indicated, check pulse, repeat 1 min of CPR, check pulse again, and then reanalyze. After three "no shock indicated" messages, repeat "analyze" period every 1–2 min.

d. For hypothermic patients limit shocks to 3. (See hypothermia algorithm Fig 11-3, Chapter 11.)

e.
If VF persists after 9 shocks, repeat sets of three stacked shocks with 1 min of CPR between each set until "no shock indicated" message is received. Shock until VF is no longer present or the patient converts to a perfusing rhythm.

FIGURE 6-4 Algorithm for automated external defibrillation. Adapted with permission. *Journal of the American Medical Association*, October 28, 1992, Volume 268, No. 16, *Guidelines for Cardiopulmonary Resuscitation and Emergency Cardiac Care.* ©1992 American Medical Association.

- A patient with an AED (or manual defibrillator, for that matter) who has been defibrillated into a perfusing rhythm may refibrillate. In this case, verify pulselessness, immediately resume the analysis mode, and deliver additional defibrillations as necessary.

Emergency Synchronized Cardioversion

As stated in the chapter introduction, there may be certain dysrhythmias in which the unstable patient is decompensating so rapidly that there may not be the luxury of time to wait for a specific drug therapy to exert its action. Or, on occasion, the patient may display a rhythm that is not responsive to routine drug therapy but has the potential to decompensate into a fatal dysrhythmia. It is in these instances that synchronized cardioversion may be the best option available.

Synchronized cardioversion is actually a "controlled" form of defibrillation that is reserved for those patients who still have organized cardiac activity with a pulse. Within the defibrillator, there is a synchronizing circuit that, when activated, will interpret the QRS cycle and deliver the electrical discharge during the "R" wave of the QRS complex. This reduces the likelihood of delivering the cardioversion on the vulnerable period of the QRS cycle, which is known to precipitate ventricular fibrillation. Additionally, synchronizing also permits the use of lower energy levels and reduces the potential for secondary dysrhythmias.

Indications for Synchronized Cardioversion

Synchronized cardioversion is used for tachydysrhythmias that, as discussed above, are unstable or unresponsive to traditional drug therapy. Table 6-2 outlines the indications for synchronized cardioversion.

Procedure for Synchronized Cardioversion

Essentially, the procedure for defibrillation and synchronized cardioversion are the same, with the exception of activating the synchronizing circuit during synchronous cardioversion. As with defibrillation, transthoracic resistance can result in subtherapeutic energy levels reaching the myocardium in synchronized cardioversion. To reduce this problem, take the necessary measures to reduce transthoracic resistance so that you may increase the potential for success in terminating the dysrhythmia.

TABLE 6-2 INDICATIONS FOR SYNCHRONIZED CARDIOVERSION

Tachydysrhythmias necessitating emergency synchronized cardioversion:

- Hemodynamically unstable* ventricular tachycardia with a pulse
- Hemodynamically unstable* supraventricular tachycardia
- Tachydysrhythmias unresponsive to drug therapy

* *Hemodynamically unstable* is defined as a patient presenting with one or more of the following findings:
  - altered mental status
  - severe chest pain
  - hypotension
  - pulmonary edema

FIGURE 6-5 Algorithm for synchronized cardioversion. Adapted with permission. *Journal of the American Medical Association, October 28, 1992, Volume 268, No. 16, Guidelines for Cardiopulmonary Resuscitation and Emergency Cardiac Care*, p. 2224. ©1992 American Medical Association.

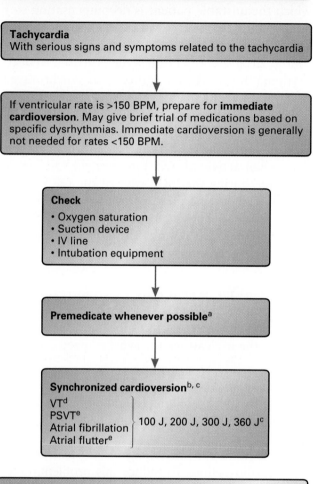

ALGORITHM: ELECTRICAL (SYNCHRONIZED) CARDIOVERSION

Tachycardia
With serious signs and symptoms related to the tachycardia

↓

If ventricular rate is >150 BPM, prepare for **immediate cardioversion**. May give brief trial of medications based on specific dysrhythmias. Immediate cardioversion is generally not needed for rates <150 BPM.

↓

Check
• Oxygen saturation
• Suction device
• IV line
• Intubation equipment

↓

Premedicate whenever possible[a]

↓

Synchronized cardioversion[b, c]

VT[d]
PSVT[e]
Atrial fibrillation   } 100 J, 200 J, 300 J, 360 J[c]
Atrial flutter[e]

---

a. Effective regimens have included a sedative (e.g., **diazepam, midazolam, barbiturates, etomidate, ketamine, methohexital**) with or without an analgesic agent (e.g., **fentanyl, morphine, meperidine**). Many experts recommend anesthesia if service is readily available.

b. Note possible need to resynchronize after each cardioversion.

c. If delays in synchronization occur and clinical conditions are critical, go to immediate unsynchronized shocks.

d. Treat polymorphic VT (irregular form and rate) like VF: 200 J, 200–300 J, 360 J.

e. PSVT and atrial flutter often respond to lower energy levels (start with 50 J).

The following steps are necessary to successfully and safely provide synchronized-cardioversion to a patient:

1. Confirm the symptomatic tachydysrhythmia on the monitor.
2. Place the patient in a safe environment if initially in contact with some electrically conductive material (e.g., water, metal).

3. Time permitting, administer a sedative agent.

4. Apply electrode gel to paddles, or place gel pads on the patient's exposed thorax.

5. Activate the synchronizing circuit by depressing the "synch" button before each cardioversion. Assure proper capture of the QRS complex.

6. Turn on and charge the capacitor to the appropriate energy level.

7. Ensure appropriate placement and pressure of electrodes on the patient's thorax.

8. ENSURE THAT NO ONE IS IN CONTACT WITH THE PATIENT. Verbally and visually clear everybody prior to any cardioversion attempt (including yourself).

9. Deliver synchronized cardioversion by depressing and holding both red buttons on the paddles simultaneously. (Depressing only one will result in no shock being delivered.) You may experience a brief pause while the unit identifies the appropriate moment to discharge. Keep the paddles firmly placed on the chest until the energy is discharged.

10. Reconfirm the rhythm on the monitor screen; if still present, recharge and repeat steps 5 to 7, using higher energy levels.

Refer to Figure 6-5 for the algorithm for synchronized cardioversion.

Special Situations Involving Electrical Therapy

Manual defibrillation, AED defibrillation, and synchronized cardioversion all share the same fundamental principle of operation. The following section discusses specific situations in which the care provider may need to slightly alter the treatment regimen or care for the device in a certain way. While these situations are not that frequently encountered, their importance makes them worthy of mention.

Defibrillation of Hypothermic Patients

Chapter 12 specifically discusses cardiac arrest in a hypothermic patient, but a few points should be mentioned here. A hypothermic heart is more likely to go into ventricular fibrillation from the cold temperature; however, it is much less responsive to defibrillation. The monitor or AED should be applied as usual, and the rhythm analyzed. However, if ventricular fibrillation or pulseless ventricular tachycardia is present and a shock is indicated, provide only the first three defibrillations. If defibrillation is unsuccessful, resume CPR, airway management, and rewarming efforts, and transport the patient to a more advanced medical facility, ideally one with cardiac bypass capabilities. Defibrillation should be continued only after adequate rewarming has been achieved.

AED Use in Pediatric Patients

As mentioned earlier in the chapter, rarely will the health care provider find a pediatric patient in cardiac arrest secondary to ventricular fibrillation. Rather, an infant or child is more likely to be in arrest secondary to hypoxia from a respiratory emergency. Therefore, the emphasis of treatment should be concentrated on correcting the respiratory problem. Additionally, an AED is not capable of the low energy levels required in pediatrics. If however, the patient is over 12 years of age, the AED can be applied and operated as usual.

Defibrillation of Patients with Automatic Implantable Cardioverter/Defibrillator (AICD)

An AICD is, in essence, a mini version of a fully automated AED that is implanted and attached to the heart. AICDs are implanted in persons at high risk for cardiac arrest due to VF or VT. These devices continually analyze the heart rhythm via electrodes attached to the heart and, upon identification of ventricular fibrillation or ventricular tachycardia, they will deliver a specific amount of energy to the heart. With regard to this, you should know the following:

- If the unit discharges while you are in contact with the patient, you may feel the current flow, but it is not dangerous. If the AICD is in the process of shocking a patient, allow it 30 to 60 seconds to complete its treatment cycle.
- If VF or VT is present despite the AICD, external transthoracic defibrillations are still warranted. In these instances, the AICD has either malfunctioned or exhausted its preprogrammed number of countershocks.
- Since the AICD electrodes are attached to the myocardium by patches, the patches may block the conventional defibrillation and reduce the amount of electricity that reaches the myocardium. If you find a patient with an AICD who is in ventricular fibrillation that is unresponsive to defibrillatory shocks at 360 J, consider changing from anterior-apex electrode placement to anterior-posterior placement (or vice versa), and attempt defibrillation again. By doing this, you may avoid the area of the myocardium covered by the AICD patches.

Interruption of CPR

During patient transport, considerable patient-handling and moving may have to take place. It is imperative that there be a concerted effort to avoid unnecessary delays in or interruption of CPR during these movements. As a guideline, CPR should not be interrupted more than 5 seconds at a time. The only exception to this is while the AED is analyzing and charging for each of its stacked shocks. During this time period, not to exceed 90 seconds, the benefits of the AED unit providing defibrillation to a fibrillating heart outweigh the negative effects of temporarily stopping CPR.

Monitor/Defibrillator and AED Maintenance

While the ACLS provider will probably not have the biomedical technical expertise to troubleshoot and repair a broken defibrillator, there are basic maintenance steps that should be completed daily to ensure the unit is operating at peak performance when it is needed. While a specific checklist is provided in AHA's *Advanced Cardiac Life Support* text, and is also available from the device manufacturer, the following highlights the points that should be checked daily.

- No breaks or cracks in the casing or wires
- Paddles are clean, non-pitted, release easily from housing
- Adequate defibrillation supplies are available (batteries, gel, strip paper, and so on)
- Device works properly on AC or battery power
- All indicator lights work
- Paper recorder works (if present)
- Device charges appropriately on AC and battery power

Emergency Cardiac Pacing

Emergency cardiac pacing is a concept that has been around in a variety of forms since the 19th century. However, the "modern age" of cardiac pacing began about 40 years ago, and this therapy has rapidly developed into one of the mainstay treatments for certain bradydysrhythmic and tachydysrhythmic patients over the past 10 years.

Its concept is simple: The heart is a muscle that will contract when stimulated with an electrical impulse. The heart is not particularly interested in where the impulse originated. Therefore, delivering an artificial electrical impulse to a heart that is mechanically capable should result in a contraction and propulsion of blood.

There are actually several different types of cardiac pacemakers; their names reflect the impulse delivery mode. Table 6-3 lists the various types. Of these, the type of pacing used most often in emergency cardiac care is transcutaneous pacing because of its minimal complications, speed of initiation, and effectiveness.

Components of a Cardiac Pacemaker

The first portion of a cardiac pacemaker is the pulse generator. This is the device that initiates the impulse and controls its rate and strength. Its location will either be outside the body or implanted within the body, depending on the type of pacemaker. The impulse created by the cardiac pacemaker then travels through the electrodes. The impulse exits the electrode and enters the

TABLE 6-3   TYPES OF CARDIAC PACEMAKERS

Name	Electrode Location	Pulse Generator Location	Synonyms
Transcutaneous	Skin (anterior chest wall and back)	External	External Noninvasive
Transvenous	Venous (venous catheter with tip in right ventricle or right atrium or both)	External	Temporary transvenous Permanent transvenous
Transthoracic	Through the anterior chest wall into the heart	External	Transmyocardial
Transesophageal	Esophagus	External	
Epicardial	Epicardium (electrodes placed on the surface of the heart during surgery)	External or Internal	
"Permanent"	Venous or epicardial	Internal	Implanted Internal

Reproduced with permission. *Textbook of Advanced Cardiac Life Support*, 1994. ©American Heart Association.

body tissue at the site where the electrode is positioned. Again refer to Table 6-3 to review various electrode locations.

Indications for Emergency Cardiac Pacing

Although there are numerous pathological changes to the conduction system of the heart that may necessitate placement of an internal pacemaker, here we will only be concerned with emergency transcutaneous cardiac pacing. Primarily, emergency cardiac pacing is indicated for those individuals who are decompensating physiologically from poor cardiac output secondary to a slow or absent heart rate. Typically, in these situations, the primary problem is simply the inability of the heart to maintain a sufficient heart rate to sustain normal cardiac output and systolic blood pressure.

Unless there is previous damage to the myocardium, stimulation of the heart to contract with an artificial rate and impulse will increase the cardiac output. Put another way, pacing is most effective in those patients who have a primary rate problem but whose myocardial contractility is effective.

Symptoms of a hemodynamically unstable patient secondary to a rate problem include hypotension (systolic <80 mmHg), pulmonary edema, alterations in mentation, and chest pain. If these signs and symptoms of hypoperfusion are present, emergency cardiac pacing can be considered either prior to drug therapy, or in conjunction with drug therapy, or in bradycardia, which is refractory to traditional drug therapy. As mentioned earlier, transcutaneous pacing is the preferred method for pacing in emergency cardiac care because it can readily be applied, is non-invasive, doesn't interfere with other treatments being rendered, has minimal complications, and is usually effective.

Transcutaneous pacing has also been used in the past to terminate tachydysrhythmias. While not the preferred treatment for rate control (drug therapy still is), by pacing the heart at a faster rate (termed "overdrive" pacing) than the intrinsic tachydysrhythmia, you can achieve "capture" of the rhythm, and then slow down the pacer rate with hopes that the normal conduction system will eventually take over.

Finally, pacing has been shown to have some limited success in capture for patients who have been in asystolic cardiac arrest for less than 10 minutes. However, survival numbers did not change. The problem is that by the time the heart is asystolic, it has suffered prolonged periods of hypoxia and acidosis, which limits the heart's ability to contract. In patients with prolonged periods of asystole (>10 minutes), some studies have indicated no benefit whatsoever to emergency transcutaneous pacing, especially in the out-of-hospital environment.

Transcutaneous Pacing Equipment

Many of the newer cardiac monitor/defibrillators have a built-in cardiac pacing device. This allows the device to be portable enough so that pacing can be conducted at the patient's bedside. While various manufacturers of pacing units offer different features, the following list illustrates basic components of a transcutaneous pacemaker.

- External pulse generator (typically housed within the monitor)
- Cables that connect the pacer to the electrodes on the thorax
- Self-adhesive pacing electrodes, some of which are capable of serving several functions (i.e. cardiac monitoring, pacing, "hands-off" defibrillation)

- Fixed-rate or demand-mode pacing option
- Adjustable amperage control
- Adjustable rate control

Procedure for Transcutaneous Pacing

After you provide oxygenation, ventilation, and intravenous access, you can then ready the patient for transcutaneous pacing.

1. If the patient has excessive body hair that interferes with adhesion of the pads, rapidly shave or clip off hair at points of contact. (Clipping of hair rather than shaving will reduce the likelihood of irritation from small nicks to the skin.)

2. Attach the pacing electrodes to the patient's thorax by placing the anterior electrode to the left of the sternum, as close to the point of maximal impulse as possible (approximately the fifth intercostal space, midclavicular line). Place the posterior electrode directly behind the anterior electrode, lateral to the spine on the left thorax.

3. Set the rate to the desired number, typically 80/min.

4. Set the unit to either the demand or the asynchronous mode. In demand mode, the pacemaker operates whenever the intrinsic heart rate drops below the designated rate; the asynchronous mode delivers pacemaker impulses regardless of the intrinsic rate of the heart. The demand mode is beneficial when performing standby pacing (discussed below).

5. Turn the unit on, and adjust the milliamps (mA):
   - For bradycardia, start at 0 mA, and slowly increase in increments of 5–10 mA until capture occurs.
   - For asystolic hearts, start at maximal mA, and decrease mA if capture is achieved.

6. Assess for capture two ways:
   - First, look for the characteristically wide QRS following the pacer spike (Figure 6-6).
   - Assess the carotid pulse to see if the artificial rhythm is producing a pulse.

7. Continue pacing at an mA level about 10% higher than needed minimally for capture.

8. Consider an analgesic or sedative for possible pain should the patient be responsive.

9. Monitor vitals and level of consciousness, and constantly assure capture.

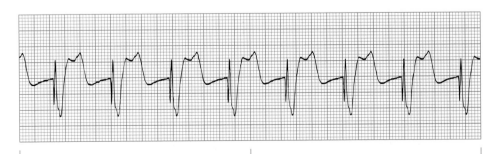

FIGURE 6-6 Normal capturing pacer rhythm.

If the unit fails to capture (Figure 6-7), the failure may be related to electrode placement or the characteristics of the patient's thorax. Be sure that you are using as many methods as possible to reduce transthoracic resistance.

Standby Pacing

Standby pacing is indicated for the patient who is hemodynamically stable but is displaying a bradydysrhythmic rate with the potential for rapid deterioration. Table 6-4 lists those rhythms requiring emergency cardiac pacing and those rhythms needing standby pacing in case the patient deteriorates before the dysrhythmia can be eliminated. By setting up the pacer and momentarily switching it on to assure capture, you will be ready to immediately institute transcutaneous pacing should the patient suddenly decompensate (become symptomatic) while emergency care is being rendered. As preparation, you should become familiar with the asystole and bradycardia algorithms, Figures 10-4 and 10-5, in Chapter 10.

Complications of Transcutaneous Pacing

The most common complication of transcutaneous pacing is pain. Fortunately, with more current revisions in pacing technology, the discomfort created by pacing is usually tolerable. If not tolerable, then it may be controllable by administration of analgesics.

Two other complications are failure to recognize if the pacemaker spike is capturing, and failure to recognize ventricular fibrillation due to the influence of the pacer spikes. These two problems can be eliminated if the monitoring is done with a special filtration process that will allow the care provider to accurately assess the underlying rhythm.

Ventricular fibrillation is a potential complication once pacing is instituted, but it is probably rare since the energy level necessary to disrupt the conduction system is greater than the energy delivered by the pacing device. Be cautious, however; that potential does exist.

Contraindications to Transcutaneous Pacing

As discussed earlier, asystolic cardiac arrest is not ordinarily responsive to external transcutaneous pacing. For this reason, it is considered to be a relative contraindication. If, during the cardiac arrest management, there are adequate personnel to apply the pacer while CPR, intubation, IV access, and drug therapy are being done concurrently, then it may be attempted. However, do not withhold these interventions in the asystolic patient in an attempt to pace the heart.

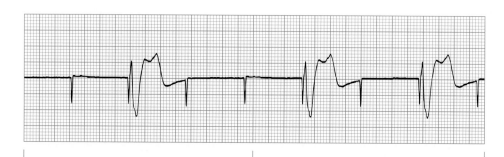

FIGURE 6-7 Abnormal pacer function: loss of capture.

TABLE 6-4 INDICATIONS FOR EMERGENCY PACING AND PACING READINESS

Emergency Pacing

Hemodynamically compromising bradycardias* (Class I)
(Blood pressure <80 mmHg systolic, change in mental status, angina, pulmonary edema)

Bradycardia with escape rhythms (Class IIa)
(Unresponsive to pharmacologic therapy)

Overdrive pacing of refractory tachycardia (Class IIb)
Supraventricular or ventricular
(Currently indicated only in special situations refractory to pharmacological therapy or electrical cardioversion)

Bradyasystolic cardiac arrest (Class IIb)
Pacing not routinely recommended in such patients. If used at all, pacing should be used as early as possible after onset of arrest.

Pacing Readiness

Anticipatory pacing readiness in setting of acute myocardial infarction (Class I)

- Symptomatic sinus node dysfunction
- Mobitz type II second-degree heart block†
- Third-degree heart block†
- Newly acquired left, right, or alternating bundle branch block or bifascicular block

* Including complete heart block, symptomatic second-degree heart block, symptomatic sick sinus syndrome, drug-induced bradycardias (i.e. digoxin, β blockers, calcium channel blockers, procainamide), permanent pacemaker failure, idioventricular bradycardias, symptomatic atrial fibrillation with slow ventricular response, refractory bradycardia during resuscitation of hypovolemic shock, and brady-dysrhythmias with malignant ventricular escape mechanisms.

† In patients with an inferior myocardial infarction, relatively asymptomatic second- or third-degree heart block can occur. Pacing in such patients should be based on symptoms or deteriorating bradycardia.

Reproduced with permission. *Textbook of Advanced Cardiac Life Support*, 1994. ©American Heart Association.

Hypothermia causes diminished responsiveness of the myocardium to the pacing impulse as with the defibrillation stimuli discussed earlier. Remember also that bradycardia is thought to be a protective function as the general metabolic activity decreases in hypothermia. Management of hypothermic patients is aimed toward rewarming and ensuring adequate ventilation. Since the heart becomes unstable due to hypothermia, the irritation caused by the pacing impulse could result in ventricular fibrillation.

Pediatric bradycardia results from hypoxia and hypoventilation and responds favorably when the hypoventilation is corrected with oxygenation and adequate alveolar ventilation. Therefore, initial management of bradycardia in pediatric patients is aimed at reversing the hypoxia. Only when the bradycardia exists within known congenital defects, drug overdose, or recent heart surgery should external pacing be considered.

Other Pacing Techniques

Several other methods are available to achieve emergency cardiac pacing in the symptomatic patient. These methods include transvenous pacing, transmyocardial transthoracic pacing, transesophageal pacing, and epicardial pacing, as listed in Table 6-3. The first three have been shown to be beneficial in specific situations; however, transcutaneous pacing should be performed until these methods are implemented. The last method (epicardial pacing) is performed under direct visualization of the heart during open chest surgery, so it is not a viable option in the vast majority of emergency-care instances.

CASE STUDY FOLLOW-UP

Assessment

During your initial assessment of Mr. Griffiths, your impression is of a middle-aged male experiencing a cardiac emergency. In addition to the vitals you obtained (blood pressure 102/62, heart rate 220 and regular, respiratory rate 36 with slight retractions), you also hear fine inspiratory crackles upon lung auscultation. You recall that extremely tachycardic rates can diminish cardiac output and drop coronary artery perfusion—both of these contributing to the chest pain.

You reassure Mr. Griffiths as you administer high-flow oxygen.

Treatment

Since Mr. Griffiths is dyspneic and has chest pain, you elect to administer 100% oxygen via a nonrebreather face mask and apply the pulse oximeter. You turn to roll the heart monitor tray closer while you ask your coworker to initiate an IV.

While monitoring Lead II, you identify an extremely rapid narrow-complex rate. Currently, there are no P waves distinguishable from the T waves, but the QRS complex is narrow and regular at 220/min. Since you consider Mr. Griffiths to be an unstable patient in supraventricular tachycardia, you ask your coworker to administer 6 mg of adenosine while you retrieve the defibrillation paddles. At this point, Mr. Griffith's orientation is diminishing and his respiratory distress is increasing. You call for the on-call physician, stat!

With no effect from the adenosine, you elect to administer a synchronized countershock at 100 joules. You place the gel pads in the anterior apex position on the thorax, apply about 25 lbs. of pressure to the paddles, and charge the unit. While assuring that the synchronizing circuit is activated, and after being sure everyone else is clear, you cardiovert the patient during exhalation.

With no success from the initial cardioversion, you rapidly administer a subsequent synchronized countershock at 200 joules. After this countershock, Mr. Griffiths becomes apneic and pulseless. Ventricular fibrillation is identified on the monitor.

You charge the paddles to 200 joules and deliver an asynchronous countershock to the patient. With no change in the rhythm, you complete the "stacked three" shocks by administering asynchronous defibrillations at 300 joules, then 360 joules. CPR is initiated, the airway is intubated, and 1 mg epinephrine is administered.

Approximately 2 minutes later, ventricular fibrillation persists on the monitor. You again defibrillate at 360 joules, and fortunately this converts the patient into a third-degree block with a pulse and low blood pressure. The external pacer is applied and it captures, causing both the rate and the systolic pressure to increase.

As you prepare Mr. Griffiths for movement to CCU and wipe the sweat off *your* face, the on-call physician walks in and says, ". . . So, is everything under control here?"

SUMMARY

Within this chapter we have covered diverse medical interventions necessary to emergency cardiac care. However diverse the methods discussed, the common thread is that they all utilize electricity therapeutically to eliminate a dysrhythmia.

A fundamental understanding of defibrillation, synchronized cardioversion, AED use, and external pacing allows the health care provider to appropriately and safely use these interventions in the symptomatic patient.

However beneficial these therapies are when used appropriately, they can certainly be fatal if used inappropriately. It is the responsibility of the health care provider, then, to be thoroughly familiar with the indications for and proper uses of these therapies. It is equally important to stay abreast of the changes and developments in the usage of electrical therapy in emergency cardiac care.

REVIEW QUESTIONS

1. Defibrillation is used to manage
   a. life-threatening bradydysrhythmias.
   b. asystolic dysrhythmia.
   c. ventricular fibrillation.
   d. chronic atrial fibrillation.
   e. c and d are both correct

2. Which of the following scenarios will most likely result in immediately successful cardioversion?
   a. applying the electrical therapy 25 minutes after onset of symptoms
   b. cardioverting after epinephrine and/or other drugs have been administered
   c. timing the cardioversion with the end-expiration phase of ventilations
   d. utilizing synchronous cardioversion for a patient in VF

3. Which of the following statements about asynchronous cardioversion is true?
   a. It is also known as defibrillation.
   b. It is the preferred method to terminate symptomatic tachydysrhythmias.
   c. The initial energy level is 50-100 joules.
   d. It does not require the use of gel pads or electrode paste.
   e. It is never used in pediatric patients.

4. Defibrillating an asystolic heart may
   a. initiate spontaneous rhythms.
   b. make the heart more susceptible to the effects of the IV drugs.
   c. be performed only after assuring the heart is in asystole in two leads.
   d. inhibit the natural pacemakers of the heart.

5. Which of the following energy dose regimes is correct for defibrillation?
   a. 50–100 joules, 200 joules, 360 joules
   b. 100 joules, 200 joules, 300 joules, 360 joules
   c. 200 joules, 200–300 joules, 360 joules
   d. 50–100 joules, 200 joules, 300 joules, 360 joules

6. AEDs are used for
   a. cardiac arrest victims in VF.
   b. cardiac arrest victims in asystole.
   c. cardiac arrest victims over 1 hour away from the hospital.
   d. cardiac arrest victims suffering from severe trauma only.

7. The difference between the countershocks delivered by the AED and those administered manually is:
   a. The AED repeatedly delivers "stacked shocks" of three, whereas manually they are delivered only one at a time.
   b. The AED uses lower energy levels than manual defibrillators.
   c. The AED uses higher energy levels than manual defibrillators.
   d. The AED is not as effective as manual defibrillation.

8. Synchronized cardioversion delivers the countershock
   a. during expiration.
   b. during the R wave of the cardiac cycle.
   c. during the T wave of the cardiac cycle.
   d. immediately upon depressing the discharge buttons of the paddles.

9. The greatest benefit of using synchronous versus asynchronous countershocks for an unstable patient in supraventricular tachycardia is
   a. lowest possible chance for causing VF.
   b. faster delivery of energy.
   c. lower risk of damage to the myocardium.
   d. a and c are correct.
   e. a, b, and c are correct.

10. Which of the following findings would indicate a hemodynamically unstable patient in ventricular tachycardia with a pulse?
    a. extreme diaphoresis   d. cyanosis
    b. chest pain   e. tachycardia
    c. mild respiratory distress

11. You have just delivered a synchronous cardioversion at 300 joules, and the patient goes into VF. You should immediately
    a. resume CPR.   d. administer epinephrine.
    b. defibrillate at 200 joules. e. administer lidocaine.
    c. intubate the trachea.

12. AED utilization for pediatric patients less than age 12 is acceptable.
    a. true
    b. false

13. It is inappropriate to defibrillate a patient with an AICD.
    a. true
    b. false

14. External cardiac pacing is the preferred treatment for
    a. bradycardia.   d. ventricular fibrillation.
    b. asystole.   e. a and b are correct
    c. tachycardia.

15. How do you confirm that the external pacemaker is "capturing"?
   a.   Assess for a QRS complex after the pacer spike.
   b.   Palpable pulse in conjunction with the pacemaker.
   c.   The presence of a blood pressure.
   d.   The patient will complain of pain or discomfort.
   e.   a and b are correct

Chapter**Seven**

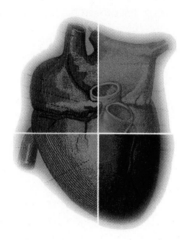

Pharmacological Therapy

In conjunction with proper oxygenation, ventilation, compressions, and defibrillation, pharmacological therapy is an integral component of successful cardiac arrest management. Additionally, caring for patients experiencing any one of many non-arrest cardiovascular emergencies will certainly include the administration of cardioactive drugs. This chapter will provide an introduction to the drugs that are most commonly used during advanced cardiac life support.

Topics to be covered are:

Cardiovascular Pharmacology

Part One: Oxygen
Part Two: Sympathomimetics
Part Three: Sympatholytics
Part Four: Antidysrhythmics
Part Five: Analgesics and Antianginal Agents
Part Six: Diuretics
Part Seven: Antihypertensives
Part Eight: Thrombolytics
Part Nine: Other Cardiovascular Drugs

Note: An index to the drugs discussed in this chapter appears on page 169.

CASE STUDY

One night you are relaxing at home after a hard day's work. And, as on every other Tuesday night, you find yourself in front of the TV so you can watch your favorite program from 9:00 to 10:00 PM. This show, which you never miss, is titled *Code Blue, Stat!*. It is a show about the heroic efforts of health care providers in a hospital emergency department as they do battle with cardiovascular disease, trauma, and death on a daily basis. Your interest in the show stems from your knowledge of emergency care—and your curiosity about the appropriateness of their treatment.

This week's program immediately catches your attention, since the first patient is a middle-aged man with chest pain and bradycardia—almost the identical presentation to the man you treated just a few hours ago at work. You lean back in your recliner and say to the TV screen, "OK, folks, impress me."

The TV character, Mr. Hedger, has arrived at the hospital because of severe chest pain, diaphoresis, and dizziness. As the TV nurses put him on the cot, the first-year ER resident applies the pulse oximeter and monitor. The TV screen flashes a saturation of 91% with a sinus brady-dysrhythmic rate. Appropriately, the doctor orders oxygen administration and the initiation of an IV of 0.9% sodium chloride.

How would you proceed to assess and care for this patient? This chapter will describe the assessment and pharmacologic treatment of patients experiencing a cardiovascular emergency. Later, we will return to the case and apply the procedures learned.

Introduction: Cardiovascular Pharmacology

Pharmacological therapy is an integral part of advanced cardiac life support, and the health care provider must become completely familiar with the most common drugs used. Admittedly, this is not an easy task, nor one of the most pleasant portions of this text to read, but it is a necessity for optimal patient outcome. The need is obvious: Quality patient care depends on the health care provider, who is therefore obligated to learn and stay abreast of current medications and their dosages.

What you must *not* do is allow yourself to become complacent and rely on charts or pocket references to guide your drug therapy during patient management. Books and charts cannot interpret the special circumstances that are part of every cardiac emergency, nor can they offer all the differential approaches to drug therapy that may be required. Proper management of the patient will only occur when the care provider understands the pathophysiology behind the patient's condition, understands the physiological actions of drugs, and can then apply this knowledge to provide the appropriate pharmacological care for the patient.

To aid the learning process, the authors of this text have made every effort to present the information about each drug in a logical, easy-to-read format. However, it will take an investment of time on your part to comprehend and apply the information. One word of advice: Do not try to simply "memorize" the indications, side effects, and contraindications. Information learned by rote memory is likely to be lost from lack of use or as a result of stress during an emergency. Rather, by learning and understanding *how a drug works*, its indications, side effects, and contraindications become obvious. Thus, the only thing left to memorize is the specific drug dose—*and there is no shortcut to memorizing drug doses.*

Take the time necessary to become familiar with the drugs discussed in this chapter. They are integral to successful resuscitation, and any one of them has the potential to help, or harm, the patient.

Organization of This Chapter
The drugs in this chapter are arranged in nine categories (chapter parts) according to their common actions and indications. This classification is designed to help you comprehend the information.

However, you will note that certain drugs found in one category may also have indications in another category (for example, oxygen or lidocaine). Also be aware that while a given drug may have numerous applications (for example, the use of epinephrine in cardiac arrest or anaphylaxis), *only the indications in cardiovascular care will be discussed here.* It is the authors' contention that arranging the drugs in these categories and keeping the information specific to cardiac emergencies will help you grasp how these drugs apply in advanced cardiac life support.

As a further aid to comprehension, the information about each drug is presented in a consistent format. First you will read about the drug's *action*, followed by the *indications, side effects/precautions, contraindications,* and finally *dosage.*

On page 169 is an index of the drugs discussed in this chapter to aid you in finding and reviewing the information for any specific drug.

PART ONE: OXYGEN

Oxygen is one of the most important and most-often-administered drugs for the patient experiencing a cardiovascular crisis. Oxygen is an essential requirement for the body to maintain its metabolic activities. Since any cardiovascular crisis can result in inadequate oxygenation at the cellular level, you must be acutely aware of the need to initiate oxygen therapy or to increase the amount and concentration of oxygen already being administered.

OXYGEN

Oxygen: Mechanism of Action
Oxygen is a colorless and odorless gas that is necessary for life. Oxygen rapidly diffuses across the alveolar walls and binds to hemoglobin in the red blood cells. After hemoglobin saturation, the blood circulates the oxygen throughout the body, and it is taken into the cells where it promotes the breakdown of glucose into adenosine triphosphate (ATP), a usable energy substance. (This process is known as *aerobic* metabolism, meaning metabolism that occurs in the presence of oxygen.) Without oxygen, glucose is broken down improperly, resulting in the development of lactic acidosis. (This process is known as *anaerobic* metabolism, or metabolism that occurs in the absence of oxygen.)

Oxygen: Indications
Oxygen is indicated whenever there is known or suspected hypoxia, regardless of the etiology. Therefore, oxygen should be administered to any patient with

INDEX BY CATEGORIES

Oxygen, 168

Sympathomimetics
epinephrine, 171
norepinephrine, 174
isoproterenol, 176
dopamine, 177
dobutamine, 179
amrinone, 180

Sympatholytics
beta blockers, 182

Antidysrhythmics
Rhythm Control
lidocaine, 184
procainamide, 187
bretylium tosylate, 189
magnesium sulfate, 191
Rate Control
atropine sulfate, 192
adenosine, 196
calcium channel blockers: verapamil
and diltiazem, 197
digitalis glycosides, 200

Other Drugs for Rate Control
dopamine, 202
epinephrine, 202
isoproterenol, 202

Analgesics and Antianginal Agents
morphine sulfate, 203
nitroglycerin, 205

Diuretics
furosemide, 206

Antihypertensives
sodium nitroprusside, 207
Other Antihypertensive Drugs
beta blockers, 208
nitroglycerin, 208

Thrombolytics
anistreplase, 210
alteplase, 210
streptokinase, 211
urokinase, 211

Other Cardiovascular Drugs
sodium bicarbonate, 211
calcium chloride, 213

ALPHABETICAL INDEX

adenosine, 196
amrinone, 180
anistreplase, 210
atenolol, 183
alteplase, 210
atropine sulfate, 192
beta blockers, 182, 208
bretylium tosylate, 189
calcium channel blockers, 197
calcium chloride, 213
digitalis glycosides, 200
diltiazem, 197
dobutamine, 179
dopamine, 177, 202
epinephrine, 171, 202
esmolol, 183

furosemide, 206
isoproterenol, 176, 202
lidocaine, 184
magnesium sulfate, 191
metoprolol, 183
morphine sulfate, 203
nitroglycerin, 205, 208
norepinephrine, 174
oxygen, 168
procainamide, 187
propanolol, 183
sodium bicarbonate, 211
sodium nitroprusside, 207
streptokinase, 211
urokinase, 211
verapamil, 197

chest pain, a medical emergency, a traumatic or surgical emergency, respiratory distress, or in any instance where you believe that the patient is or has the potential to become hypoxic.

Oxygen: Side Effects/Precautions

The major precaution with administering high concentrations of oxygen is to ensure that there is sufficient gas available to meet the patient's inspiratory volume.

There is some concern that patients with chronic obstructive pulmonary disease (COPD) may experience depressed ventilations with the administration of high flow oxygen. (COPD patients' respiration tends to be regulated by a "hypoxic drive"—in which respiration is stimulated by the brain's perception of a low oxygen level, rather than by a high CO_2 level, as in normal patients. Therefore, there is concern that the COPD patient will react to the administration of oxygen with depressed respiratory effort.) However, even high flow oxygen to these patients will not have a clinically significant effect on ventilatory effort during the brief time it is used during acute cardiopulmonary resuscitation.

Additionally, there is a fear that neonates may suffer retinal damage from high flow oxygen; but again, this is not a concern in the acute situation in view of the short period of time that oxygen will be administered.

Oxygen toxicity, as a side effect, usually does not occur until a patient has spent days on high flow oxygen and ventilatory support. But the emergency patient may complain of nasal irritation from drying the mucosa or may experience epistaxis (a nose bleed) if non-humidified oxygen is administered for a long period of time.

Oxygen: Contraindications

In the emergency setting, there are no contraindications to the use of oxygen. Additionally, despite the known side effects and precautions, OXYGEN SHOULD NEVER BE WITHHELD FROM ANY PATIENT KNOWN (OR SUSPECTED) TO BE HYPOXIC.

Oxygen: Dosage

There is no concern about overdosing with oxygen. It can be administered relatively liberally.

The general guidelines about administration of oxygen during the initial phase of an emergency are as follows: Administer oxygen in the highest concentration available. The means by which the oxygen will be administered should be based upon the patient's clinical condition and ventilatory status. (Review the Chapter 3 discussion of oxygenation devices.) Eventually, as pulse oximetry and capnography indicate proper oxygenation and normal levels of expired CO_2, administration of oxygen may be decreased.

Arterial blood gases (ABGs) may also guide administration of oxygen, but be cautious about contemplating an arterial puncture for a patient who may receive thrombolytic drug therapy, because of the potential for uncontrollable bleeding at the site. (See the discussion of thrombolytics later in this chapter.).

PART TWO: SYMPATHOMIMETICS

By definition, a *sympathomimetic* is a substance that "mimics" the actions of the sympathetic nervous system. As such, these drugs either directly stimulate the adrenergic receptors of the sympathetic nerve fibers, or indirectly stimulate the sympathetic nervous system by causing certain hormones (catecholamines) to be released within the body (Figure 7-1). These agents may either be naturally occurring in the body (endogenous), or synthetically derived.

The final result of either mechanism is an increase in sympathetic tone. (Recall that the autonomic nervous system has two divisions: the sympathetic and the parasympathetic. The sympathetic nervous system is responsible for the excited effects of the "fight or flight" response. The parasympathetic system tends to have opposite, calming effects. See Figure 7-2.)

Administered sympathomimetics have effects that are similar to the actions of the sympathetic nervous system. Two common effects of sympathomimetic drugs are *positive inotropic effects* (increasing the heart's contractile force) and *positive chronotropic effects* (increasing the heart rate).

EPINEPHRINE

Epinephrine: Mechanism of Action

Epinephrine is an endogenous catecholamine. This means it is a hormone that is normally produced, secreted, and utilized by the body. A catecholamine is a substance that acts on the autonomic nervous system. Administered epinephrine has effects that result from stimulation of the sympathetic nervous system.

Epinephrine (known casually as *epi*) achieves its therapeutic benefits by stimulating the alpha and beta adrenergic receptor sites of the autonomic nervous system. (If these concepts are unfamiliar to you, any physiology text should explain them in detail. Understanding how the autonomic nervous system, hormones, and alpha and beta adrenergic receptors work is integral to an appreciation of the complex actions of epinephrine.) By stimulating the

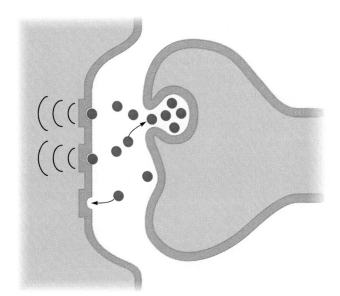

FIGURE 7-1 Activity at nerve synapses (spaces) of the sympathetic nervous system. Catecholamines are released from pre-synaptic nerve endings, travel across the synapse, and stimulate receptors on the post-synaptic nerves. Subsequently, the catecholamines are either deactivated by enzymes in the synapse or taken up by the pre-synaptic nerve.

FIGURE 7-2 Organization of the nervous system. Many drugs stimulate or mimic actions of the sympathetic or parasympathetic nervous system.

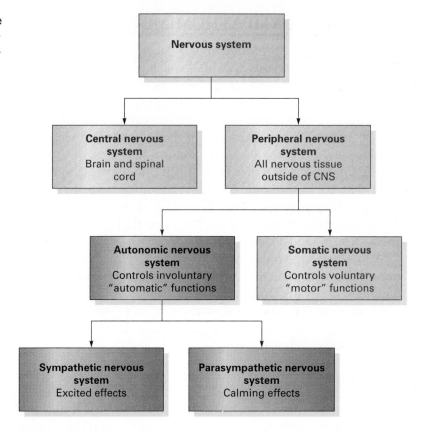

beta 1 and beta 2 receptor sites, epinephrine increases the activity of the heart and causes dilation of the bronchioles. By stimulating alpha receptor sites, epinephrine increases vascular tone, which helps increase blood pressure. The cardiac effects of epinephrine are summarized below.

Cardiac Effects of Epinephrine

- Increased heart rate (positive chronotropic effect)
- Increased contraction strength (positive inotropic effect)
- Increased conduction velocity
- Increased arterial tone (i.e., vascular resistance)
- Increased blood pressure
- Increased coronary and cerebral perfusion during CPR
- Increased electrical activity in the heart
- Increased myocardial oxygen demand

In the cardiac emergency setting, the alpha properties are the chief reason for the use of epinephrine: Because it increases vascular tone, it will selectively increase blood flow to the heart and brain during compressions. But its beta effects are also beneficial, since it may initiate electrical activity in a heart that has none. In addition, epinephrine is also thought to increase the coarseness of ventricular fibrillation.

A final important consideration is that epinephrine normally degrades rapidly in the body. For this reason, it is necessary to administer epinephrine to the patient at continuous short intervals to keep the blood levels in a therapeutic range.

Epinephrine: Indications

Epinephrine is indicated in any patient who requires extensive cardiopulmonary resuscitation. And since the alpha properties are so desirable, it is the first drug (after oxygen) that is administered to every patient in complete cardiac arrest—regardless of the underlying rhythm causing the arrest.

Epinephrine: Side Effects/Precautions

As mentioned in the beginning of this chapter, when you understand how a drug works, you can also understand the potential side effects and/or precautions. If you bear in mind the strong alpha and beta effects of epinephrine, it will be obvious why the side effects are those that are typical of strong sympathetic stimulation. The awake patient may demonstrate palpitations, tremors, anxiety, headache, dizziness, even nausea and vomiting. More severely, the patient may complain of chest pain if the sympathetic effects of epinephrine increase myocardial oxygen demands beyond the ability of the coronary arteries to supply oxygenated blood. There are few side effects from epinephrine in the cardiac arrest patient. The post-arrest patient may experience hypertension and tachycardia.

Epinephrine, like other catecholamines, can be deactivated if mixed with an alkaline solution. Thus, do not mix epinephrine with drugs like sodium bicarbonate. Also be aware of other medications the patient is taking or receiving. For example, if the patient takes an antidepressant, the effects of epinephrine may be intensified by the synergistic actions of the two drugs.

Since epinephrine increases the work load of the heart it may precipitate additional cardiac dysrhythmias and/or ischemia. Be prepared to manage these emergencies if they should occur.

Epinephrine: Contraindications

Since the administration of epinephrine is mainly reserved for the patient with severe cardiovascular instability, there are no real contraindications in the emergency setting when it is administered via intravenous bolus. Be aware, however, that epinephrine may also be given via infusion, and with that mode of administration there are additional considerations.

Epinephrine: Dosages

There is a very important delineation to make here: Parenteral epinephrine is commonly packaged in two strengths, each containing the same amount of drug. The 1:10,000 concentration has one milligram of epinephrine in 10 ml of solution in a prefilled syringe. This is the common packaging for intravenous use. Epinephrine also comes packaged as a 1:1,000 ampule, which is one milligram of drug in 1 ml of solution. Obviously then, the latter packaging has the same dose but is more concentrated (1 mg in 1,000 parts of water versus 1 mg in 10,000 parts of water.)

The 1:1,000 ampule form gives the care provider the ability to administer the same amount of drug with less fluid, or high amounts of the drug with relatively small amounts of fluid. For example, if you were to administer 10 mg of epinephrine using the 1:1,000 concentration, you would administer a total of 10 ml of fluid. Administering the same dose of epinephrine with 1:10,000 would mean administering 100 ml of fluid. As stated above, 1:10,000 is the common strength for intravenous administration. Epinephrine 1:1,000 is more commonly used for administration by endotracheal tube when higher dosages are given and when additional fluid may be undesirable.

As mentioned earlier, there are enzymes in the body that constantly degrade epinephrine and decrease its effects. For this reason, epinephrine boluses must be repeated frequently. Increased dosages of the drug are used with repeat administrations, because current research indicates that "high-dose" epinephrine may have beneficial effects in cardiac arrest.

The following list identifies the dosing regimen of epinephrine in cardiac arrest. Please note when the different concentrations are applicable.

Cardiac Arrest

- 1 mg every 3–5 minutes intravenous push, or endotracheal instillation using 1:10,000 concentration. Consider higher doses of epinephrine if several attempts of the traditional dose fail. This is administered according to one of the following schedules:

  - escalating: 1, 3, 5 mg 3–5 minutes apart
  - intermediate: 2–5 mg 3–5 minutes apart
  - high dose: 0.1 mg/kg 3–5 minutes apart

When administering the drug via IV push, follow the dose with a 20 cc flush and raise the arm to speed venous return to the core circulation. If doses are administered via the endotracheal route, use 2–2.5 times the normal IV dose. A 1:1,000 concentration should be used, diluting the dose to 10 cc prior to administration. If possible, use the endotracheal route only when no IV is available and only until a patent IV is established.

Symptomatic Bradycardia

- 1 µg/min titrated to the desired hemodynamic response (2 to 10 µg/min).

NOREPINEPHRINE

Norepinephrine: Mechanism of Action
Norepinephrine is an endogenous catecholamine similar to epinephrine. Norepinephrine is a potent vasoconstrictor (arterial and venous) that achieves this effect by profoundly stimulating the alpha receptors of the sympathetic nervous system. Norepinephrine also exhibits some stimulation of the beta receptors and may, therefore, increase the heart rate and contractility of the myocardium. However, such stimulation is slight and is not considered the primary action of norepinephrine.

Norepinephrine: Indications
Norepinephrine is indicated in hypoperfusion states that are refractory to other means of stabilization. As a result of norepinephrine's ability to promote arterial and venous vasoconstriction, norepinephrine facilitates a desirable increase in blood pressure. Norepinephrine is considered in cases of cardiogenic shock or hypotension that does not respond to other agents such as dopamine or fluid challenges.

Norepinephrine: Side Effects and Precautions
It is paramount to monitor the blood pressure throughout administration of norepinephrine (every 5 to 10 minutes) so as to prevent a dangerous

hypertensive state. In the case of hypertension, the norepinephrine should be titrated down to a dosage that results in a more desirable blood pressure.

Norepinephrine stimulates the sympathetic nervous system. Side effects include nervousness, anxiety, tremors, headache, dizziness, nausea, and vomiting.

Through a complex chemical reaction, norepinephrine is deactivated when mixed in any alkaline solution. The alkaline solution most commonly used in ACLS is sodium bicarbonate. Be careful to avoid mixing norepinephrine with sodium bicarbonate.

Conversely, the effects of norepinephrine can be potentiated when administered with other drugs that promote similar action. For example, a dangerous state of hypertension can be induced when delivering norepinephrine concomitantly with beta blockers. Recall that blocking the beta receptors located on the arterial blood vessels will cause vasoconstriction and increase blood pressure. As norepinephrine accomplishes the same effect through a different mechanism, administration of both agents can prove devastating.

Norepinephrine predominantly stimulates the alpha receptors, but some beta receptor stimulation may occur. While this is not the primary mechanism of action, it may promote an increased myocardial workload. Consequently, it is prudent to administer supplemental oxygen with norepinephrine to counteract any myocardial ischemia that might result from an increase in heart rate and contractility. Similarly, dysrhythmias may also occur and should be addressed on an individual basis.

Norepinephrine: Contraindications

As discussed under "Indications," norepinephrine is a *late* intervention used in the treatment of hypoperfusion. This means that more appropriate, less invasive means of treating hypotension should be attempted prior to the administration of norepinephrine. Norepinephrine is never used in the long-term treatment of hypoperfusion.

Volume depletion should be addressed with volume replacement. Decreased vascular tone is first treated by the administration of dopamine rather than norepinephrine. If these interventions fail, norepinephrine can then be tried. Some authorities allow for the use of norepinephrine in cases of volume-related hypotension, but only as a temporary measure until adequate volume replacement is achieved.

Norepinephrine: Dosage

Norepinephrine is delivered by intravenous infusion. Norepinephrine may cause tissue necrosis (tissue death) and should be administered into the largest vein possible so as to avoid infiltration.

Norepinephrine should be given within the dose range of 0.5–30 µg/kg per minute. Mixing 1 mg of norepinephrine in 250 cc of D_5W yields a concentration of 16 µg/cc. Initially, norepinephrine should be initiated at 0.5–1.0 µg/kg per minute. From this beginning point, the dosage can be titrated upwards to the desired effect.

If more than 20–30 µg/kg per minute are needed, using dopamine with norepinephrine is permissible. A mechanical infusion pump should be used to achieve precise delivery of norepinephrine.

ISOPROTERENOL

Isoproterenol: Mechanism of Action

Although falling from favor in current ACLS recommendations, isoproterenol is a sympathetic agonist used in the treatment of bradycardic emergencies. As a synthetic catecholamine, isoproterenol primarily stimulates the beta 1 and beta 2 receptors of the sympathetic nervous system.

When stimulated, beta 1 receptors produce an overall increase in the rate and contractile strength of the heart. In response, cardiac output increases and improved perfusion should ensue. Isoproterenol also affects the beta 2 receptors located in the bronchiole and vascular smooth muscle. Stimulation of the beta 2 receptors promotes vasodilation and relaxation of the pulmonary bronchioles. Characteristically, this permits more oxygen to flow through the pulmonary tree. The increase in cardiac output is usually enough to offset the slight drop in vascular resistance that results from the peripheral vasodilation.

In the treatment of bradycardic emergencies, isoproterenol has generally been replaced by more reliable agents with fewer negative side effects. Such agents include atropine, dopamine, dobutamine, amrinone, and transcutaneous pacing.

Isoproterenol: Indications

After other interventions prove ineffective, isoproterenol should be used in the temporary treatment of hemodynamically significant bradycardia. Direct stimulation of the cardiac beta 1 receptors will increase the rate and stroke volume of the heart and facilitate a greater cardiac output.

Isoproterenol has shown some promise in the treatment of bradycardia as it pertains to the transplanted heart. A problem with transplanted hearts is a relative lack of innervation from the autonomic nervous system. In this situation, giving a drug that will directly stimulate the heart rather than stimulating the autonomic nervous system may be beneficial. Also as a result of its direct stimulatory properties, isoproterenol may be effective in the stabilization of bradycardia that occurs secondary to a more serious heart block. However, it must be emphasized that other interventions have proven more reliable and must be tried prior to the administration of isoproterenol.

Isoproterenol: Side Effects/Precautions

Any drug that increases the workload of the heart also increases the heart's oxygen demands. Isoproterenol is no different. By increasing rate and contractility, isoproterenol causes the heart to require more oxygen to function. If oxygen is not available, myocardial ischemia can present itself. For this reason, be cautious about administering isoproterenol to anyone with ischemic heart disease, in whom it is prone to promote dysrhythmias. Also, isoproterenol can lead to the loss of potassium resulting in hypokalemia. If profound, this electrolyte disturbance can manifest itself with dysrhythmias. This is most likely to occur with protracted use of the drug in the non-acute setting. Therefore, when isoproterenol is delivered, the electrical rhythm of the heart must be monitored. Should a dysrhythmia develop, deal with it by reducing the dosage of isoproterenol and administering the appropriate drug therapy.

As stated above, beta 2 stimulation can cause vasodilation and drop blood pressure. A drop in blood pressure leads to a decrease in coronary artery perfusion. Hence, there is an increased possibility of cardiac arrest. Consequently, it is paramount to remain vigilant to blood pressure when isoproterenol is used.

Isoproterenol: Contraindications

As with any bradycardia, the slow rhythm should never be treated pharmacologically unless it is hemodynamically significant. Treat the patient, not the monitor! Additionally, isoproterenol should *never* be used as a *first-line* intervention in the treatment of hemodynamically significant bradycardia. Newer agents and interventions with fewer negative side effects than isoproterenol have proven more effective in the treatment and stabilization of bradycardic emergencies.

Isoproterenol: Dosage

Isoproterenol is administered as an IV infusion and is constituted by mixing 1 mg of the drug in 250 cc of D_5W. This mixture yields a concentration of 4 µg/cc and should be delivered through a microdrop administration device.

Isoproterenol should be administered within the range of 2–10 µg/minute. The higher the dosage, the greater opportunity for adverse side effects. Therefore, the administered dosage should be titrated to the lowest possible amount that achieves the desired hemodynamic effect. Often, this equates to a heart rate of approximately 60 beats per minute or a blood pressure of >90 mmHg. As with other infusions, administration of isoproterenol must be precise and requires an infusion pump for exact delivery.

DOPAMINE

Dopamine: Mechanism of Action

Dopamine is a naturally occurring catecholamine that is a chemical precursor to norepinephrine. Dopamine stimulates the sympathetic nervous system by interacting with the dopaminergic, alpha, and beta 1 receptor sites. By doing so, dopamine promotes vasoconstriction and increased myocardial contractility without producing tremendous increases in the heart rate. The net result is an increase in blood pressure without straining the heart by significantly raising its rate. In addition, dopamine promotes perfusion of the kidneys and abdominal organs through stimulation of dopaminergic receptors. Because of these properties, dopamine is the most commonly used agent in symptomatic states of hypoperfusion.

Dopamine: Indications

The etiology of hypoperfusion (<90 mmHg) must always be considered prior to treatment. If hypovolemia exists due to fluid depletion, volume replacement should be attempted first. If the hypotension exists secondary to bradycardia, the first attempts must address correcting the slow rhythm so as to establish an acceptable cardiac output and blood pressure (>90 mmHg). If hypoperfusion is the result of decreased myocardial contractility or loss of vascular tone or does not respond to the previous measures, then a dopamine infusion should be started.

In addition, dopamine should be administered for residual hypotension following the return of spontaneous circulation post cardiac arrest.

Dopamine: Side Effects/Precautions
Side effects with dopamine depend on the dose. (See the detailed discussion of dosages below.) At moderate to high dosages, cardiac dysrhythmias may occur. The drug should be used cautiously if there are preexisting tachydysrhythmias. Dysrhythmias or an acceleration of the heart rate will increase oxygen demand and, with an already-impaired heart, myocardial ischemia becomes an issue. It may be necessary to increase the inspired concentration of oxygen (FiO_2) in this setting.

Since dopamine directly stimulates the sympathetic nervous system, many side effects related to the sympathetic nervous system may become evident. These include:

- Nervousness
- Headaches
- Palpitations
- Chest pain
- Dyspnea
- Nausea/vomiting

Also, because it causes vasoconstriction, dopamine can worsen pulmonary congestion. As the heart is presented with a greater preload and afterload, it may not be able to eject all the blood. Consequently, an increase in hydrostatic pressure in the pulmonary vessels may increase the difficulty in breathing.

Dopamine can cause adverse reactions when administered with some other medications. Dopamine and Dilantin®, when used simultaneously, can cause acute hypertension. When administering dopamine with a monoamine oxidase (MAO) inhibitor, a type of antidepressant, administer one-tenth the normal dose of dopamine. Furthermore, as with norepinephrine, dopamine is chemically inactivated when combined with an alkaline substance such as sodium bicarbonate. When discontinuing a dopamine infusion (as with any vasoactive infusion), gradually taper off the administration so as to avoid acute hypotension.

Dopamine: Contraindications
In symptomatic hypotension, dopamine is always contraindicated before an attempt has been made to correct the underlying abnormality. However, if an attempt has been made and proven ineffective, dopamine should be considered.

Dopamine is relatively contradicted in the presence of symptomatic hypotension with pulmonary congestion. In such situations the fear is that, as mentioned above, dopamine will worsen pulmonary congestion and inhibit the exchange of oxygen and carbon dioxide at the alveolar-capillary interface. However, this must be weighed against the benefits of improved myocardial contractility. As a practical matter, dopamine is often used in patients with pulmonary edema. Carefully think through the effects of dopamine and, if it is applicable, use the drug at the lowest possible dose that proves effective.

Dopamine: Dosages
Dopamine is administered through an IV infusion within the range of 2–20 µg/kg/minute. As stated earlier, the effects that dopamine produce are extremely dose-dependent. Simplistically, dopamine dosages can be broken down into the following ranges:

- *2–5 µg/kg/minute: Renal dose*—At this dosage, dopamine stimulates dopaminergic receptors in the kidneys and abdomen. Subsequently, arteries in these regions dilate and increase the perfusion of the kidneys and abdominal organs. At this dosage, renal output can be greatly increased.
- *5–10 µg/kg/minute: Cardiac dose*—Dopamine administered at this level predominantly interacts with the cardiac beta receptors. The net effects are an observable increase in contractility with a slight increase in heart rate. Through an increase in cardiac output, blood pressure is also increased. In addition, some stimulation of alpha receptors occurs, causing some vasoconstriction. This action enhances an increase in blood pressure.
- *10–20 µg/kg/minute: Vasopressor dose*—At this higher dose of dopamine, alpha receptors are primarily stimulated. In response, there is an overwhelming constriction of the arterial and venous vasculature amounting to an increase in blood pressure.

To prepare an infusion, mix 800 mg of dopamine in 500 cc of D_5W. This mixture yields a concentration of 1600 µg/cc, which should be titrated to the lowest possible dose that achieves the desired effect. At dosages greater than 20 µg/kg/minute, norepinephrine can be added to the dopamine for an increased effect. Because dopamine is so dose dependent, an infusion pump should be used for precise delivery.

DOBUTAMINE

Dobutamine: Mechanism of Action

Dobutamine is another drug used in the treatment of hypotension and low cardiac output. Similar to dopamine, dobutamine stimulates the sympathetic nervous system. However, unlike dopamine, dobutamine is a synthetic agent that primarily stimulates the beta 1 receptors located within the myocardium and beta 2 receptors located on the smooth muscle of the bronchioles and peripheral blood vessels.

While dobutamine does stimulate the alpha receptors also found on the myocardium and peripheral blood vessels, this stimulation is insignificant when compared with the beta stimulation that predominates. For this reason, dobutamine produces a greater myocardial contraction with a mild vasodilatory response. Consequently, the heart's work load is eased as increased contractility is balanced by a reduced afterload.

Dobutamine will characteristically induce production of endogenous norepinephrine as the dose increases. When released, the norepinephrine stimulates the sympathetic nervous system in a profound manner. For this reason, at higher dosages, dobutamine may produce an accelerated heart rate and increased peripheral resistance. An accelerated response can strain the myocardium and increase its oxygen demands. Therefore, be cognizant of the need for constant monitoring and supplemental oxygen.

Dobutamine: Indications

The ability of dobutamine to increase contractility while dilating the peripheral vascular system makes dobutamine an ideal choice for patients who have pulmonary congestion with symptomatic hypotension. In this situation, dobutamine serves to increase the cardiac output while ejecting blood through a lower resistance in the vascular system. The dilated vascular system also serves as a reservoir. Consequently, blood is shifted from the pulmonary vessels into the peripheral vascular system.

For similar reasons, dobutamine finds application in the short-term management of patients with congestive heart failure (CHF) or those with left ventricular failure who are unable to tolerate potent vasodilators.

Dobutamine: Side Effects/Precautions

As previously mentioned, dobutamine at higher dosages may produce tachy-dysrhythmias. A faster heart rate demands more oxygen and, if additional oxygen is not readily available, myocardial ischemia can occur. Additionally, high-dose dobutamine has been known to induce nervousness, hypertension, chest pain, and nausea and vomiting.

Dobutamine: Contraindications

Similar to norepinephrine and dopamine, dobutamine is not indicated in the treatment of symptomatic hypotension until after other treatments have been executed that are geared directly toward correcting the underlying abnormality. And even when volume replacement or correction of a slow heart rate have proven ineffective at increasing cardiac output, dopamine is more reliable and therefore preferred over dobutamine in the stabilization of hypoperfusion.

Dobutamine: Dosage

While possibly being effective at lower doses, the standard dose range for this drug is 2–20 μg/kg/minute. And, as with other vasoactive infusions, the smallest dose possible to maintain desired hemodynamic effects should be administered. When possible, limit the increase in heart rate to only 10% over initial values if the patient has a history of coronary artery disease.

To prepare the infusion, mix 500–1000 mg of dobutamine into 250 ml of D_5W or normal saline. As with other infusions, a volumetric infusion pump should be used to assure a precise and consistent administration of the drug.

Amrinone

Amrinone: Mechanism of Action

Amrinone is a positive inotropic agent. In addition, amrinone has vasodilatory properties that serve to decrease myocardial workload by reducing the resistance against which the heart must pump. As a result of the increased contractility and decreased resistance, the heart is able to eject more blood with each contraction. Amrinone is particularly helpful in improving myocardial output when there is fluid in the pulmonary vessels and lung fields.

Amrinone: Indications

In light of its actions, amrinone is a drug considered in the treatment of congestive heart failure that has proven refractory to other and usually more reliable means of intervention. Such interventions would include vasodilators, diuretics, and other inotropic agents like dobutamine. After such interventions prove ineffective, amrinone can be administered in the short-term management of CHF or severe left ventricular dysfunction.

Amrinone: Side Effects/Precautions

Because of its propensity to increase contractile strength, amrinone increases myocardial oxygen demand and may precipitate myocardial ischemia. Therefore, the lowest possible dose of amrinone must be used, and constant monitoring of the heart and its hemodynamic effects must be undertaken.

In addition, higher doses of amrinone have been shown to decrease the number of circulating platelets. Decreased platelets can precipitate hemorrhage, which must be considered when treating a patient with a history of bleeding or platelet disorders. Furthermore, general (noncardiovascular) side effects that can be expected with amrinone include muscular pain, fever, and liver dysfunction.

Amrinone: Contraindications

Amrinone contains bisulfate, a sulfuric acid salt. Therefore, anyone with a declared sensitivity to sulfa compounds must *not* receive this drug! Also, amrinone is not indicated as a first-line agent in the emergent treatment of acute CHF or left ventricular failure. Vasodilators and diuretics often achieve better results than does amrinone.

Amrinone: Dosage

Amrinone is administered as an IV infusion. Because of chemical incompatibility, amrinone must *never* be mixed in a dextrose-containing solution such as D_5W! Rather, normal saline of 0.9% or 0.45% is preferred.

Amrinone is administered as a loading dose followed by an infusion. The loading dose can be administered in either of two ways, depending on the urgency of the situation. Generally, a therapeutic level and desired inotropic effect are quickly achieved by administering the loading dose of 0.75–1.0 mg/kg over 10–15 minutes. In an extremely urgent situation, the same dosage can be administered more rapidly, over 2–5 minutes.

To maintain the serum levels, an infusion should be established within the range of 2–5 µg/kg/minute, increased as needed to a level of 10–15 µg/kg/minute. The dose should be titrated to patient response with the lowest possible dose utilized, as side effects become more prevalent at higher levels. As with other infusions, an infusion pump is necessary to deliver precise levels of the medication.

PART THREE: SYMPATHOLYTICS

The suffix -*lytic*, commonly means to block or inhibit. So when combined with the root word *sympatho*-, the literal meaning is to block the effects of the sympathetic nervous system. Sympatholytics are a unique class of drug which does not exert a specific physiologic action itself; rather it merely inhibits the effects of the catecholamines by occupying the alpha or beta receptor sites of the sympathetic nervous system. This "antagonistic" effect may be exerted on both alpha and beta receptors, on alpha receptors only, or on beta receptors only. The drugs discussed next are known as "beta blockers"; that is, they are sympatholytics that specifically antagonize the beta receptor sites of the sympathetic nervous system.

BETA BLOCKERS

Beta Blockers: Mechanism of Action

Beta blockers antagonize and block the stimulation of the beta receptors. This decreases the heart rate, myocardial contractility, and blood pressure and also decreases the overall workload and oxygen consumption of the myocardium.

Beta blockers also reduce electrical conduction through the AV node and are thus useful in controlling ventricular responses to detrimental atrial rhythms. In addition, since many dysrhythmias occur in response to increased sympathetic activity, beta blockers help prevent the occurrence of such dysrhythmias by blocking the uptake of sympathomimetic catecholamines.

Beta Blockers: Indications

Beta blockers are used in the control of recurrent ventricular fibrillation, ventricular tachycardia, or PSVTs. In that these disturbances are often related to the circulation of endogenous catecholamines, the blockage of beta receptors can prevent the occurrence of such dysrhythmias.

Beta blockers are also useful in the long term treatment of a myocardial infarction. As stated above, beta blockers decrease the overall workload and oxygen consumption of the heart. Because an infarction occurs secondary to a mismatch between myocardial oxygen supplies and demands, beta blockers are quite effective in the reduction of mortality following an MI.

Beta Blockers: Side Effects/Precautions

Beta blockers can have adverse effects. If the heart rate and contractility are decreased excessively by these agents, hypotension and pulmonary congestion can ensue.

Also recall that there are beta receptors on the bronchiole smooth muscle. Inhibiting stimulation of these receptors can precipitate serious bronchospasm. Therefore, you must be aware of any history of asthma, COPD, or congestive heart failure when you contemplate using beta blockers for cardiac situations. As with many other drugs, the effects of beta blockers can be potentiated when combined with drugs of a similar nature.

Beta Blockers: Contraindications

Beta blockers are contraindicated in situations where beta receptor stimulation is necessary for normal function. Such situations would include:

- Preexisting bradycardia
- History of asthma
- History of COPD
- Congestive heart failure

Blocking the beta receptors may worsen the above situations and cause detrimental complications.

Beta Blockers: Dosages

There are several different types of beta blockers commonly used in modern medicine. The routes of administration and dosages vary. Some of the more common beta blockers, and their dosages, include:

Atenolol

- *IV administration*—5 mg IV push over 5 minutes. If the patient requires it, another 5 mg over 5 minutes can be given 10 minutes later.
- *Oral administration*—10 minutes after the second IV dose, assuming adequate patient toleration, an oral dosage of 50 mg twice a day can be implemented.

Metoprolol

- *IV administration*—5 mg IV push over 2–5 minutes. The drug can be readministered twice at 5-minute intervals for a total dose of 15 mg.
- *Oral administration*—Following the IV administration, the patient should take an oral dose of 50 mg twice a day, increased to 100 mg twice a day after 24 hours.

Propanolol

- *IV administration*—1–3 mg IV push over 2–5 minutes. This dose should be repeated after 2 minutes to a total dose of 0.1 mg/kg.
- *Oral administration*—The oral follow-up should range between 180–320 mg/day and be given in divided dosages.

Esmolol

Esmolol, a rapidly acting beta blocker with a relatively short duration, is administered via an IV infusion. After the drug has achieved the desired result, it can be titrated and eventually eliminated. As an IV infusion, it must be prepared with a final concentration of 10 mg/ml. This is best accomplished by placing 2.5 grams of the drug (one 10-ml ampule), into a 250 ml bag of D_5W. The general administration procedure is as follows:

- *IV administration*— loading infusion of 250–500 µg/kg over one minute. Follow with a maintenance infusion at 25–50 µk/kg/min over the next 4 minutes. Titrate the maintenance infusion up by 25–50 µg/kg/min at 5–10-minute intervals to a maximum of 300 µg/kg/min as clinically indicated.

PART FOUR: ANTIDYSRHYTHMICS

Antidysrhythmics is the general classification for those drugs that help to correct disturbances in the heart's electrical activity. First, they may be used to eliminate cardiac conduction disturbances that interfere with the heart's normal rhythm (i.e., rhythm control). Secondly, they may be used to correct some abnormality in the heart's rate if it becomes too fast or too slow (i.e., rate control). Under "Rhythm Control" and "Rate Control," you will find a series of agents that may or may not exert a similar action, but have a common physiologic result.

FIGURE 7-3 Conduction through ischemic myocardial tissue. White areas are islands of tissue that are severely depressed and no longer excitable. Gray areas surrounding these islands are also depressed but still excitable. They conduct electrical impulses at reduced velocities. In (A), before lidocaine administration, the electrical impulse, though conducted at reduced velocity, is able to continue through the ischemic area and re-emerge into the normal myocardial tissue. In (B), lidocaine has been administered and has further depressed conduction velocity to the extent that the electrical impulse is blocked and unable to re-emerge into normal myocardial tissue.

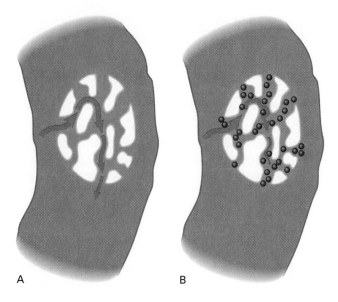

A   B

Rhythm Control

LIDOCAINE

Lidocaine: Mechanism of Action

Of the drugs available, lidocaine is probably the most commonly used ventricular antidysrhythmic drug administered to patients with ventricular irritability. Ventricular irritability is evident by the fr
premature ventricular contractions or independent ventricular rhythms on the ECG tracing.

Lidocaine exerts numerous actions to achieve its antidysrhythmic effects. It depresses the conduction velocity through ischemic tissue and depresses the increased automaticity seen with ischemic tissue. These effects can inhibit ventricular rhythms by blocking the conduction wave in areas of ischemia (so it can't re-emerge to excite surrounding tissue) as depicted in Figure 7-3, and it can eliminate ventricular rhythms caused by changes in automaticity of ischemic tissue by depressing phase 4 of spontaneous depolarization as shown in Figure 7-4.

Lidocaine also raises the ventricular fibrillation threshold, thus making it harder for the heart to go into ventricular fibrillation. This is analogous to raising a dam against water flow. As the dam gets higher (raising the threshold), it blocks the water from overflowing; as lidocaine increases the threshold, V-fib is less likely to occur. Finally, lidocaine has little effect

FIGURE 7-4 Phase 4 cardiac depolarization. (A), before lidocaine administration, shows normal phase 4 depolarization. (B), after lidocaine administration, shows depressed phase 4 depolarization.

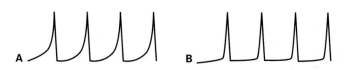

A   B

on atrial tissue, nor on SA and AV node function, at therapeutic doses. As such, lidocaine does not harm atrial or AV activity when used for ventricular irritability, nor is it useful for atrial dysrhythmias.

Lidocaine: Indications

As mentioned above, lidocaine is the drug of choice for ventricular irritability in need of suppression. PVCs can be a normal consequence of degeneration in the conduction system as a person ages. However, there are also numerous acute causes of PVCs which must be corrected so that the PVCs do not interrupt the normal conduction of the heart. The following list identifies the appropriate uses for lidocaine:

- Suppression of malignant PVCs
  - \>6 unifocal PVCs/minute
  - multifocal PVCs
  - couplet PVCs
  - R on T phenomena
- Ventricular tachycardia (with and without a pulse)
- Ventricular fibrillation

Since ventricular irritability is typically the result of some other cause (e.g., hypoxia, MI, rate disturbances, drug), often lidocaine is not administered until after treatment has been instituted to correct the underlying etiology. This will be explained in more detail under "Dosage," below.

Lidocaine: Side Effects/Precautions

Side effects become more evident as the amount of drug administered increases. At therapeutic doses, lidocaine has minimal side effects of concern. However, at greater dosages lidocaine toxicity manifests itself, primarily in the central nervous system (CNS). The patient may display:

- Drowsiness
- Irritability
- Disorientation
- Muscle twitching
- Seizures
- Coma (including death)

Precaution should be taken when administering lidocaine to a patient who may have depressed liver function. Regardless of the cause of the dysfunction (e.g., age over 70 years, hepatic disease, hypoperfusion, acute MI), there will be a delay in clearing the lidocaine from the body. This will result in serum levels increasing to toxic levels should the drug be administered continually. In this instance, the maintenance infusion of lidocaine should be reduced by 50%. The loading dose remains the same, since the body still requires that amount of drug to achieve initial therapeutic levels.

Exercise caution as well with the administration of lidocaine concurrently with procainamide, phenytoin, quinidine, and beta blockers.

Lidocaine: Contraindications

Lidocaine is contraindicated in second degree Type II and third degree (infranodal) heart blocks. Many times there is a ventricular rhythm in conjunction with these conduction blocks. It is important for the health care provider to realize that these contractions (albeit abnormally wide) are the only perfusing beat the patient has! If they are abolished by lidocaine, the patient may well go into cardiac arrest. This is also true for ventricular escape rhythms.

The same applies for extreme bradycardia with frequent PVCs. The PVCs may be the body's attempt to maintain cardiac output in the face of the bradycardic rhythm, and abolishing them with lidocaine will worsen the cardiac output. Always remember to treat the rate first with atropine and pacing, then take care of the ventricular rhythms if they persist with a heart rate >60/minute.

Lidocaine: Dosages

As mentioned under "Indications," there are numerous instances when lidocaine can be administered. It is important to remember that the drug is initially given and repeated as an IV bolus until the ventricular abnormality is corrected. Only after the abnormality is suppressed should a maintenance infusion be initiated. Since lidocaine undergoes hepatic degradation, a constant infusion is necessary to maintain therapeutic blood levels, but only after the boluses achieve the desired effect. The following outlines the administration of lidocaine by IV bolus or via an endotracheal tube to a symptomatic patient with ventricular irritability:

Suppression of Malignant PVCs (IV Loading Bolus)

- Administer 1.5 mg/kg IVP or ETT (increase ETT dose 2–2.5 times). Repeat every 5–10 minutes at half the initial dose (0.5–0.75 mg/kg). Follow this dosing schedule until 3 mg/kg total cumulative dose has been administered.

Ventricular Tachycardia with a Pulse (Stable and Unstable)

- Administer 1.5 mg/kg IVP or ETT (increase ETT dose 2–2.5 times). Repeat every 5–10 minutes at half the initial dose (0.5–0.75 mg/kg). Follow this dosing schedule until 3 mg/kg total cumulative dose has been administered.

Ventricular Fibrillation and Pulseless Ventricular Tachycardia

- Administer 1.0–1.5 mg/kg IVP or ETT (increase ETT dose 2–2.5 times). Repeat every 3–5 minutes at the same dose. Follow this dosing schedule until 3 mg/kg total cumulative dose has been administered.

As you have probably noticed, lidocaine administration varies, depending on the hemodynamic status of the patient. Allow the following guidelines to help you simplify the administration of lidocaine when appropriate:

If the Patient Has a Pulse

- Give 1.0–1.5 mg/kg, repeat at 0.5–0.75 mg/kg every 5–10 minutes to maximum of 3 mg/kg.

If the Patient Does Not Have a Pulse

- Give 1.5 mg/kg, repeat once at same dose after 3–5 minutes.

After the IV bolus(es) of lidocaine have achieved the desired effect, and the patient has a relatively stable rhythm and hemodynamic status, it

TABLE 7-1 LIDOCAINE IV ADMINISTRATION

Amount Given IV Bolus	Infusion Rate	Drops per Minute
1.0 mg/kg	2 mg/min	30
1.5–2.0 mg/kg	3 mg/min	45
2.25–3.0 mg/kg	4 mg/min	60

becomes necessary to institute a maintenance infusion of lidocaine to keep the blood serum levels in an acceptable range. You should start by mixing 2 grams of lidocaine into 500 ml of D_5W to yield a 4 mg/ml concentration. Premixed lidocaine is also available, typically packaged as 2 grams in 500 ml of D_5W. This should be administered with a microdrip infusion set at 2–4 mg/min, based upon the total amount of lidocaine given via IV push, as shown in Table 7-1.

PROCAINAMIDE

Procainamide: Mechanism of Action

Procainamide is yet another ventricular antidysrhythmic drug useful in the suppression of ventricular irritability. Somewhat like lidocaine, it achieves its desired action by depressing phase 4 of the depolarization sequence, which will slow automaticity. In addition, procainamide can depress the slope of phase 0 of cardiac depolarization, which will naturally slow conduction velocity and possibly block an impulse in an already slowed ischemic tissue, which avoids reentry dysrhythmias. As will be discussed shortly, depression of phase 0 may also result in a negative inotropic effect.

In summary, procainamide can reduce ventricular irritability by slowing automaticity and/or conduction velocity.

Procainamide: Indications

Procainamide is another drug in the arsenal for combating ventricular dysrhythmias. However, due to its mechanism of action, it may precipitate additional undesirable side effects. Also, it is administered as an infusion, so it may take longer to exert an action compared to the IV bolus of lidocaine. As such, it is not preferred as an antidysrhythmic drug over lidocaine. But as a general rule, procainamide is a drug that can be considered for ventricular problems after the administration of lidocaine has failed to control the problem. The following list identifies ventricular problems that procainamide may be useful for when lidocaine is unsuccessful:

- Persistent malignant PVCs
- Persistent ventricular tachycardia with a pulse
- Persistent ventricular fibrillation/pulseless ventricular tachycardia
- May be considered for supraventricular dysrhythmias (due to its ability to slow conduction velocity by depressing phase 0)

Procainamide: Side Effects/Precautions

One of the most significant side effects of procainamide is its negative inotropic effect, which results from depression of phase 0 of depolarization. This slowing of conduction speed has the tendency to also weaken the contraction force, which results in reduced ejection from the ventricles and possibly hypotension. (Hypotension is exacerbated by the fact that procainamide also has a vasodilatory effect.) If hypotension ensues, the procainamide infusion should be eliminated.

Additionally, the depressive effects of procainamide on the cardiac conduction system may result in a widening of the QRS complex. (As phase 0 is flattened, the QRS will be widened and the force of contraction weakened.) Therefore, during procainamide administration, the QRS, PR, and QT intervals should be monitored for widening. If any interval widens by >50% from its pretreatment width, the procainamide infusion should be stopped.

Procainamide: Contraindications

As with lidocaine, procainamide should not be used if the ventricular dysrhythmia exists with bradycardia. In these instances, the slow rate should be normalized by atropine and pacing first. Additionally, since procainamide has the ability to slow conduction speed, its use in a patient with a conduction disturbance (e.g., second degree Type II or third degree block) should be avoided. As well, preexisting hypotension should be a reason to avoid procainamide.

Procainamide: Dosage

Procainamide is administered via infusion, unlike lidocaine which is given as an IV bolus. This typically results in a slower onset of action for procainamide; effects should be seen in about 15 minutes. When treating a patient with ventricular dysrhythmias refractory to lidocaine and other appropriate treatment, a procainamide loading infusion should be initiated at 20–30 mg/min until a maximum dose of 17 mg/kg is achieved. The following outlines a simple approach to procainamide administration:

1. Compute the total amount of drug allowed (multiply the patient's weight in kilograms by 17).
2. Add that amount of drug to a small amount of D_5W (50–100 ml). This places the maximum amount of drug into the D_5W. The benefit is that once the bag is empty you know the maximum dose has been administered.
3. Compute the math for administering the drug at 20–30 mg/min.
4. Stop the loading infusion when one of the following occurs:
   - Maximum dose is achieved (17 mg/kg—or bag is emptied).
   - Ventricular dysrhythmia is abolished.
   - QRS, QT, or PR interval widens by 50% of pretreatment width.
   - Hypotension ensues.

Assuming the rhythm is abolished by the procainamide loading infusion, a maintenance infusion needs to be initiated to maintain therapeutic blood levels. This is achieved the same as lidocaine's maintenance infusion was: 2 grams of procainamide can be mixed into 500 ml of D_5W to yield 4 mg/ml. This is then attached to a microdrip administration set and infused at 1–4 mg/min (15–60 drops/minute) to maintain suppression of the ventricular dysrhythmia. An alternative mixing is 1 gram of procainamide into 500 ml D$_5$W, to yield 2 mg/ml. With the latter mixing, the infusion would need to run at 30–120 drops/min to achieve 1–4 mg/min. Never should the loading infusion and the maintenance infusion be running at the same time.

BRETYLIUM TOSYLATE

Bretylium Tosylate: Mechanism of Action

Bretylium is the third ventricular antidysrhythmic drug used in the management of ventricular abnormalities. Like procainamide, bretylium exerts its ventricular suppressive action somewhat differently than lidocaine. It can be used as an alternative drug when lidocaine is unsuccessful in converting a ventricular dysrhythmia.

Bretylium has been described as exerting a "biphasic" response in the myocardium. Bretylium works initially (in its first phase) by promoting the release of the adrenergic neurotransmitter norepinephrine into the synaptic cleft of the post-ganglionic nerve endings of the myocardium. Subsequently, when the norepinephrine has been depleted, bretylium (in its second phase) blocks the uptake of norepinephrine, which then results in adrenergic blockade—thus its desired effects. The adrenergic blockade results in prolongation of the action potential of *normal* tissue. Since *ischemic* and *infarcted* tissue already have a prolongation of the action potential, bretylium's effects may equalize the two, resulting in a suppression of the reentry phenomenon (Figure 7-5). Bretylium is also thought to have other depressive effects on the myocardium, not yet fully understood.

The biphasic response of bretylium usually follows a characteristic sequence. Initially, due to the release of norepinephrine, there is a sympathomimetic response with an increase in heart rate, blood pressure, and cardiac output. This phase lasts about 15–20 minutes. Subsequently, with inhibition of norepinephrine, adrenergic blockade prevails with possible hypotension (particularly orthostatic hypotension). Adrenergic blockade begins about 20 minutes after the drug is administered, peaks at about 45 minutes, and lasts several hours (Figure 7-6).

Bretylium Tosylate: Indications

Presently, bretylium is not considered to be a first line antidysrhythmic for ventricular abnormalities, since it is no more effective than lidocaine and has side effects not seen with lidocaine. However, its actions may be beneficial in those patients whose ventricular abnormality is unresponsive to oxygen and lidocaine, and occasionally to electrical therapy and procainamide. The following list identifies those rhythms in which bretylium may prove beneficial:

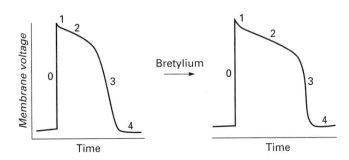

FIGURE 7-5 Bretylium acts to prolong the action potential in normal tissue, thus tending to prevent reentry from ischemic or infarcted tissue. (Left) Normal Purkinje fiber potential before bretylium administration. (Right) Normal Purkinje fiber potential after bretylium administration.

FIGURE 7-6 The biphasic effects of bretylium. In the first phase, bretylium stimulates release of the catecholamine norepinephrine from pre-synaptic nerve endings. The norepinephrine stimulates receptors on the post-synaptic nerves, causing a sympathomimetic response. However, the bretylium blocks the normal subsequent taking up of the norepinephrine by the pre-synaptic nerves, causing second-phase adrenergic blockade with possible hypotension.

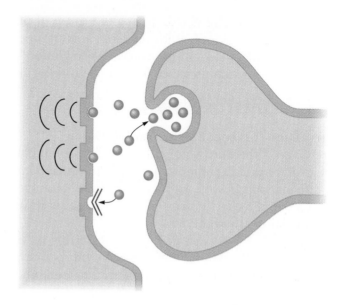

- Persistent malignant PVCs
- Persistent ventricular tachycardia with a pulse
- Persistent ventricular fibrillation/pulseless ventricular tachycardia

Bretylium Tosylate: Side Effects/Precautions

The side effects of bretylium are consistent with the drug's biphasic action. The initial side effects are a response to the first-phase sympathomimetic actions of bretylium. (Ensure that the patient is well oxygenated in view of the anticipated increase in myocardial workload during this norepinephrine depletion phase.) Subsequently, hypotension and orthostatic hypotension are commonly reported as the second-phase adrenergic blocking effect prevails. Additionally, nausea and vomiting are commonly reported in the conscious patient receiving bretylium. Other side effects may include dizziness, seizures, and angina.

Care should be exercised when administering bretylium to the patient also receiving digitalis, since the sympathomimetic phase of bretylium will potentiate digitalis toxicity. As well, other sympathomimetic drugs administered in conjunction with bretylium may have an enhanced or prolonged effect since the adrenergic blocking action of bretylium may allow the other drugs to accumulate in the synaptic cleft.

Bretylium Tosylate: Contraindications

There are no real contraindications to the use of bretylium in the emergency setting with a patient suffering from myocardial compromise. Remember that it is administered not as a first line agent but rather in cases with refractory rhythms. However, the aforementioned side effects and precautions should always be kept in mind when you consider administering bretylium.

Bretylium Tosylate: Dosages

Depending on the patient's status and the presenting dysrhythmia, the dose and method of bretylium administration may change. The differing approaches to administering bretylium are important to remember since they minimize the potential side effects. The following outlines the administration of bretylium:

Malignant PVC Suppression

- Administer 5–10 mg/kg of bretylium by diluting the dose into 50 ml of D_5W and administering it by slow IVP over 8–10 minutes. Faster injection will lead to nausea, vomiting, and hypotension. Repeat at 10 mg/kg after 10–30 minutes, and thereafter every 6–8 hours if necessary.

Refractory Ventricular Tachycardia with a Pulse

- Administer 5–10 mg/kg of bretylium by diluting the dose into 50 ml of D_5W and administering it by slow IVP over 8–10 minutes. Faster injection will lead to nausea, vomiting, and hypotension. Repeat at 5–10 mg/kg after 10–30 minutes, and thereafter every 6–8 hours if necessary.

Ventricular Fibrillation/Pulseless Ventricular Tachycardia

- Administer a 5 mg/kg dose via rapid IV push. Repeat in 5 minutes at 10 mg/kg rapid IV push. Any subsequent doses are at 10 mg/kg every 5–30 minutes until 35 mg/kg is achieved. Defibrillation and epinephrine should be administered concurrently with the bretylium administrations.

MAGNESIUM SULFATE

Magnesium Sulfate: Mechanism of Action

Magnesium is an important component of numerous biochemical activities within the body. It is integral to the normal functioning of the sodium-potassium pump which, among other things, helps maintain cellular wall stability. Magnesium has also been identified as a "physiological" calcium channel blocker and a blocker of normal neuromuscular nerve transmission. Finally, it plays a role in the movement of potassium across the cellular wall during cellular depolarization.

Magnesium Sulfate: Indications

Research has shown that some patients with a deficiency in magnesium may also suffer from certain cardiac abnormalities. Hypomagnesemia has been associated with life-threatening cardiac emergencies such as ventricular fibrillation, ventricular tachycardia, torsades de pointes, cardiac insufficiency, and sudden cardiac death. As mentioned earlier, these problems have been observed in patients with low levels of magnesium; therefore, its replacement by IV administration may help terminate and/or prevent these occurrences.

Magnesium Sulfate: Side Effects/Precautions

Magnesium sulfate has few serious side effects. It has been documented that rapid administration of this drug can result in a drop in the heart rate, diaphoresis, flushing of the skin, and a possible drop in blood pressure. Magnesium should be administered slowly via IV push to minimize these effects. Toxicity associated with higher doses, however, carries with it the more severe side effects of flaccid muscle paralysis (remember that it can block normal neuromuscular transmission), depression of the deep tendon reflexes, respiratory paralysis, and circulatory collapse.

There are some significant drug interactions noted between magnesium and digitalis. Conduction defects may result if magnesium is administered with digitalis. As well, the patient should be continuously reassessed during administration of magnesium. If side effects become severe, or signs of toxicity are present, calcium chloride should be immediately available to administer as an antidote.

Magnesium Sulfate: Contraindications

Magnesium should not be administered to patients in shock or with a heart block, since its physiological "blocking" capability (discussed earlier) may worsen this condition. Magnesium should not be administered to a dialysis patient, or to a patient known to have a lowered calcium level (hypocalcemia).

Magnesium Sulfate: Dosages

The appropriate dose of magnesium sulfate will be defined by the patient's particular ECG rhythm and myocardial status. Alternative dosing regimens are:

Prophylactic for Prevention of Post-MI Dysrhythmias

- 1 gram to 2 grams of magnesium can be diluted into 100 ml of D_5W. Administer over a 5–30 minute period as a loading infusion.

Ventricular Fibrillation and Ventricular Tachycardia

- 1 gram to 2 grams of the drug should be mixed in 10 ml of D_5W, and administered via IV push slowly, over a 1–2 minute period.

Torsades de Pointes

- An increased dose is typically required to be effective with this particular dysrhythmia. Mix 5 to 10 grams of the drug into a 100 ml bag of D_5W. This should then be administered at a rate of 1 gram/minute, until the dysrhythmia is abolished or the total amount has been administered.

Rate Control

ATROPINE SULFATE

Atropine Sulfate: Mechanism of Action

The heart is innervated by branches of the sympathetic and parasympathetic nervous system. The sympathetic nervous system stimulates the heart; the parasympathetic system reduces cardiac activity. The parasympathetic system achieves this by releasing the neurotransmitter acetylcholine (Figure 7-7), which causes a decrease in the heart rate and conduction velocity—without really influencing the strength of ventricular contraction.

Occasionally, you may hear this parasympathetic-mediated reduction in heart rate and conduction velocity referred to as "vagal tone." V*agal* relates to the vagus nerve, the tenth cranial nerve, which is the primary nerve of the parasympathetic nervous system. Stimulation of the vagus nerve causes the release of acetylcholine and the associated depression of cardiac activity.

Occasionally, excessive vagal tone may be present in a diseased or an ischemic heart. This increase in vagal tone can result in excessive slowing of the heart and/or conduction disturbances. Excessive vagal tone may also be observed secondary to parasympathomimetic overdoses.

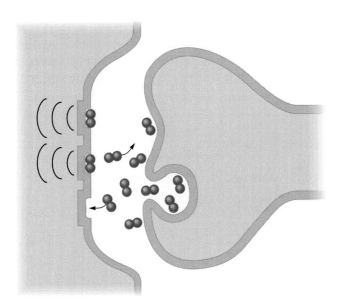

FIGURE 7-7 Activity at nerve synapses of the parasympathetic nervous system. Acetylcholine is released from pre-synaptic nerve endings, travels across the synapse, and stimulates receptors on the post-synaptic nerves. Subsequently, the catecholamines are broken down and the products taken up by the pre-synaptic nerve.

Atropine is known to be a *parasympatholytic* drug (*parasympatho-* refers to the parasympathetic branch of the autonomic nervous system, and *-lytic* means to block or stop). Other common names for this drug class include "vagolytic" and "anticholinergic." Atropine exerts its action by blocking the acetylcholine receptors, thereby inhibiting the effect of the neurotransmitter, and diminishing or preventing the influence of vagal tone on the heart. An important distinction is that atropine is not a sympathomimetic drug, as is epinephrine. Atropine increases the heart rate by blocking vagal tone, not by stimulating beta receptor sites as epinephrine would.

Atropine Sulfate: Indications

Since atropine has the ability to counteract vagal tone in the heart, its benefits would be desirable in a patient who is suffering cardiovascular compromise from an excessively slow heart rate. Bradycardias cause instability in the patient because of a drop in cardiac output. This drop, when severe, results in arterial hypotension, organ hypoperfusion, and a decrease in coronary artery perfusion.

Patients who may respond to atropine include those who present with sinus bradycardia and certain conduction blocks of the AV node. Research has shown that individuals with a first degree AV conduction block or a second degree Type I AV conduction block may benefit from atropine. These blocks have more recently been labeled as "nodal" blocks, located exactly at the level of the AV node. Patients with second degree Type II and third degree ("infranodal") heart blocks should be given special consideration prior to atropine administration, as atropine has been reported to be harmful in some of these patients. This consideration will be discussed more under "Contraindications," below.

One important delineation needs to be made regarding the administration of atropine for bradycardia. Atropine should only be administered when the patient has been identified as symptomatic or unstable from the bradydysrhythmia. (Administration of atropine to a patient who is not symptomatic may have adverse consequences.)

"Absolute bradycardia" occurs when the patient displays a heart rate below 60 beats per minute (for example 55) with signs of hemodynamic compromise. "Relative bradycardia" occurs when the patient displays a heart rate above 60 (for example 65), but still has signs and symptoms consistent with hypoperfusion.

Absolute Bradycardia

- A spontaneous heart rate < 60 beats/min
  and
- Concurrent signs/symptoms of hemodynamic compromise:
  - shortness of breath
  - chest pain
  - altered mental status
  - hypotension
  - pulmonary edema
  - myocardial infarction

Relative Bradycardia

- A spontaneous heart rate > 60 beats/min
  and
- Concurrent signs of poor cardiac output:
  - acute myocardial infarction
  - symptomatic hypotension

Atropine has been cited as beneficial in a bradyasystolic heart secondary to excessive vagal tone. Ongoing research results are controversial regarding the appropriateness of atropine in the asystolic heart. However, since the asystolic heart has a poor prognosis for resuscitation, atropine administration is not viewed as harmful. Also, some cases of asystole are thought to result from massive parasympathetic tone. For this reason, asystolic cardiac arrests should routinely receive atropine administration.

Atropine Sulfate: Side Effects/Precautions

Since the effect of atropine is to increase the heart rate, naturally the myocardial oxygen demand will also increase. This is of concern in a patient with an MI or myocardial ischemia, since the imbalance between myocardial oxygen supply and demand may be worsened. This is especially true in a patient with coronary artery disease. Finally, excessive doses of atropine may result in an anticholinergic syndrome characterized by the following symptoms:

Anticholinergic Syndrome

- Tachycardia
- Blurred vision
- Flushed and hot skin
- Coma (alterations in mentation)
- Muscle incoordination
- Dilated pupils
- Dry mouth

Atropine Sulfate: Contraindications

As mentioned earlier, atropine should be avoided in patients who are in a symptomatic Type II or third degree heart block, which are considered "infranodal" (located below the AV node, actually at the level of the ventricle). The reason to avoid atropine in infranodal blocks is logical. There is very little parasympathetic innervation at the level of the ventricles, so in the absence of parasympathetic fibers there cannot be excessive parasympathetic tone, and thus atropine can exert no benefits of increased conduction speed.

Instead, there can be an adverse effect from atropine: If atropine is administered and causes the sinus discharge rate above the conduction block to increase, it may further irritate the conduction defect and worsen the block. A simple analogy would be to take an old wooden covered bridge, only able to support a single lane of traffic, and widen the road that leads to the bridge into a superhighway. As the vehicular traffic increases (i.e., the sinus discharge rate increases), the old bridge will start to break down under the added weight and strain—until it collapses (i.e., the conduction block becomes irritated by the additional electrical traffic from the sinus node until the block is complete).

Since researchers still argue about the exact appropriateness of atropine administration in infranodal blocks, some protocols may still recommend considering a single atropine bolus. However, if atropine is administered to an infranodal block, watch closely for paradoxical slowing of the ventricular rate. Be prepared to artificially pace the rhythm should the conduction defect worsen.

Atropine Sulfate: Dosages

Atropine is administered via an intravenous line. It can also be administered down the endotracheal tube when no IV line is present. When the endotracheal route is used, the dose should be 1 to 2 mg diluted with no more than 10 cc of solution. However, when administering more than one dose of atropine, do not rely on the endotracheal tube as the sole route, since excessive amounts of fluids will be instilled into the respiratory tree. The following outlines the administration of atropine for the patient suffering from cardiovascular instability:

Hemodynamically Unstable Bradycardia

- Initial dose of 0.5–1.0 mg given IVP or ETT (1–2 mg via ETT). Repeat atropine at 0.5 mg–1.0 mg every 3–5 minutes to a maximum dose of 0.03 mg/kg. Up to 0.04 mg/kg has been used in some extreme instances of severe bradycardia.

Cardiac Arrest (Asystole or PEA with Extreme Bradycardia)

- Initial and repeat doses are at 1.0 mg every 3–5 minutes until the full vagolytic dose of 0.04 mg/kg is achieved.

As you will notice, the amount you administer is standard (either 0.5 mg or 1.0 mg), but the maximum cumulative dose is based upon the weight of the patient. There is an easy way to determine the maximum dose at 0.04 mg/kg. For every 25 kg of patient weight, administer 1 mg of atropine to achieve the maximum allowance. For example, if the patient weighed 165 pounds, that would convert into 75 kg (divide weight in pounds by 2.2), which results in 3 mg as the maximum amount of drug to be administered. A patient who weighs 100 kg would receive a maximum of 4 mg of atropine.

Also be cautious not to administer less than a 0.5 mg bolus of atropine. At low doses, there has been a documented paradoxical effect worsening the bradycardia, which may possibly lead to V-fib.

ADENOSINE

Adenosine: Mechanism of Action

Adenosine is a "purine nucleoside," a naturally occurring body protein. It is a substance found in all body cells. When administered parenterally, it has numerous effects which include slowing of conduction through the AV node and interruption of reentry pathways which may be the underlying etiology of PSVT rhythms.

Adenosine will not convert atrial tachydysrhythmias such as atrial tachycardia, atrial flutter, multifocal atrial tachycardia, or atrial fibrillation into a sinus rhythm. The benefits of adenosine result from its ability to slow conduction through the AV node. In essence, you are creating a form of heart block. For example, if a patient presents with atrial flutter with a 1:1 conduction and a heart rate of 270 prior to adenosine, after adenosine the *atrial* rate may still be 270/minute—but the *ventricular* response may now be 90/minute with a 3:1 conduction block of the atrial flutter. The immediate goal of treating a hemodynamically unstable PSVT is to control the rapid ventricular response. After initial stabilization, the underlying cause of the PSVT can be identified and managed.

Adenosine: Indications

Adenosine is the drug of choice for symptomatic tachydysrhythmias that are supraventricular in nature. Oftentimes with a tachycardic rate, it is impossible to identify the exact cause of the rhythm because the atrial activity and T waves are superimposed on each other. But as noted earlier, this distinction is unnecessary since adenosine will have no effect on atrial tissue; rather it slows AV conduction.

Adenosine is also effective in terminating tachycardias from a reentry pathway. This is probably the most common cause of PSVT. Adenosine is also appropriate for PSVT rhythms associated with Wolff-Parkinson-White (WPW) syndrome. (WPW will be discussed in more detail under "Verapamil and Diltiazem.") Instances when adenosine administration would be appropriate are:

• Symptomatic PSVT associated with WPW
• Atrial dysrhythmias resulting in a rapid ventricular response
• Wide complex tachycardia of unknown etiology

Adenosine: Side Effects/Precautions

Side effects after adenosine administration occur often but, fortunately, are short lived, because its half-life is extremely short, lasting only about 5 seconds. The following list identifies the side effects that the patient should be forewarned about, again remembering that they are of a short, often inconsequential, duration:

• Facial flushing
• Nausea
• Dizziness

- Headache
- Dysrhythmias
- Dyspnea
- Chest pain

Adenosine does, however, have important drug interactions that must be given special attention. Methylxanthines (aminophylline) block the receptor sites where adenosine exerts its therapeutic action, so that larger doses may be required for the desired effect. Conversely, dipyridamole (Persantine) blocks the uptake of adenosine and thus potentiates its effects. In this instance, the dose should be decreased. These interactions are extremely important, and the presence or potential use of any of these drugs needs to be determined prior to administration of adenosine.

Adenosine: Contraindications
As with any other drug, an absolute contraindication is known hypersensitivity to the drug. Adenosine should be avoided in patients with a second or third degree heart block, since the actions of this drug include delaying AV node conduction. This drug should not be used in patients known to have sick sinus syndrome, especially in the absence of a pacemaker.

Adenosine: Dosage
Successful conversion from the tachydysrhythmia is greatly enhanced if the adenosine administration procedure is strictly followed. Since adenosine has such a short half-life, improper administration could result in the drug being metabolized by the body before it ever reaches the coronary circulation and the myocardium. Adenosine should be administered in the closest medication port to the IV site, preferably in a large antecubital vein, and should be followed by a rapid flush of 20 cc of saline each time it is administered. The proper dose and administration procedure are:

Hemodynamically Significant Tachycardia
- Initial bolus of 6 mg via rapid IV push over 1–3 seconds. After 1–2 minutes, if the rhythm did not convert, administer 12 mg, then another 12 mg if still unresponsive. The maximum dose of adenosine is 30 mg.

CALCIUM CHANNEL BLOCKERS: VERAPAMIL AND DILTIAZEM

Verapamil and Diltiazem: Mechanism of Action
Calcium ions are necessary for normal nerve propagation and smooth muscle contraction. Therefore, a drug that alters the normal movement of calcium would also interfere with conduction velocity and smooth muscle contraction.

Verapamil and diltiazem are known as "calcium channel antagonists," or "calcium channel blockers." They act by blocking the movement of calcium across cellular membranes. Although they differ slightly in the degree of effect, verapamil or diltiazem slows conduction velocity through the AV node and relaxes vascular smooth muscle. These benefits would be desirable for patients experiencing a tachydysrhythmia in which the ventricular rate needs to be slowed. Additionally, since these drugs exert negative chronotropic (rate) and inotropic (contractile force) effects on the heart, they will lessen myocardial oxygen demand. These are desirable anti-ischemic effects. Finally, verapamil and diltiazem result in coronary artery dilation which assists in the treatment of angina.

Although they both are calcium channel blockers, verapamil and diltiazem exert slightly different effects. Table 7-2 identifies the differences in their actions.

Verapamil and Diltiazem: Indications

Because both verapamil and diltiazem slow conduction and prolong refractoriness by interfering with calcium movement across the cellular membrane, it is only logical that they are used in treating tachydysrhythmias. Verapamil was previously the drug of choice in treatment of PSVT rhythms; however, since adenosine can accomplish the same result more reliably with fewer side effects, calcium channel blockers are now used less frequently in the management of symptomatic tachydysrhythmias.

Specifically, verapamil and diltiazem are used when a symptomatic but stable patient has a need for rate control that is unresponsive to adenosine but does not require electrical cardioversion. It is important to remember that the calcium channel blockers should be used with narrow-complex tachydysrhythmias. If used in tachydysrhythmias with a wide QRS (e.g., V-tach, wide complex, with unknown etiology), severe hemodynamic compromise could result, since these drugs have negative inotropic effects.

Experience with IV administration of diltiazem is more limited than with verapamil. But both appear effective in the elimination and prevention of narrow complex PSVT rhythms. Lastly, IV administration of diltiazem in the patient with known atrial fibrillation or atrial flutter may be more appropriate than verapamil since diltiazem produces less myocardial depression than verapamil.

Verapamil and Diltiazem: Side Effects/Precautions

Precautions associated with the use of calcium channel blockers stem logically from the mechanism of action. Impeding calcium movement exerts a negative inotropic effect. Additionally, vasodilation in peripheral blood vessels occurs. The combination of the side effects may result in the possibility of precipitating hypotension. In fact, the blood pressure must be closely monitored for evidence of hypotension during the administration of calcium channel blockers. For this reason, avoid the use of verapamil, and be cautious about administering diltiazem, in patients with known left ventricular dysfunction. If hemodynamic compromise becomes apparent after the administration of the calcium channel blocker, consider administering calcium

TABLE 7-2 VERAPAMIL AND DILTIAZEM: COMPARATIVE ACTIONS

	Effect on AV Conduction	Effect on Smooth Muscle Relaxation
Verapamil	Potent negative inotropic and chronotropic effect	Lesser effect on vascular and smooth muscle relaxation
Diltiazem	Mild negative inotropic but potent negative chronotropic effect	Greater effect on vascular and smooth muscle relaxation

TABLE 7-3 CALCIUM CHANNEL BLOCKERS (VERAPAMIL/DILTIAZEM): DRUG INTERACTIONS

Calcium channel blockers such as verapamil and diltiazem should not be administered with certain drugs with which they will have negative interactions. These drugs and their interactive effects with calcium channel blockers are listed below.

Drug	Interaction with Calcium Channel Blockers
Digitalis	Conduction disturbance, CHF
Beta blockers	Possible CHF, bradycardia, asystole
Furosemide	Do not simultaneously administer: incompatible

intravenously, as this may help restore blood pressure without disturbing the electrical activity of the myocardium.

Significant drug interactions occur with the administration of calcium channel blockers. Typically, you may find that a patient with a PSVT rhythm may already be on certain antidysrhythmic drugs for that problem. If so, your administration of either verapamil or diltiazem may have a synergistic effect, potentiating the seriousness of the side effects. It is not only important to be aware of these possible drug interactions, but you must actively *look for* usage of these drugs while taking the patient's history or by searching the patient's medical records. Table 7-3 identifies these drug interactions.

Finally, just as many other drugs do, calcium channel blockers can have some systemic side effects that may be uncomfortable for the patient, but are generally not dangerous.

Minor Side Effects
- Nausea
- Vomiting
- Headache
- Dizziness

More Serious (but Less Frequent) Side Effects
- Bradycardia
- Heart block
- Asystole

Verapamil and Diltiazem: Contraindications
A major contraindication to the use of calcium channel blockers is a medical condition known as Wolff-Parkinson-White (WPW) syndrome. This is a condition in which there is an abnormal conduction pathway between the atria and ventricles of the heart. This pathway, when active, allows for a cyclic depolarization wave to move rapidly from the atria to the ventricles and back again. In other words, it allows the impulse to "run in circles" through the upper and lower chambers of the heart. Verapamil or diltiazem administration may actually increase the conduction velocity in the abnormal

pathway and allow the rate to increase further. (Fortunately, adenosine does not have this effect and can be used safely in patients with WPW.)

Another contraindication to use of calcium channel blockers results from their ability to slow AV node conduction. Calcium channel blockers should not be administered to someone with a conduction defect (heart block) since it may only worsen the block. Verapamil and diltiazem should be avoided in the patient with severe hypotension and/or cardiogenic shock, because its negative inotropic effects will worsen the cardiac compromise. And finally, remember that these drugs are not indicated for tachydysrhythmias with a wide complex QRS.

Verapamil and Diltiazem: Dosages

Although effective in controlling rapid ventricular rates in patients with PSVT or A-fib/A-flutter, both verapamil and diltiazem are relatively dangerous to administer. It is critical to administer the appropriate dose, at the appropriate rate, at the appropriate timing intervals to avoid disastrous complications. Remember also that, unlike adenosine, verapamil and diltiazem must be administered by slow IV push. This means: *Administer the medication over at least a 2 minute time period every time it is given.*

Verapamil

- *For PSVT and A-fib/flutter with rapid ventricular response*, administer 2.5 mg to 5.0 mg initial bolus IVP over 2 minutes, followed by a 5 mg to 10 mg bolus after 15–30 minutes have lapsed. Repeat it again in 5 mg to 10 mg doses every 15–30 minutes until a maximum dose of 30 mg has been administered.

Diltiazem

- *For PSVT* administer 0.25 mg/kg initial bolus IVP over 2 minutes, followed by a repeat dose of 0.35 mg/kg in 15 minutes if the PSVT has not yet resolved.
- *For A-Fib and A-Flutter with a rapid ventricular response*, administer an initial bolus of 0.25 mg/kg over 2 minutes, after which you should initiate a maintenance infusion at 5 mg/hour. You can titrate the maintenance infusion until you achieve the desired heart rate as long as the infusion does not exceed 15 mg/hour.

DIGITALIS GLYCOSIDES

Digitalis Glycosides: Mechanism of Action

Digitalis glycoside preparations are commonly used in the control of ventricular responses to rapid atrial dysrhythmias. By inducing vagal tone at the level of the AV node, electrical impulses traveling from the atria to the ventricles are substantially slowed. This slowing action allows for an increased diastolic period in which greater ventricular filling can occur and adequate coronary artery perfusion is achieved. The lengthened diastole also allows for an improvement in left ventricular preload.

Depending upon dose, digitalis also acts as a positive inotrope. By increasing the uptake of cellular calcium, a more forceful contraction is produced.

However, the positive inotropic activity of digitalis is negligible compared to that of other inotropic agents, and digitalis is generally not used in situations where positive inotropic activity would be beneficial, e.g., acute CHF. Also, it is not titratable, nor does it have as rapid an onset as other agents.

Digitalis Glycosides: Indications

Digitalis glycosides are useful in two situations: First, digitalis can counteract or correct rhythm disturbances that interfere with ventricular filling. Second, digitalis can have positive hemodynamic effects in the long-term treatment of congestive heart failure.

The first category includes ventricular response to atrial fibrillation or atrial flutter. Generally, a ventricular response of greater than 100 beats per minute is considered uncontrolled. The danger with an uncontrolled ventricular response is that, as it increases, ventricular filling time will be shortened and cardiac output will be reduced. In addition, coronary artery perfusion occurs during diastole, and as diastolic filling decreases, so does the coronary artery perfusion. Therefore, regulation of the ventricular response is paramount in cases of atrial fibrillation, atrial flutter, and PSVT. Digitalis preparations, usually used to achieve long-term control, must be considered for stabilization of PSVT after adenosine, verapamil, and electrical conversion have proven unsuccessful for this purpose.

The second category is long-term treatment of CHF. As stated previously, digitalis glycosides have positive inotropic effects, the ability to bring about a more forceful contraction of the heart. While other medications are more effective in the treatment of *acute* CHF and left ventricular failure, digitalis is useful in the *long-term* treatment of heart failure. The positive inotropic activity is dose dependent and occurs more frequently at lower doses.

Digitalis Glycosides: Side Effects/Precautions

Toxicity is a major potential side effect of digitalis and must be closely monitored. Levels of digitalis that exceed the therapeutic range may produce many different signs and symptoms. These include:

Cardiovascular
- Bradydysrhythmias
- Tachydysrhythmias
- Premature beats
- Hypotension
- Heart blocks
- Cardiac arrest

Non Cardiac
- Anorexia
- Nausea/vomiting
- Abdominal pain
- Yellow vision
- Headache
- Dizziness

- Rash
- Sweating

Patients suffering an acute myocardial infarction or electrolyte disturbances (particularly hypokalemia) are more prone to develop digitalis toxicity. In addition, toxicity can be promulgated through concurrent administration of other medications. For instance, digitalis administered with beta blockers might produce profound bradycardia, or the depletion of potassium by a diuretic can alter the electrolyte balance. Also, quinidine and calcium channel blockers serve to increase overall levels of digitalis.

In any case of toxicity, current levels of administration must be discontinued and the underlying abnormality corrected. In cases of massive toxicity, digoxin antibodies may prove effective in reversal.

Digitalis Glycosides: Contraindications
Digitalis glycosides are commonly used and are only contraindicated in the presence of digitalis toxicity.

Digitalis Glycosides: Dosages
The dosage at which digitalis is administered determines the effect of the medication. Digitalis administered at higher dosages influences the ventricular response, while lower dosages tend to elicit an inotropic response. Digitalis preparations can be administered either orally or via intravenous access.

- *Oral administration*—Oral administration pertains to long-term management of CHF or atrial dysrhythmias.
- *IV administration*—IV administration is generally geared toward the immediate control of ventricular activity secondary to rapid atrial dysrhythmias. Digitalis is administered at a loading dose of 10–15 µg/kg of the patient's lean body weight. The maintenance infusion is dependent upon body size and must be calculated on an individual basis.

Because medications such as quinidine, verapamil, and amrinone diminish the body's ability to eliminate digitalis, patients who are on these medications are more at risk for the accumulation of toxic levels of digitalis. In these situations, a 50% reduction in the dose of digitalis is considered the general rule of thumb.

Other Drugs for Rate Control
As mentioned in the opening to this chapter, some drugs may have more than one application in the treatment of a patient with cardiovascular instability. The drugs listed below are sympathomimetic agents that will increase the heart rate directly by stimulation of the heart or indirectly by stimulation of the sympathetic nervous system. For this reason, they are considered to be drugs that are appropriate for rate control. To understand more fully how these drugs work, review the information about them under "Sympathomimetics" earlier in the chapter.

- dopamine
- epinephrine
- isoproterenol

PART FIVE: ANALGESICS AND ANTIANGINAL AGENTS

Analgesic agents are used to alleviate pain. The most commonly used analgesics would be morphine (an opiate derivative) or a synthetic narcotic. They are used for pain associated with a myriad of medical or traumatic causes; however most often they are used for the treatment of chest pain from a cardiovascular crisis.

Antianginal agents have similar indications. This drug class includes agents, such as nitroglycerin, that will help alleviate the ischemic chest pain characteristic of a hypoxic heart. Typically, when cardiac pain is not relieved by administered oxygen and nitroglycerin, more potent analgesics are used.

MORPHINE SULFATE

Morphine Sulfate: Mechanism of Action

Morphine sulfate, a narcotic, is a derivative of the opiates, which are substances that occur naturally in the environment. When administered, morphine interacts with the opiate receptors in the brain where it causes central nervous system effects.

Morphine promotes hemodynamic changes. There is a drop in systemic vascular resistance and an increase in venous capacitance. These hemodynamic changes will lower preload as a result of decreasing venous return and will reduce myocardial afterload (and intramyocardial-wall tension) by dilating the arterial side of the circulation. These changes, in turn, will reduce myocardial workload and oxygen requirements.

Secondly, morphine serves as an analgesic, thereby diminishing the pain and apprehension associated with an acute MI. This is beneficial since sympathetic nervous system activity is heightened during an MI with an increased demand made on the heart. Morphine will help blunt that effect.

Morphine Sulfate: Indications

The role of morphine sulfate in the management of an MI and other cardiovascular emergencies has been well documented. In general, it is useful whenever there is severe pain (e.g., chest pain) that is compounding the medical emergency, or whenever cardiovascular instability results in pulmonary edema (with or without pain). The use of morphine should be considered only after an appropriate physical assessment and patient interview, as long as the vital signs (especially the blood pressure) are within acceptable limits. Typically, you will find yourself considering morphine either after nitroglycerin has failed to relieve the chest pain or as part of the treatment regimen for acute pulmonary edema.

Morphine Sulfate: Side Effects/Precautions

Since it is a narcotic drug with a potential for addiction and abuse, morphine has since been regulated under the 1970 Controlled Substances Act, as a Schedule II drug. This requires care providers using this drug to adhere to specific documentation and security measures.

Morphine acts as a CNS depressant. It can cause profound respiratory depression and possible hypotension. These effects may be pronounced in

TABLE 7-4 MORPHINE INTERACTIONS
The CNS depressive effects of morphine can be enhanced if administered concurrently with any of the drugs listed below.
• Other sedatives • Hypnotics • Antihistamines • Antiemitics • Barbiturates • Alcohol

individuals who already have some type of respiratory impairment or who are receiving CNS-depressant drugs. It is always best to administer morphine in several small incremental doses rather than as large boluses to avoid these complications. Table 7-4 lists potential drug interactions that should be considered prior to morphine use.

As a narcotic drug, morphine can be reversed by naloxone (Narcan®). Undesirable complications of excessive narcosis or respiratory depression can be reversed by administering 0.4 to 0.8 mg of naloxone. Naloxone administration is typically titrated to allow the analgesic and sedative effects to predominate while maintaining a sufficient ventilatory and circulatory status.

Other possible side effects of morphine that should be anticipated include nausea and vomiting, abdominal cramping, blurred vision, altered mental status, constricted pupils, and headaches.

Morphine Sulfate: Contraindications
Morphine should not be administered to anyone with a known hypersensitivity to narcotics (a situation, incidentally, that is rather common). Additionally, because of the hemodynamic effects described earlier, morphine should not be administered to anyone who is hypotensive or thought to be volume-depleted. And due to its vasodilatory effects and depression of the mental status, it should also be avoided in head-injury patients and those with undiagnosed abdominal pain.

Morphine Sulfate: Dosage
Morphine can be administered via the intravascular, intramuscular, and subcutaneous routes. In emergency situations morphine is preferentially given via small intravenous boluses to avoid precipitating excessive respiratory depression and/or cardiovascular collapse.

* *IV administration*—The dose should be started at 1 mg to 3 mg and given slowly (over 1-5 minutes) via IV push. The dose can be repeated at 5-minute intervals until the desired effect is achieved.

You should always have the narcotic reversal agent naloxone (Narcan®) readily available when morphine is administered.

NITROGLYCERIN

Nitroglycerin: Mechanism of Action

Nitroglycerin is a nitrate that lowers blood pressure by relaxing vascular smooth muscle. Through its actions, nitroglycerin dilates the vasculature, thereby reducing the pressure against which the heart must eject blood (afterload) and the amount of blood that is returned to the heart for pumping (preload).

The heart constantly requires an adequate oxygen supply. In situations where oxygen supply is depleted—such as a myocardial infarction—myocardial ischemia and subsequent necrosis may result. A reduction in workload results in a reduction in the demand for oxygen. The heart works less because it is pumping against a reduced systemic vascular resistance and has a lower left ventricular filling volume. Nitroglycerin improves the balance between workload and available oxygen. As a result, ischemic pain is alleviated and the possible infarct size limited.

It is also thought that nitroglycerin may dilate coronary arteries and promote collateral circulation to ischemic regions where the normal blood flow is interrupted.

Nitroglycerin: Indications

Ischemic tissue produces pain. If the ischemia can be alleviated, as through the action of nitroglycerin, the pain will most likely resolve. Therefore, nitroglycerin is commonly prescribed for any type of ischemic myocardial pain. This includes pain occurring secondary to angina or as a result of acute myocardial infarction.

Nitroglycerin is also indicated in the emergent treatment of acute congestive heart failure. By increasing capacitance in the venous system, nitroglycerin reduces pressure in the pulmonary vessels and enables a more effective cardiac output, thereby improving respiration and the exchange of gases.

Nitroglycerin: Side Effects/Precautions

Since nitroglycerin can produce a drop in blood pressure, it can also limit the amount of blood available for perfusion of the myocardium. Decreased coronary perfusion worsens myocardial ischemia. For this reason, no more than a 10% reduction in the mean arterial blood pressure is recommended.

Again as a result of the reduction in blood pressure, the patient may experience syncope, dizziness, weakness, and tachycardia. In addition, headache, dry mouth, nausea, and vomiting may occur.

Nitroglycerin should be administered with the patient sitting or lying down due to the potential for a sudden drop in blood pressure. If systemic hypotension does occur, the patient should be immediately placed in the Trendelenburg position (supine, with feet elevated) to facilitate blood flow to the brain and myocardium.

Nitroglycerin: Contraindications

Nitroglycerin should be avoided if preexisting hypotension is present. In addition, nitroglycerin dilates the cerebral veins and can elevate intracranial pressure. Therefore, if increased intracranial pressure exists, nitroglycerin should be used with caution. Finally, anyone with declared sensitivity to nitroglycerin should not be given the drug.

Nitroglycerin: Dosages

Nitroglycerin can be administered through several different routes in varying dosages. These include:

- *Sublingual spray or tablet*—The sublingual administration of nitroglycerin is a rapid route for administration in the emergent situation. A 0.3 to 0.4 mg starting dose is given and can be repeated at 5-minute intervals, until discomfort is relieved, or a total of 3 tablets or sprays is achieved.
- *Transcutaneous paste or patch*—For a continuous administration of nitroglycerin, the transcutaneous route is advantageous. Slow absorption through the skin promotes a consistent delivery of nitroglycerin into the body. Paste is usually applied in a ½-to-1-inch strip. Patches are typically applied to the chest.
- *Intravenous*—Intravenous administration is the fastest and most potent route of delivery of nitroglycerin. A loading dosage of 12.5–25 µg should be given initially. Following the loading dose, a maintenance infusion at a concentration of 200–400 µg/ml can be administered at a rate of 10–20 µg/min. If needed, the maintenance infusion should be increased 5–10 µg/minute every 5–10 minutes until the desired clinical response has been achieved and appropriate blood pressure maintained.

PART SIX: DIURETICS

A diuretic agent is one that will enhance the body's ability to eliminate excess fluid via the renal system. This can be desirable in a patient with congestive heart failure or acute pulmonary edema. These emergencies result from a buildup of fluid caused by failing ventricles. If the fluid backs up as a result of right ventricular failure, peripheral edema, jugular vein distention (JVD), and ascites may be present along with a positive hepato-jugular reflex. If fluid backs up because of left ventricular failure, the fluid becomes displaced into the alveoli, resulting in diminished diffusion of gases. In either instance, furosemide (Lasix) will reduce the circulating volume by ridding the body of excess fluid. And since the volume is less, there is a drop in preload, which allows the heart to more efficiently pump the remaining fluid.

FUROSEMIDE

Furosemide: Mechanism of Action

Furosemide is a potent diuretic that works to reduce vascular volume. In doing so, it removes excess volume from within the lungs, as is seen with acute congestive heart failure or pulmonary edema.

Furosemide exerts its influence in the kidneys where it promotes the excretion of sodium and, ultimately, the water that follows sodium. As volume is removed from the intravascular space, fluid from the extravascular space shifts and is excreted accordingly. This promotes removal of fluid from the lungs, resulting in enhanced gas exchange at the alveolar capillary membrane.

In addition, furosemide exerts a venodilatory effect and increases cardiac output by reducing preload.

Furosemide: Indications

In light of its mechanisms of action, furosemide is applicable in the emergency treatment of pulmonary congestion associated with left ventricular failure.

Furosemide: Side Effects/Precautions

As with any diuretic, you must be aware of possible electrolyte disturbances, especially of potassium. Electrolyte disturbances can manifest as electrical dysrhythmias and prove difficult to correct unless the underlying abnormality is targeted. Chronic use of furosemide may precipitate electrolyte disturbances.

Also, severe fluid depletion can result in dehydration and hypotension. Blood pressure and fluid status must be monitored closely during the use of furosemide.

Furosemide: Contraindications

As furosemide is a derivative of sulfamide, it should be withheld from anyone declaring sensitivity to sulfas. Also, preexisting hypotension or dehydration should discount the use of furosemide.

Furosemide: Dosage

In the emergency setting, furosemide should be given intravenously.

- *IV administration*—Administer an initial dosage of 20–40 mg or 0.5–1 mg/kg. Delivery should be slow, occurring over 1–2 minutes. If there is failure to respond, an infusion of furosemide can be initiated at a rate of 0.25–0.75 mg/kg/hr.

With use of furosemide, fluid intake and urinary output should be strictly monitored.

PART SEVEN: ANTIHYPERTENSIVES

Another relatively common cardiovascular emergency is hypertension. Well known as the "silent killer," hypertension may also present as an acute emergency requiring immediate reduction in blood pressure. Although the extent and rate at which you should reduce systolic pressure is still disputed by the experts, all agree that if the indicators of a hypertensive crisis are present, reduction of blood pressure should be a priority.

SODIUM NITROPRUSSIDE

Sodium Nitroprusside: Mechanism of Action

Sodium nitroprusside is a potent and rapid-acting vasodilator that quickly decreases symptomatic hypertension. Sodium nitroprusside dilates the arterial and venous vasculature, thereby dropping blood pressure and reducing myocardial workload.

Sodium Nitroprusside: Indications

Because of its ability to reduce blood pressure rapidly, sodium nitroprusside is useful in a hypertensive crisis. Sodium nitroprusside is titratable and can be used in the management of left ventricular failure or CHF.

Sodium Nitroprusside: Side Effects/Precautions

Because its vasodilatory effects are so rapid, you must be careful not to over-administer sodium nitroprusside and create a state of hypotension.

Hepatic and renal dysfunction can slow the clearance of nitroprusside from the body. Since the elderly typically suffer a gradual degradation of hepatic and renal function, the dose of nitroprusside for an elderly patient should be reduced.

The effects of sodium nitroprusside can be severely potentiated by administration with other hypertensive agents. Also, because of the possibility of reduced perfusion, administration of sodium nitroprusside can result in dizziness, hypotension, chest pain, palpitations, nausea, and vomiting.

Be aware that sodium nitroprusside is susceptible to light and can be severely deactivated after exposure.

Sodium Nitroprusside: Contraindications

In the emergency setting, there are no contraindications to the use of sodium nitroprusside.

Sodium Nitroprusside: Dosage

Sodium nitroprusside is administered as an infusion and is constituted by combining 50–100 mg of the drug in 250 cc of D_5W or 0.9% normal saline. The bag should be immediately wrapped in an opaque material such as aluminum foil to protect it from the light.

- *IV administration*—Initial infusion should consist of 0.1 µg/kg/minute and titrated to the desired blood pressure. Typically, the range of administration is between 0.5–8.0 µg/kg/minute. For precise delivery, it is best to use an infusion pump.

Other Antihypertensive Drugs

The following drugs may also be considered as alternative agents for reducing the blood pressure. Remember, however, to use more appropriate methods first. A more detailed explanation of these drugs can be found earlier in the chapter.

- beta blockers
- nitroglycerin

PART EIGHT: THROMBOLYTICS

Thrombolytics are one of the newest developments for the management of a myocardial infarction. Thrombolysis is the process of dissolving a blood clot in patients with myocardial infarction where the clot resides in a coronary vessel (Figure 7-8). If detected early enough, thrombolysis of the clot will prevent cellular death. For this reason, numerous hospitals across the country are instituting protocols within the emergency department to allow the myocardial infarcted patient to receive a thrombolytic drug within 30 minutes of arriving at the hospital.

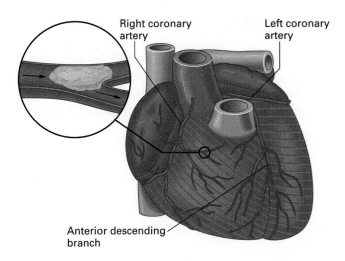

Right coronary artery

Left coronary artery

Anterior descending branch

FIGURE 7-8 A clot or embolism forming in a coronary artery prevents oxygenation of a portion of the myocardium, causing ischemia, injury, and infarction. If administered early enough, thrombolytic drugs dissolve the clot and prevent further myocardial tissue injury.

THROMBOLYTIC THERAPY

Thrombolytic Therapy: Mechanism of Action

Thrombolytic therapy has revolutionized the treatment and decreased the mortality rate of the acute myocardial infarction. Through a chemical conversion, thrombolytics activate the enzyme plasmin which proceeds to dissolve the thrombus or clot that is occluding the coronary artery.

When the thrombus or clot is dissolved, a reperfusion of the oxygen-starved myocardium occurs. Consequently, the process of infarction can be halted and areas of ischemic myocardium salvaged.

Thrombolytic Therapy: Indications

Thrombolytics should be initiated as soon as possible to anyone who is under 70 years of age, satisfies predetermined criteria, and does not exhibit any contraindications to the therapy. The age limit is currently under discussion. Predetermined criteria include a history compatible with a myocardial infarction and ST elevation that suggests acute infarction. Contraindications to thrombolytic treatment are identified and discussed below.

Thrombolytic Therapy: Side Effects/Precautions

As thrombolytics promote the dissolution of blood clots, bleeding is a major complication of thrombolytic therapy. This is a major concern with trauma induced by CPR, excessive venipuncture attempts, and the propensity an individual may have toward intracranial hemorrhage. In addition, caution must be exercised when thrombolytics are administered to anyone with a history of GI bleeding or cardiovascular problems that may result in internal hemorrhage.

Hypotension has been reported with certain agents. If hypotension occurs, the infusion should be reduced and careful monitoring of the blood pressure undertaken. In addition, allergic reactions have been known to occur and should be treated with the appropriate medications such as steroids and diphenhydramine.

Also, it must be noted that the process of thrombus formation is an ongoing process. After a clot is dissolved, it may start to reform. Therefore, adjunctive therapy, such as aspirin and heparin, is often used in conjunction with thrombolytic agents.

Furthermore, as clots are dissolved, residual pieces can break free and travel throughout the body as emboli. The emboli can then create other occlusive problems such as pulmonary embolism or cerebrovascular accident. Therefore, vigilant patient monitoring for such complications is a must.

Thrombolytic Therapy: Contraindications
In the administration of thrombolytics, many contraindications and relative contraindications are based on the danger of promoting deadly hemorrhage.

Absolute Contraindications
- Active internal hemorrhage
- Suspected aortic aneurysm
- Known trauma from CPR such as rib fractures or pneumothorax, or traumatic endotracheal intubation
- Persistent hypertension despite pain relief and initial drugs
  systolic > 180 mmHg
  diastolic > 110 mmHg
- Recent head trauma or known intracranial tumor
- History of CVA in the past 6 months
- Pregnancy

Relative Contraindications
- Recent trauma or surgery within the past 2 months
- Initial blood pressure of >180 mmHg systolic and/or > 110 mmHg diastolic pressure that is controlled by medical treatment
- Active bleeding ulcers
- History of CVA, tumor, injury, or brain surgery
- Known bleeding disorder or use of warfarin (Coumadin)
- Significant kidney or liver dysfunction
- Previous use of the thrombolytic agents streptokinase or anistreplase within the past 12 months
- Known cancer with possible thoracic, abdominal, or intracranial abnormalities
- Prolonged CPR efforts

Thrombolytic Therapy: Dosages
Currently, several thrombolytic agents exist and are administered intravenously.

Anistreplase
- 30 U IV over 2–5 minutes

Alteplase
- 100 mg IV (60 mg in first hour, then 20 mg/hr over the next 2 hours)
- **Note:** An accelerated regimen is used by some clinicians as follows:*
  - Give 15 mg bolus
  - Then 0.75 mg/kg over next 30 minutes (not to exceed 50 mg)
  - Then 0.50 mg/kg over next 60 minutes (not to exceed 35 mg)
  Total dose <100 mg

Streptokinase

- 1.5 million U in a 1-hour infusion

Urokinase

- 1.5 million U IV over 2 minutes, then 1.5 million U IV over 90 minutes *

* FDA approval pending

PART NINE: OTHER CARDIOVASCULAR DRUGS

The remaining two drugs, used in specific cardiovascular emergency situations, do not readily fit into any of the aforementioned categories. As such, they have been placed here at the end of the chapter under a general heading. But be aware that this placement is not meant to imply that these drugs are unimportant or ineffective. It is actually quite the opposite: When these drugs are called for, they are often the only option you have to correct the abnormality.

SODIUM BICARBONATE

Sodium Bicarbonate: Mechanism of Action

Cardiac arrest produces a lack of adequate perfusion and oxygenation at the cellular level. The body rapidly uses up all the residual oxygen in the blood while allowing the accumulation of waste products. After all the oxygen has been depleted in the cells, and in an attempt to maintain normal activity, the metabolism will change from aerobic to anaerobic.

Anaerobic metabolism, however, creates important waste products, mainly hydrogen ions (H^+) and carbon dioxide (CO_2), which accumulate in the body to toxic levels. This profound acidosis has a negative impact on cellular function, myocardial activity, and survivability from cardiac arrest.

Normally, the body can handle the acid production by combining the "strong" hydrogen acid waste product with a base (alkaline) substance. This in turn yields a "weak" acid, carbonic acid, which in turn dissociates into carbon dioxide and water (see below). The carbon dioxide is eliminated through the respiratory system, while the water is eliminated by the kidneys.

hydrogen ion [plus] bicarbonate ion [equals] carbonic acid
[which yields] carbon dioxide and water

Or, as a chemical formula:

$$H^+ + HCO_3^- \rightleftarrows H_2CO_3 \rightleftarrows H_2O + CO_2$$

This process is known as "blood buffering" of hydrogen ions, the process by which the body maintains acid-base balance.

Unfortunately the body's compensatory mechanism, the buffering process, is overwhelmed in cardiac arrest because excessive amounts of hydrogen and carbon dioxide are produced. This propels the process in the opposite direction to produce hydrogen ions and increased acidosis. Sodium bicarbonate may be useful when this occurs.

Sodium bicarbonate is nothing more than a "salt" which will dissociate into sodium (Na^+) and the bicarbonate ion (HCO_3^-). The bicarbonate ion liberated during this process is then available to bind the excess hydrogen waste products, which will help lower the acidity of the blood. Integral to the success of this process, however, is adequate pulmonary blood flow and ventilation to eliminate CO_2 produced at the end of the reaction.

Sodium Bicarbonate: Indications

Years ago, sodium bicarbonate was one of the cornerstone medications used in cardiac arrest. The theory was that profound metabolic acidosis accompanies cardiac arrest, and sodium bicarbonate administration would correct that abnormality. Subsequent studies have not supported the routine use of sodium bicarbonate in cardiac arrest.

The poor tissue perfusion that accompanies CPR does not allow for sufficient elimination of the CO_2 that is produced by the bicarbonate buffering process. The produced CO_2 accumulates, pushing the buffering reaction in the reverse direction to re-produce hydrogen ions. Since carbon dioxide diffuses easily into the cells, there is a resultant worsening of intracellular acidosis. This finding has been associated with many adverse reactions.

As a result, sodium bicarbonate has a less important role in the management of cardiac arrest. Effective ventilations and chest compressions have been shown to adequately limit the accumulation of acid in cardiac arrests of short duration. This is because most acidosis in early cardiac arrest states is caused by respiratory insufficiency. Thus, in the early phases of CPR, a buffering agent is unnecessary.

Under certain circumstances, sodium bicarbonate may still play a role in cardiac arrest management. For example, if there is confirmed preexisting metabolic acidosis or hyperkalemia, sodium bicarbonate administration may be beneficial. During routine cardiac arrest management, however, bicarbonate administration should be considered only after the other interventions—CPR, defibrillation, intubation, ventilation, and epinephrine administration—have failed to produce successful results.

Sodium Bicarbonate: Side Effects/Precautions

As alluded to earlier, a major concern with sodium bicarbonate administration is the worsening of intracellular acidosis when carbon dioxide is rapidly produced from buffering hydrogen ions. This high level of CO_2 is actually more immediately damaging to the myocardium than the accumulation of the hydrogen ions, since they do not pass through the cellular walls as rapidly as CO_2 does. This serves as the first precaution when using sodium bicarbonate.

Also, since the bicarbonate is attached to a sodium ion that is liberated upon administration, hypernatremia and hyperosmolarity are also concerns when larger quantities of sodium bicarbonate are used. Excessive metabolic alkalosis caused by bicarbonate overutilization also impedes the release of oxygen from hemoglobin at the tissue level.

Lastly, as a general rule, do not administer sodium bicarbonate when sympathomimetic drugs are being given. Sympathomimetics (e.g., epinephrine, dopamine) can be deactivated in an alkaline environment. If you are administering sodium bicarbonate and other drugs through the same IV line, be sure to properly flush out the line after each medication administration.

Sodium Bicarbonate: Contraindications

Actually, there are no absolute contraindications to the use of sodium bicarbonate as long as the precautions identified above are understood and followed. But again, remember that sodium bicarbonate is not a first line agent in the treatment of metabolic acidosis in cardiac arrest. It should only be administered after the interventions described above have been completed.

Sodium Bicarbonate: Dosage

When sodium bicarbonate is to be used, it should not be administered for the first 10–20 minutes of cardiac arrest management unless hyperkalemia or pre-existing acidosis is present. Administer sodium bicarbonate only after other interventions have been proven unsuccessful.

- *IV administration*—Administer 1 milliequivalent per kilogram (1 mEq/kg) IV bolus. The dose can be repeated at half its initial amount (0.5 mEq/kg) every 10 minutes thereafter.

Preferentially, use arterial blood gas analysis to guide the administration of sodium bicarbonate.

CALCIUM CHLORIDE

Calcium Chloride: Mechanism of Action

Calcium, like magnesium, is an elemental ion that is necessary for numerous physiological activities of the body. Calcium chloride replaces calcium in cases of hypocalcemia. Its main role in the management of cardiovascular emergencies, is its influence on muscle contraction. Calcium ions increase the force of myocardial contractions. They do this by entering the portion of the cell where actin and myosin filaments interact. Here, calcium can initiate and strengthen the myofibril shortening. Calcium may also aid in peripheral vasoconstriction, which will allow for a rise in blood pressure when coupled with its myocardial effects.

Calcium Chloride: Indications

Although it is well established that calcium plays a critical role in myocardial performance, studies have so far not shown administration of calcium chloride in cardiac arrest to be beneficial. This may be due to the excessively high levels of calcium that develop with its administration. Therefore, it has a limited (albeit important) role in the management of the patient experiencing a cardiovascular emergency.

Listed below are specific conditions in which calcium administration would be desirable.

- Acute hyperkalemia (elevated potassium)
- Acute hypocalcemia (decreased calcium)
- Calcium channel blocker toxicity

In these instances, the main role of calcium is to prevent the negative effects of the initial disturbance (e.g., changes in potassium or calcium levels). (Remember to try to guide the administration of calcium chloride by documented abnormalities in blood lab values.)

Calcium Chloride: Side Effects/Precautions

One of the most important considerations when administering calcium chloride is to first ascertain if the patient is on digitalis. Calcium can cause digitalis toxicity and ventricular irritability. Additionally, be sure to administer calcium through a secure IV line, since extravation of this drug can result in local tissue necrosis.

Also important are the precautions pertaining to drug interactions for calcium chloride. If calcium chloride and sodium bicarbonate are simultaneously administered into an IV line, mixing the two will result in the formation of a precipitate.

Be sure to also administer the drug dose over the appropriate amount of time. Administering calcium chloride too quickly has been associated with a slowing of the cardiac rate. Other side effects relating to the drug itself include:

- Nausea
- Vomiting
- Syncope
- Bradycardias
- Dysrhythmias
- Cardiac arrest

CASE STUDY FOLLOW-UP

On your favorite Tuesday night TV show, *Code Blue, Stat!*, a patient named Mr. Hedger has arrived at the hospital with severe chest pain, diaphoresis, and dizziness. You are especially interested in this episode, because you had a patient just like Mr. Hedger only a few hours ago at work. You settle back to match wits with the fictional emergency department team and to second-guess the assessment and care the scriptwriters have thought up for this patient.

Assessment

From the assessment performed by the TV doctors and nurses, you believe that the patient is most likely experiencing either myocardial ischemia or infarction complicated by bradycardia. In this instance, just like the one you saw at work, the goals of treatment are to decrease anxiety, ensure oxygenation, normalize the rate, and limit or reverse the myocardial ischemic process. Before getting too involved in the way the TV team is managing this patient, however, there are certain assessment parameters that you would like to know about.

Your mind drifts back to the assessment you performed on your patient, including a full set of vitals, airway and breathing patency, lung sounds, 12-lead ECG, skin characteristics, and associated signs and symptoms.

The TV nurse gives the doctor the "bullet": 45-year-old male with substernal chest pain radiating into the left arm, started 2 hours ago, lungs clear, abdomen benign, no peripheral edema, skin cool and diaphoretic, 12-lead shows early ischemia in the inferior leads, vitals are BP 122/76, HR 42, RR 26.

Treatment

You are pleased by the appropriateness of the TV show demonstrating that these assessment findings were completed prior to the main treatment. However, the new TV resident seems to be having some trouble deciding what to administer to the patient. He hesitates as the emergency room monitors and gadgets flash and blink and fill the air with a chorus of hums, clicks, beeps, and rings. You talk to the TV as if the young physician can hear you. "OK, pal, you already have the patient oxygenated and an IV initiated. Let's get the ball rolling so this guy doesn't go farther down the tubes."

Calcium Chloride: Contraindications

Since the complications that result from promoting digitalis toxicity are so severe, the use of calcium should be avoided in those patients concurrently receiving a digitalis preparation.

Calcium Chloride: Dosages

Of the different preparations available, it is best to use the 10% calcium chloride solution, since this has been shown to be the most effective in increasing plasma levels of calcium. Based upon the need for the calcium administration, the dosage may vary.

Prophylaxis when Administering Calcium Channel Blockers

- Using the 10% solution of calcium chloride, administer 2 mg/kg to 4 mg/kg via slow IV push. If the desired effects are not seen, you can repeat the drug administration at the same dose after 10 minutes.

Hyperkalemia and Calcium Channel Blocker Overdose

- In these instances, the dose of calcium needs to be increased in order to receive the desired benefit. As such, administer 8 mg/kg to 16 mg/kg via slow IV push. If, however, there is no clinical response after 10 minutes, you can repeat administration at the same dose.

(continued)

You decide to give the TV doctor some more advice. You remind him that certain drugs, like nitroglycerin and morphine, have the ability to decrease the workload on the heart, which is appropriate to help reduce ischemia. As well, Mr. Hedger is bradycardic, and for this you advise starting with atropine at 1 milligram IV push, since it is a parasympatholytic that will increase the heart rate with only a small increase in the workload. If this doesn't work, you point out, transcutaneous pacing is always an option.

The TV doctor? Well, he mumbles out something about giving nitroglycerin sublingual at 0.3 mg. "Good boy," you say. "That may help reduce the ischemic pain and decrease the ischemic area." Next the doctor wants to administer dopamine. "What???" you yell to the TV. "How about finishing out the administration of atropine before using such a strong sympathomimetic?!" Well, the physician doesn't seem to be listening to you. He orders 10 mg/kg/min intravenously. "No, no!" you groan. "Start at 5 mils per kilogram per minute with an infusion!"

The TV nurse chimes in that the blood pressure is starting to drop, and now Mr. Hedger is in a heart block. The young resident orders an increase in dopamine to 20 mils per kilogram, and you yell, "Fluid bolus, fluid bolus!!"—recalling that careful administration of a fluid bolus can increase preload and myocardial stretch, which enhances contractility. "By the way," you ask the TV team, "has the chest pain resolved? If not," you urge, "try some morphine—cautiously—perhaps 2 mg IV push. That will help with the ischemia, as long as the systolic blood pressure isn't too low." This time, fortunately, the doctor seems to have heard you. He orders the morphine after the patient continues to complain of chest pain.

Suddenly you're pulled away from the TV show because your telephone is ringing. It's your friend Dawn. You and she got off work at the same time tonight. She says, "Hey, switch to Channel 3. *Code Blue, Stat!* is on and they are really botching up this MI guy with bradycardia and hypotension. They didn't even *think* about preparing this guy for aspirin or thrombolytics." "I know," you tell her. "I'm watching it....I'm just glad we didn't treat our MI patient like that today. We would probably both be mopping the ED floor if we did!"

SUMMARY

Pharmacological therapy is an integral component of successful cardiac arrest management. The health care provider must become completely familiar with the most common drugs used. There are no short cuts. You must learn and stay abreast of current medications. For each drug, you must learn the mechanisms of action, indications, side effects and precautions, contraindications, and dosages. You must *not* rely on pocket references and charts. In the heat of an emergency, there is no time to look things up and, unless you already have a thorough understanding of *how each drug works*, mistakes are easy to make.

REVIEW QUESTIONS

1. While treating a patient experiencing a cardiovascular emergency, which of the following drugs is most likely to be initially administered?
   a. atropine
   b. nitroglycerin
   c. oxygen
   d. 0.45% sodium chloride

2. Why is atropine beneficial in the management of a patient with sinus bradycardia?
   a. Atropine mimics the effects of enhanced parasympathetic stimulation.
   b. Atropine blocks the effects of enhanced parasympathetic stimulation.
   c. Atropine mimics the effects of sympathetic stimulation.
   d. Atropine blocks the effects of sympathetic stimulation.

3. Epinephrine administered via IV push during cardiac arrest increases coronary and cerebral perfusion by
   a. dilating coronary and cerebral blood vessels.
   b. constricting coronary and cerebral blood vessels.
   c. reducing systemic vascular resistance.
   d. increasing systemic vascular resistance.

4. What type of adrenergic stimulation accounts for the changes in coronary and cerebral perfusion identified in Question 3?
   a. alpha
   b. beta
   c. dopaminergic
   d. synaptic

5. Which of the following drugs could alter the pupillary findings in a patient?
   a. atropine
   b. lidocaine
   c. oxygen
   d. nitroglycerin

6. Lidocaine can suppress ventricular dysrhythmias by
   a. eliminating the reentry phenomenon.
   b. depressing automaticity of ischemic tissue.
   c. inhibiting calcium ion movement across the cellular membrane.
   d. a and b are both correct

7. Which of the following correctly contrasts lidocaine and bretylium?
   a. Lidocaine is a ventricular antidysrhythmic agent while bretylium is an atrial antidysrhythmic agent.
   b. Lidocaine depresses ventricular contractility at normal doses while bretylium does not.

    c. Lidocaine temporarily stimulates adrenergic receptor sites while bretylium only causes dysrhythmia suppression.

    d. Lidocaine and bretylium are both effective ventricular antidysrhythmics, but lidocaine has fewer side effects.

8. Verapamil and diltiazem share what common mechanism of action?
    a. Both are calcium channel blockers.
    b. Both are sympathomimetics.
    c. Both are diuretics.
    d. Both are vasoconstrictors.

9. Based on their mechanism of action, what is the major indication shared by verapamil and diltiazem?
    a. Both may be used to treat tachydysrhythmias.
    b. Both may be used to treat bradycardia.
    c. Both may be used to treat pulmonary edema.
    d. Both may be used to treat hypotension.

10. Procainamide's mechanism of action is most similar to the action of
    a. atropine.   c. lidocaine.
    b. adenosine.   d. verapamil.

11. Which of the following drugs would be most appropriate for a patient with symptomatic tachycardia and a history of Wolff-Parkinson-White (WPW) syndrome?
    a. verapamil   c. morphine
    b. diltiazem   d. adenosine

12. Of the following drugs, which is most dissimilar to the other three?
    a. magnesium sulfate   c. procainamide
    b. lidocaine   d. diltiazem

13. When appropriate, the same drug may be applicable in numerous situations. Epinephrine, for example, can be used for both
    a. bradycardia and hypertension.
    b. chest pain and ventricular irritability.
    c. cardiac arrest and bradycardia.
    d. b and c are correct

14. What is the major indication for sodium bicarbonate?
    a. symptomatic hypotension
    b. systemic hypokalemia
    c. respiratory acidosis
    d. metabolic acidosis

15. An increase in venous capacitance and a reduction in systemic vascular resistance is characteristic of which of the following drugs?
    a. dopamine   c. morphine
    b. procainamide   d. nitrous oxide

16. Which of the following drugs will have a depressive effect on the pumping action of the heart?
    a. atropine   c. diltiazem
    b. calcium chloride   d. epinephrine

17. Which of the following will **not** depress the pumping action of the heart at therapeutic doses?
    a. lidocaine
    b. diltiazem
    c. propranolol
    d. atenolol

18. Which of the following drugs is **primarily** an alpha receptor stimulator?
    a. epinephrine
    b. norepinephrine
    c. dopamine
    d. All of the above equally stimulate alpha receptor sites.

19. If you are treating a patient with diminished systemic vascular resistance, which of the following drug(s) could help restore the vascular tone?
    a. epinephrine
    b. norepinephrine
    c. dopamine
    d. All of the above could help restore vascular tone.

20. Which of the following drugs would be the most similar in action to dopamine when used to raise blood pressure?
    a. atropine
    b. dobutamine
    c. isoproterenol
    d. metaprolol

21. Amrinone exerts its action by
    a. increasing stroke volume.
    b. inhibiting calcium ion movement.
    c. decreasing systemic vascular resistance.
    d. a and c are correct

22. Based on its actions as addressed in Question 21, amrinone may be indicated for treatment of which of the following conditions?
    a. pulmonary fluid back-up
    b. a rapid heart rate
    c. hypotension
    d. b and c are correct

23. All of the following drugs can result in peripheral vasodilation except for
    a. nitroglycerin.
    b. morphine.
    c. digitalis.
    d. nitroprusside.

24. Which of the following is **not** a mechanism of action for the class of drugs known as "beta blockers"?
    a. depress contractility
    b. diminish oxygen requirements to the heart
    c. decrease the heart rate
    d. increase the blood pressure

25. You are treating a patient suffering from severe congestive heart failure (CHF). Based on the mechanisms of action of the following drugs, which would you most likely **avoid?**
    a. nitroglycerin
    b. lasix
    c. morphine
    d. verapamil

26. The initial dose of 2.5 mg IV push is appropriate for which of the following medications?
    a. oxygen
    b. verapamil
    c. adenosine
    d. diltiazem

27. **Initial** therapy for a patient with chest pain, dyspnea, and symptomatic bradycardia should include which of the following?
    a. atropine at 2.5 mg/kg
    b. oxygen via nonrebreather at 15 lpm
    c. external pacing
    d. dopamine at 2.5 μg/kg/min

28. Epinephrine is traditionally repeated at
    a. 1 mg.
    b. 3 mg.
    c. 5 mg.
    d. none of the above

29. What drug, when administered for hemodynamically unstable bradycardia, has the **maximum** dosage of 0.04 mg/kg?
    a. epinephrine
    b. isoproterenol
    c. dopamine
    d. none of the above

30. What drug has the initial dose of 1–1.5 mg/kg?
    a. lidocaine
    b. bretylium
    c. procainamide
    d. none of the above

31. Which of the following drugs does **not** have an initial dose of 1 mg?
    a. epinephrine
    b. atropine
    c. sodium bicarbonate
    d. none of the above

32. The repeat dose of bretylium for ventricular fibrillation is
    a. 1 mg/kg.
    b. 5 mg/kg.
    c. 10 mg/kg.
    d. none of the above

33. What drug, used for symptomatic paroxysmal supraventricular tachycardia (PSVT), may be administered at 5 mg IVP as an initial dose?
    a. adenosine
    b. verapamil
    c. diltiazem
    d. none of the above

34. What drug used for symptomatic PSVT is administered at 10 mg IVP as an initial dose?
    a. adenosine
    b. verapamil
    c. diltiazem
    d. none of the above

35. How much magnesium sulfate should be mixed with 10 ml of D_5W for administration in ventricular fibrillation?
    a. 1 mg
    b. 1 gram
    c. 1 mg/kg
    d. none of the above

36. Which of the following drugs is **not** usually calculated in milligrams per kilograms for the initial bolus?
    a. sodium bicarbonate
    b. lidocaine
    c. bretylium
    d. none of the above

37. What is the appropriate dose for the correct answer in Question 36?
    a. 1 mEq/kg
    b. 10 mEq/kg
    c. 5 mEq/kg
    d. none of the above

38. Morphine is administered at
    a. 2–10 mg slow IVP.
    b. 1 mg/kg slow IVP.
    c. 0.5 mg to 1.0 mg slow IVP.
    d. none of the above

39. Which of the following is an appropriate dose of calcium chloride in a patient with known hyperkalemia, or calcium channel overdose?
    a. 3 mg/kg
    b. 6 mg/kg
    c. 8 mg/kg
    d. none of the above

40. What sympathomimetic infusion can be administered within a dose range of 0.5–30 μg/kg per minute?
    a. epinephrine
    b. norepinephrine
    c. dopamine
    d. none of the above

41. To allow for stimulation of dopaminergic receptors in the kidneys and abdomen, dopamine should be run at
    a. 2 μg/kg/min.
    b. 10 μg/kg/min.
    c. 20 μg/kg/min.
    d. none of the above

42. To allow primarily for stimulation of dopaminergic receptors in the kidneys and abdomen, **dobutamine** should be run at
    a. 2 μg/kg/min.
    b. 10 μg/kg/min.
    c. 20 μg/kg/min.
    d. none of the above

43. Which of the following infusions for bradycardia does **not** have a maximum infusion rate of 10 μg/min?
    a. epinephrine
    b. isoproterenol
    c. dopamine
    d. none of the above

44. A correct loading dose of amrinone would be
    a. 0.75 mg/kg.
    b. 7.5 mg/kg.
    c. 75 mg/kg.
    d. none of the above

45. What drug is usually administered at 10 μg/kg?
    a. bretylium
    b. procainamide
    c. digitalis
    d. none of the above

46. When administering nitroglycerin sublingually for chest pain, the maximum dosage should be
    a. 1 mg.
    b. 1.2 mg.
    c. 3 mg.
    d. none of the above

47. What would be an appropriate starting dose for an **initial** infusion of nitroglycerin?
    a. 5 μg/min
    b. 20 μg/min
    c. 35 μg/min
    d. none of the above

48. What beta blocker has the initial dose of 1 mg to 3 mg IV push?
    a. metoprolol
    b. esmolol
    c. atenolol
    d. none of the above

49. What would be an acceptable loading dose of furosemide for a 55 kg patient?
    a. 55 mg
    b. 10 mg
    c. 22.5 µg
    d. none of the above

50. Which thrombolytic agent is typically dosed in milligrams?
    a. anistreplase
    b. streptokinase
    c. alteplase
    d. urokinase

Chapter**Eight**

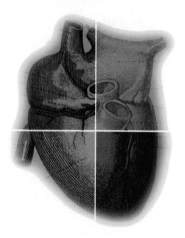

Acute Coronary Syndromes

Annually, over 900,000 people experience an acute myocardial infarction (AMI or MI), with roughly 225,000 of these lives being claimed. Furthermore, the majority of these deaths take place outside of a medical facility, with many occurring before any medical attention is ever sought. Remarkably, this figure does not account for the millions of people permanently disabled by an acute MI. From this perspective, the health care professional must develop a great appreciation of the devastating impact that the acute myocardial infarction has, not only on the individual but on society as a whole.

Topics to be covered in this chapter are:

- The Heart as a Pump
- Pathophysiology of an AMI
- Assessment of the AMI Patient
- Management of AMI: Prehospital, Emergency Department, and Hospital Considerations
- Management of Specific AMI Presentations

CASE STUDY

In a small rural urgent care center, you are working the graveyard shift as a cardiac specialist. As it is a holiday, you and two other health care providers comprise the only staff. Abruptly, the quiet night is interrupted as Kathy Miller drags her husband Steve in from the night's cold. The 48-year-old male is pale, disoriented, diaphoretic, and complaining of constant chest pain that radiates to his upper back.

You immediately take Steve into the assessment room. With much difficulty and confusion, Steve tells you that he has had this chest pain for the past day and a half. He continues on to state that he has had several episodes of "blacking out" and difficulty in breathing. In addition, you discover that Steve has a history of previous heart attacks and hypertension.

Quickly, you obtain a set of vitals which include a pulse of 52 beats per minute, respirations at 32 per minute with noted effort, and blood pressure of 78 by palpation. You inquire whether Steve has taken any medications for his present condition. Instead of replying, Steve turns slightly combative and noncompliant.

How would you proceed to assess and care for this patient? This chapter will describe the assessment and management of a patient suffering a myocardial infarction, or acute coronary syndrome. Later, we will return to the case and apply the procedures learned.

Introduction

Frequently, an acute MI occurs secondary to coronary artery disease. The magnitude of the threat of acute MI becomes quite evident when we consider the estimates that well over 6 million Americans have significant coronary artery disease! Regrettably, an acute MI and subsequent disability and/or death are often the first, and sometimes the last, sign of decades of coronary artery disease.

Advances in medicine have produced interventions that can successfully counter the adverse effects of the myocardial infarction and have made surviving an acute MI a realistic possibility. However, the process of reperfusing myocardial muscle by use of thrombolytics is extremely time dependent and may vary dramatically in response to the variety of infarct presentations. Therefore, to appropriately manage an acute MI or other coronary syndrome, you must have a strong working knowledge of the heart and its relation to the human body.

This chapter will provide a framework and basic knowledge required for effective management of the acute myocardial infarction.

The Heart as a Pump

The heart functions as a pump. Through the circulatory system, the heart pumps blood to every organ, tissue, and cell in the human body. Each of these living cells depends upon the continual circulation of blood for the delivery of oxygen and elimination of wastes. *Without sufficient circulation, the organs, tissues, cells, and subsequently the human organism will die.* Therefore, the effective pumping action of the heart is critical to the maintenance of life. Any problem with the muscular pump can result in serious disability and even death.

FIGURE 8-1 The anatomical structures of the heart.

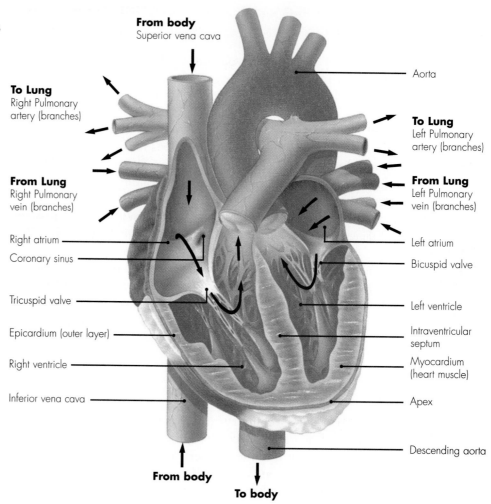

From body
Superior vena cava

Aorta

To Lung
Right Pulmonary artery (branches)

To Lung
Left Pulmonary artery (branches)

From Lung
Right Pulmonary vein (branches)

From Lung
Left Pulmonary vein (branches)

Right atrium

Left atrium

Coronary sinus

Bicuspid valve

Tricuspid valve

Left ventricle

Epicardium (outer layer)

Intraventricular septum

Right ventricle

Myocardium (heart muscle)

Inferior vena cava

Apex

Descending aorta

From body

To body

The effective circulation of oxygenated blood relies on two distinct pumping actions, one on the right side of the heart and one on the left side (Figure 8-1). Consequently, the heart must be viewed as two distinct pumps that function simultaneously.

The Right-Side Pump

The right atrium and right ventricle compose the right-side pump. The function of the right side of the heart is to eject the unoxygenated blood that has been returned to the heart by the venous system into the capillaries of the lungs for reoxygenation. This delivery is very dependent on the effective contraction of the right ventricle. *Any compromise in right ventricular contraction can cause blood to back up into the venous system, thus resulting in a reduction of blood sent to the lungs for oxygenation and, subsequently, a shortage of blood available to be distributed through the left side of the heart to the tissues and cells of the body.*

The Left-Side Pump

Similar to the right side, the left-side pump consists of the left atrium and the thick-walled left ventricle. The left-side pump works to deliver the freshly oxygenated blood that has been returned to the heart from the lungs to every cell in the human body. As the powerful left ventricle contracts, blood is ejected into the arterial system. *Any compromise in left ventricular contraction can reduce the amount of blood ejected into the arterial system and cause an increase in pulmonary vessel hydrostatic pressure, leading to a reduction in the amount of oxygenated blood for distribution to the tissues and cells of the body.*

The Cardiac Output

With each contraction of the heart, blood is ejected into the circulatory system. The quantity of blood that the heart ejects with each contraction is commonly referred to as *stroke volume*. The stroke volume is very dependent on *preload* (blood available from the right side of the heart), *afterload* (pressure against which the heart must eject the blood), and *contractility* (the muscular contraction of the ventricles). If preload is inadequate, the stroke volume will decrease. Similarly, a significantly elevated afterload will also decrease stroke volume in that it is more difficult for the heart to eject blood against high pressure.

Contractility depends on preload to fill and stretch the ventricular muscle fibers. Myocardial muscle fibers are elastic, and after incoming preload sufficiently stretches them, a mechanical stimulus causes the muscle fibers to "snap" back to original size. This is the action that provides the mechanism of contraction. The principle of this action is referred to as *Starling's Law* which states that the greater the stretching of the myocardium (to a certain point) the more forceful the subsequent contraction will be. With this in mind, it is easy to understand how an inadequate preload, and resulting inadequate stretching of the myocardial fibers, can cause a significant decrease in stroke volume.

The amount of blood pumped in one minute is referred to as the *cardiac output*. Cardiac output is dependent on both stroke volume and heart rate. In equation form:

$$\text{Cardiac Output} = \text{Stroke Volume} \times \text{Heart Rate}$$

Heart rate and stroke volume can interact in a variety of ways to determine cardiac output. If the stroke volume remains constant while the heart rate increases, the overall cardiac output will rise. However, if the stroke volume is compromised, an increase in heart rate will not result in increased cardiac output. This is a danger with paroxysmal supraventricular tachycardia (PSVT). Conversely, a bradycardic rhythm with no increase in stroke volume will result in a decreased cardiac output. And, even if the stroke volume increases, the slow heart rate will prevent it from effecting an optimal cardiac output. The interplay between stroke volume, heart rate, and cardiac output is summarized on the next page.

Unacceptable cardiac output must be examined in terms of the heart rate plus preload, contractility, and afterload (the latter three being the factors that affect stroke volume). If you know which factor or factors are at fault, you can determine which interventions are most likely to restore an adequate cardiac output.

The nervous system varies cardiac output to meet the ever-changing demands of the body. With all parameters functioning normally, the heart is able to supply a cardiac output that is in balance with the needs of every tissue

Stroke Volume/Heart Rate Changes	Cardiac Output Result
Increased stroke volume with an increased or unchanged heart rate	Increased
Increased heart rate with an increased or unchanged stroke volume	Increased
Increased stroke volume with a decreased heart rate	Unchanged
Decreased stroke volume with an increased heart rate	Unchanged
Decreased stroke volume with a decreased or unchanged heart rate	Decreased
Decreased heart rate with a decreased or unchanged stroke volume	Decreased

and cell. If a greater amount of blood is needed to provide oxygen and waste removal, the stroke volume and heart rate can be increased so as to increase the cardiac output. The reverse happens during times of rest when the cells do not require much oxygen and waste removal.

Optimal cardiac output is essential for the perfusion of the myocardium. If the cardiac output falls to dangerously low levels, the availability of oxygenated blood to the myocardial cells themselves also decreases. This represents a serious situation, in that the heart must sustain a certain level of arterial perfusion in order to continue to function as a pump.

It is important to emphasize that *myocardial workload and oxygen requirements are directly proportional to the status of the preload, contractility, afterload, and heart rate.* As these factors increase, so do the myocardial workload and oxygen demand. Conversely, the diminishment of these variables results in a heart that consumes less oxygen because it is working less.

As you might assume, *alteration in the heart's ability to pump blood is a distinct possibility in the setting of an acute MI.* Because intervention varies in relation to the presentation of the infarct, it is critical that the clinician have a commanding knowledge of the heart's role as a pumping mechanism and the many variables that affect cardiac output.

Pathophysiology of an AMI

A myocardial infarction must be viewed as a *continuing process* that starts when the heart cells are deprived of oxygen. In order to power the electrical and mechanical actions that permit the heart to pump blood, the myocardial cells must receive an uninterrupted supply of oxygenated blood. In the absence of oxygen, the affected heart cells will become *ischemic* and eventually undergo detrimental changes that promote cellular *injury*. If the provision of oxygen is still not resumed, the injured cells will eventually die and be replaced by nonfunctional scar tissue. This cellular death is termed *infarction*.

The damage inflicted by the acute MI typically arranges into three distinct regions (Figure 8-2). From the center to the outside, these regions are:

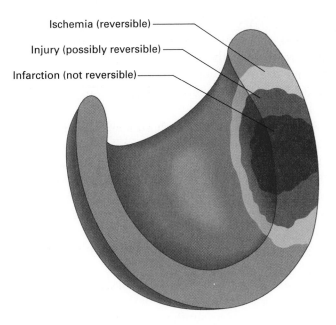

Ischemia (reversible)

Injury (possibly reversible)

Infarction (not reversible)

FIGURE 8-2 A myocardial infarction typically has three distinct regions.

- Infarcted tissue
- Injured tissue
- Ischemic tissue

The center of the infarct consists of the actually infarcted (dead) tissue. Since this tissue is nonfunctional, *electrical conduction and active depolarization do not occur*. If the infarct is of significant size, the decrease in active wall motion can seriously impair the ability of the heart to effectively pump blood.

Encircling the infarcted tissue is a ring of injured (but not yet dead) heart cells, which is immediately surrounded by a ring of ischemic heart cells (oxygen-deprived, but not yet injured). The ischemic and injured cells have the potential to *aberrantly conduct electrical impulses*. Electrical aberrancy can result in the production of *lethal* and *nonlethal dysrhythmias*. Additionally, *myocardial ischemia produces pain*. This explains the retrosternal chest pain that is frequently experienced during an acute myocardial infarction. Restoring oxygen to the ischemic cells can reverse ischemia and effectively alleviate the discomfort.

Myocardial ischemia is reversible! This is a critical concept to remember when managing the acute MI. Quick restoration of oxygen to the ischemic heart cells can halt the process of injury and infarction, thus not only alleviating ischemic pain but also preventing further damage.

With injured cardiac cells, reversal of the detrimental changes is extremely time dependent. If addressed in a timely fashion, the injury process can effectively be stopped and possibly even reversed. If a significant delay in reoxygenation occurs, the injury will become permanent and possibly result in cellular infarction.

Unfortunately, once the heart cells infarct, their function cannot be restored.

Myocardial infarction occurs secondary to an *insufficient supply of oxygenated blood* for the demanding myocardial cells. Most frequently, this inadequacy is precipitated by coronary artery disease. As the deposition of atherosclerotic plaque narrows the lumen of the coronary arteries, the amount of blood that can pass through the arteries is diminished. In addition, the atherosclerotic surface is covered with plaque, which is rough and prone to the formation of a blood clot, or *thrombus,* that can cause total occlusion with subsequent infarction.

Total occlusion can also occur secondary to a sudden rupture of the plaque, which creates a raw surface upon which a thrombus can form. Again, if the preexisting narrowing is sufficient, the thrombus can generate a total occlusion that deprives any distal cell of necessary oxygen. From this point on, the process of myocardial infarction begins.

In addition to atherosclerosis, an acute MI can be precipitated by a sudden spasm of a coronary artery. Such spasm is often an effect of cocaine or unstable angina. Other causes of infarction include microemboli, severe hypotension, and hypoxemia from acute respiratory failure.

The size and location of an infarct are directly related to the specific coronary artery that has been affected. Recall that the left side of the heart is supplied by the left coronary artery, left circumflex artery, and left anterior descending coronary artery (Figure 8-3). If one of these arteries becomes occluded, an infarct is likely to occur somewhere in the left ventricle. The more proximal the occlusion, the greater the potential damage, in that more cells beyond the occlusion are now deprived of oxygen. Because pumping blood throughout the body is harder work than pumping blood to the lungs, the left ventricle is larger and more muscular than the right ventricle. Due to its size and workload, the left ventricle is frequently the site for an acute MI.

Similarly, the right coronary artery perfuses the right side of the heart—including the inferior and posterior regions of the myocardium. If the right coronary artery or one of its branches becomes occluded, an infarct must be suspected within the right ventricular region, possibly including the inferior wall of the left myocardium. The right ventricle is affected less often than the left ventricle (Figure 8-3).

An unchecked myocardial infarction can inflict varying degrees of damage to the myocardium. This damage can extend through the entire thickness of the heart wall (*transmural*) or only affect a partial depth of muscle (*subendocardial*). Usually the innermost portion of the heart is affected first.

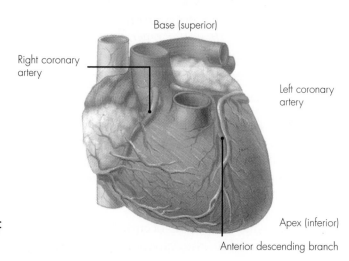

FIGURE 8-3 The coronary vessels of the heart.

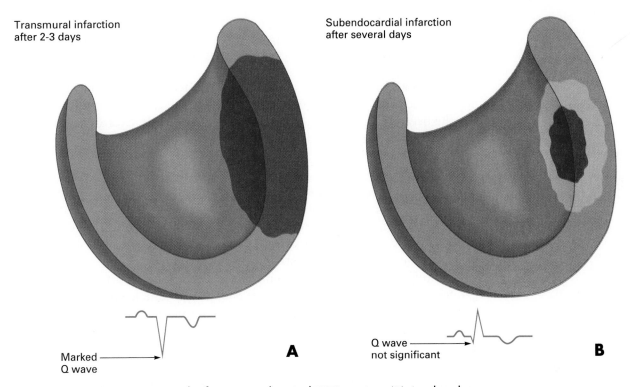

Transmural infarction
after 2-3 days

Subendocardial infarction
after several days

Marked
Q wave

A

Q wave
not significant

B

FIGURE 8-4 (A) A transmural infarction and typical ECG tracing. (B) A subendocardial infarction and typical ECG tracing.

The two types of infarct can be readily differentiated through examination of the ECG tracing. The more serious transmural infarction is identifiable by changes in the normal Q wave. If no changes in the Q wave are observed, but existence of an acute MI is otherwise confirmed, a subendocardial infarction is likely (Figures 8-4 a and 8-4 b).

Myocardial infarction is a devastating event that can produce two basic complications:

- **Abnormal electrical conduction.** *Abnormal electrical conduction arising from the ischemic and injured myocardial tissues can produce lethal and nonlethal dysrhythmias.* This electrical aberrancy indicates serious underlying problems with the myocardium. *Most deaths associated with an acute MI occur secondary to electrical instability.*

  During the early hours of infarction, *ventricular fibrillation* is the most common life-threatening dysrhythmia. Other rhythms, such as bradycardia or PVCs, warn of underlying abnormalities that may lead to an immediate life threat if not addressed. Death from electrical dysrhythmias, when it occurs within 1 hour of the onset of cardiac symptoms, is termed sudden death.

- **Mechanical pumping failure.** *Mechanical pumping failure secondary to the loss of effective depolarization and contractility is another danger that accompanies the acute MI.* Extensive infarction can result in significant myocardial wall damage. Infarcted tissue is nonfunctional and does not actively participate in contraction, thus decreasing overall pumping effectiveness and cardiac output. Also, infarcted tissue is weak and has the potential for the formation of aneurysms. If conditions are right, these aneurysms contain the inherent risk of ventricular wall rupture.

All in all, dysrhythmias and the loss of effective contraction can compromise the heart's ability to provide an adequate cardiac output that satisfies the needs of all tissues and cells within the body. If severe, the net result can be disability and even death.

Who Is at Risk?

Many risk factors greatly enhance one's chance of incurring a heart attack. As previously suggested, coronary artery disease is a frontline contributor to the increased incidence of myocardial infarction. While everyone has the potential for coronary artery disease, some individuals are more prone than others to the development of atherosclerotic arteries.

Many risk factors are unchangeable. These include genetics, age, and gender. Conversely, many factors are changeable and, when modified, can significantly reduce the risk of myocardial infarction. When combined with coronary heart disease, these factors place an increased workload on the heart—a workload for which it is not built! These modifiable risks include physical inactivity, obesity, and diets high in fat and cholesterol.

Awareness of nonmodifiable and modifiable risk factors, with relevant and appropriate life-style modification, remains the best way of preventing an acute myocardial infarction.

General Presentation of an Acute Myocardial Infarction

An acute MI can manifest itself with a variety of signs and symptoms. The specific signs and symptoms depend on the *size* and *location* of the infarct and the response of the body to ischemic pain, dysrhythmias, and possible compromise in ventricular pumping ability.

Chest Pain

Chest pain, the most common complaint in the acute myocardial infarction, can occur at rest, or with physical exertion, or as a result of emotional stress. As discussed earlier, chest pain originates from ischemic tissues. Frequently, this pain is described as "oppressive" or "crushing" and is typically located behind the lower half of the sternum.

Often, chest pain from an acute MI crescendos in intensity and can radiate to the shoulders, jaw, neck, arms, or back. However, radiation is not a constant. An MI can occur without this pain pattern. Also, myocardial ischemic pain will sometimes locate in the epigastric region, often with the unfortunate result of being dismissed as indigestion. As discussed later in this chapter, some acute MIs are painless.

Respirations

There are dramatic variations in respiratory presentation relating to factors such as pain, anxiety, electrical dysrhythmias, and pump problems. While a small infarct may result in no respiratory deficit, a large infarct of the left ventricle may cause signs of hypoxia and laborious breathing as blood backs up behind the left ventricle, engorges the pulmonary capillaries, and impairs the diffusion of oxygen at the alveolar-capillary membrane.

Edema

If there is a major pump problem, the retention of blood and disturbance of lymphatic fluid drainage may be observable in different regions of the body. Severe right-side pump failure will cause the backup of blood from the right ventricle into the body itself. Engorged neck veins, distended abdomen, pedal edema, and edema to the lower back of bed-confined patients are all indications of inadequate right-ventricle pumping. These signs may also be evident with a left ventricular failure that has caused right ventricular impairment through the massive backup of blood through the lungs into the right ventricle itself.

Skin Characteristics

Any patient who has cool, clammy skin and is complaining of chest pain must be thoroughly examined! In the presence of an acute MI, skin of either presentation (cool or clammy or both) suggests *hypoperfusion* and activation of the *sympathetic nervous system*. The sympathetic nervous system brings about an increase in heart rate and blood pressure which forces a weak heart to work harder. Therefore, the sympathetic influence upon an infarcting heart is detrimental.

Other Signs and Symptoms

A variety of other complaints may be noted when evaluating a patient with an acute MI. Such complaints can include anxiety, weakness, general malaise, nausea, vomiting, and syncope.

It must be reiterated that an acute myocardial infarction can present with a variety of signs and symptoms. Generally, the presentation is determined by the size and location of the infarct. *Ironically, some individuals suffering an acute MI may complain only of shortness of breath or a vague uneasiness without accompanying pain!* Diabetics and the elderly are more prone to this unique presentation because of nerve degeneration and a lowered ability to perceive pain. *In addition, some patients may have no complaints and suffer what is termed a "silent" MI.* Totally asymptomatic, a silent MI can only be diagnosed by observing delayed ECG changes or characteristic cardiac enzyme elevations.

Regardless of the severity or mildness of outward appearances, it must be recognized that all myocardial infarctions destroy valuable heart tissue and can produce immediate or delayed compromises in normal heart activity. Therefore, anyone with a suspected acute MI or chest pain of probable cardiac origin must be promptly examined and a definitive diagnosis made. This includes any individual with a history of angina who experiences chest pain that is unrelieved by rest and nitroglycerin or who experiences a sudden change in the pattern or duration or severity of the episodes of anginal chest pain.

Assessment of the AMI Patient

Physical examination of the patient with an acute MI focuses on the heart and its ability to pump blood. Recall that during a myocardial infarction the heart is prone to serious electrical dysrhythmias and contractile failure—both of which can adversely affect cardiac output. While not every acute MI will produce a dysrhythmia or pumping failure, the potential does exist and must be taken seriously. In consequence, a targeted assessment of the heart's electrical and hemodynamic capabilities must be rapidly initiated and completed within 7 to 10 minutes.

General Presentation

Initial evaluation focuses on the *general presentation* of the patient. Through rapid observation, an impression of the patient's current problem and level of distress can be quickly developed. Patients suffering an acute MI rarely thrash about but choose to remain still. However, keep in mind that cerebral hypoxia secondary to an inadequate cardiac output can result in a combative, confused patient. Also, pump failure tends to force patients into a sitting position, since the supine position enhances blood return to the heart and forces the strained myocardium to work harder to pump this blood.

The ABCs

Following a quick observation, *the airway, respiratory, and circulatory status* of the cardiac patient must be evaluated.

Airway

If the airway appears obstructed, rapid correction of the obstruction is necessary. Correction can occur, as indicated, through positioning, suctioning, placement of an oropharyngeal airway, or placement of an endotracheal tube. Because an infarct occurs secondary to myocardial hypoxia, it is paramount that the airway provide an unobstructed conduit for delivery of oxygen into the lungs.

Breathing

A rapid but thorough evaluation of the respiratory status is crucial. In addition to observing rate and effort, it is necessary to perform a comprehensive auscultation of all lung fields. As stated earlier a left ventricular pump problem, and consequent inability to eject blood from the ventricle, will cause an increase in the hydrostatic pressure in the pulmonary capillaries, which will result in rales and/or wheezing.

Clear lung sounds could indicate a myocardial infarction without pumping complications, or may suggest only right ventricular involvement. (Recall that right ventricular compromise will promote the accumulation of blood in the venous system, not in the lungs.) A pulse oximeter will be useful in determining the status of oxygen delivery to the tissues.

Circulation

The pumping ability of the heart can quickly be determined by palpating peripheral pulses. In states of low cardiac output, the radial and pedal pulses may be weak or not present at all. Strong distal pulses indicate a heart that is pumping and circulating blood well. Electrical dysrhythmias may cause the pulse to be irregular, fast, or slow. Finally, heart tones and the auscultation of carotid bruits can contribute valuable information as to the current status of the myocardium.

If a pump problem is suspected, *effective management is dependent upon identifying and treating the cause.* If inadequate cardiac output and hypoperfusion result from ventricular failure without dysrhythmias, the ventricle at fault must be identified.

Left Ventricular Failure   As previously discussed, a failing left ventricle can cause unejected blood to pool in the pulmonary capillaries. Depending on the severity of the left ventricular dysfunction, respiratory distress with rales and wheezing may be noted upon auscultation. In addition to dyspnea, severe failure of the left ventricle can bring about a profound decrease in cardiac output.

Right Ventricular Failure   A decrease in the efficiency of the right ventricle causes the backup of blood in the dependent areas of the body, accompanied by relatively clear lung sounds. Again, depending on the severity, failure of the right ventricle to deliver blood through the lungs to the left ventricle can also precipitate a dramatic decrease in cardiac output.

Occasionally, left ventricular failure can provoke right ventricular failure. As blood backs up through the pulmonary circulation and into the right ventricle, there will be signs of right-side failure along with pulmonary congestion.

Vital Signs

Vital signs are not reliable in the diagnosis of an acute myocardial infarction. Depending on the infarct location and severity and the nervous system response, the presenting vital signs can vary tremendously. A sympathetic response can result in a rapid heart rate, but if the parasympathetic response predominates, the result can be a bradycardic rate. Also, dysrhythmias may cause an irregular heart rate.

Blood pressure measurements can also vary. Hypotension in the presence of an acute MI is an ominous sign, suggesting that a significant decrease in cardiac output or profound parasympathetic tone now exists.

In spite of the wide variations in vital signs that can accompany an acute MI, it is important that the examiner monitor the vital signs and view them as valuable clues that can aid in determining the location of damage and the appropriate treatment.

ECG Tracings

In the acute myocardial infarction, electrical dysrhythmias originating from ischemic and injured tissues are a common complication. These dysrhythmias can prove unstable and life threatening. Of particular concern is ventricular fibrillation, which is an immediate life threat and the primary cause of cardiac arrest in the infarcting patient. *Ventricular fibrillation may occur suddenly, with no warning whatsoever.* If treated immediately with defibrillatory shocks, ventricular fibrillation is a correctable rhythm.

While not immediately life-threatening, other dysrhythmias such as PVCs and bradycardia may be a warning of underlying abnormalities. Such warning dysrhythmias must be heeded and the underlying abnormality identified and corrected. *If underlying disturbances are ignored, warning dysrhythmias can swiftly degenerate into lethal dysrhythmias with rapidly ensuing death!*

In the setting of an acute MI, electrical monitoring of the heart is paramount. Effective pumping is dependent on solid electrical conduction. Electrical monitoring of the heart is accomplished with an electrocardiograph monitoring device.

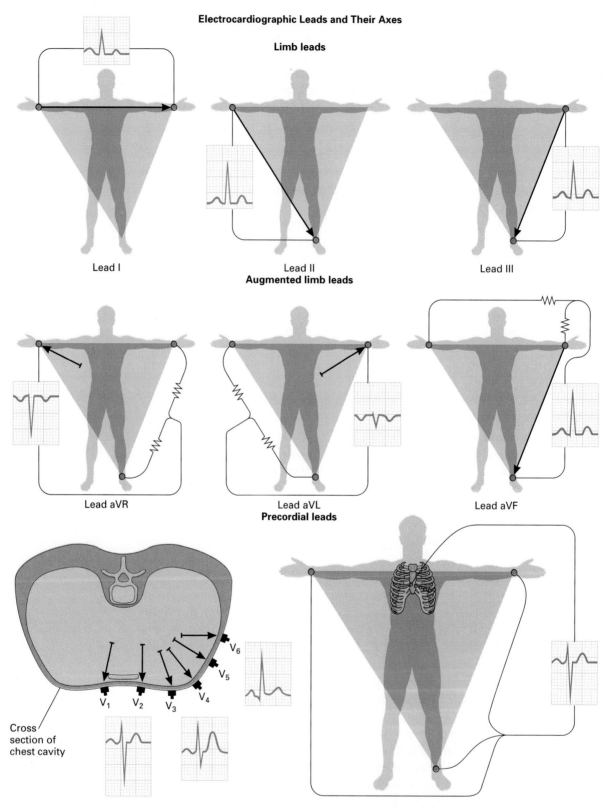

Electrocardiographic Leads and Their Axes

Limb leads

Lead I   Lead II   Lead III

Augmented limb leads

Lead aVR   Lead aVL   Lead aVF

Precordial leads

V_1 V_2 V_3 V_4 V_5 V_6

Cross section of chest cavity

When current flows toward arrowheads (axes), upward deflection occurs in ECG
When current flows away from arrowheads (axes), downward deflection occurs in ECG
When current flows perpendicular to arrows (axes), no deflection occurs

FIGURE 8-5 12-lead placement and views of the heart.

While the 3-lead ECG machine adequately illustrates the heart's rate and rhythm, the 12-lead ECG monitor provides a more comprehensive picture of the myocardium during an acute infarction. The 12-lead machine reveals 12 distinct views of the myocardium and can isolate areas of ischemia, injury, and actual infarction (Figure 8-5).

On the 12-lead ECG tracing, ischemia is illustrated by *symmetrically inverted T waves and/or ST segment depression.* Cells incurring injury exhibit an *elevation of the ST segment of more than 1 mm in height.* As stated earlier, infarcted tissue is exhibited by the presence of a *pathologic Q wave* (Figure 8-6). For a relative diagnosis, these changes must be viewed in two or more contiguous leads. This is a general description, and exceptions do apply to certain leads.

It must be remembered that ischemic and injured myocardial cells show the above-mentioned changes immediately, while the pathologic Q waves that define infarction take hours to days for development. Up to 20% of initial ECGs are normal on patients later found to have acute MI. *Therefore, the emergency health care provider must suspect an acute MI on the basis of a compatible history and ECG changes indicative of ischemia and injury.* If the clinician were to remain passive and attempt to discount an MI by the absence of the pathologic Q waves, a fatal mistake could be made.

Table 8-1 correlates the site of infarction and coronary artery with the leads that view them.

Often, the acute MI knows no boundaries. In such cases, infarcts are not exclusive to the anterior wall or lateral wall. Rather, infarcts can cover multiple areas such as the anterolateral or anteroseptal.

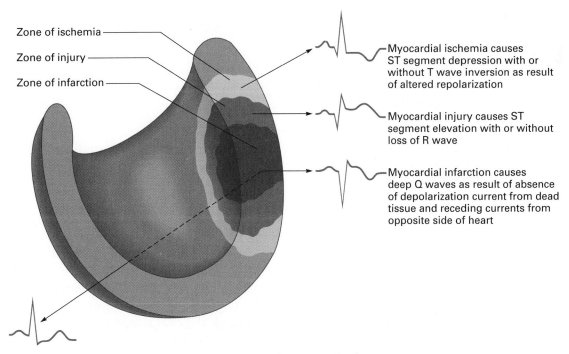

FIGURE 8-6 ECG changes reflecting ischemia, injury, and infarction.

TABLE 8-1 CORRELATION OF INFARCTION SITES AND LEADS

Site	Leads	Coronary Artery Affected
1. Anterior wall	V_1 to V_4	Left coronary artery or left anterior descending artery
2. Inferior wall	II, III, aVF	Right coronary artery
3. Right ventricle	II, III, aVF, right precordial V_{4R}	Right coronary artery
4. Lateral wall	I, aVL, V_5, V_6	Left circumflex artery

History

In addition to the physical exam, a targeted history should be rapidly attained. While suspicion of an acute infarction is based on the patient's symptoms and ECG tracings, a targeted cardiac history can reinforce this suspicion and provide a further guide for specific management.

A cardiac history should focus on the onset, nature, and duration of symptoms associated with the current emergency as well as previous cardiac history. Any symptoms that may potentially pertain to the physiological actions of the heart should be discussed. Questions should address the presence and location of chest pain, radiation of pain, shortness of breath, orthopnea (difficulty breathing if not in an upright position), diaphoresis, syncope, weakness, and so forth. The examiner should also establish the patient's actions at the time of onset, past medical history, and a list of all medications used within the last 6 months.

If the history reinforces suspicion of an acute MI, the interviewer should attempt to determine the patient's eligibility for thrombolytic therapy. This information centers on:

- History of trauma, surgery, or bleeding
- History of CVA within the last 6 months
- Pregnancy
- Any bleeding problems

See the discussion of indications and contraindications to thrombolytic therapy later in this chapter under "Management of the Uncomplicated AMI," subsection "Thrombolytic Therapy."

Conclusions

Suspicion of an acute myocardial infarction is based on a compilation of the information obtained through the patient presentation, clinical evaluation, and supportive history. The definitive diagnosis of an acute myocardial infarction is made upon serum enzyme changes and the development of pathologic Q wave changes. In that pathologic Q waves are not immediate, presumption is further reinforced through the characteristic changes noted with ischemia and injury. *However, let the clinician beware: Even if all aspects of the physical and electrical exam appear unremarkable, an individual still may be actively infarcting!*

Management of AMI: Prehospital, Emergency Department, and Hospital Considerations

The location and size of an acute myocardial infarction will determine the manner in which it outwardly presents. The acute MI can present with a variety of signs and symptoms indicating complications such as (but not limited to) dysrhythmias, pump failure, or absolutely no complications other than chest pain.

For instance, an infarct of the anterior left ventricle will present differently than an infarct of the posterior right ventricle. Along the same lines, an occlusion high in the left coronary artery will affect the heart differently than an occlusion low in the left anterior descending artery. Regardless of size and location, any infarct represents a serious situation in which early and aggressive intervention must be deployed.

The following discussion outlines the management essentials for an acute MI, followed by additional information identifying specific steps and interventions that should be taken by health care providers as the patient moves from the prehospital environment to the hospital's cardiac care unit.

Halting the process of infarction is the overriding goal in the emergency management of the acute MI. This can be achieved through several different interventions that must be tailored to the particular presentation. Essentially, these interventions work toward the following goals:

- Alleviation of pain and apprehension
- Prevention and management of dysrhythmias
- Limitation of the infarct size
- Initiation of thrombolytic therapy

All of these serve to reduce the cardiac workload and myocardial oxygen consumption, ward off electrical or mechanical complications, and protect the healthy myocardium from greater infarct. The underlying purpose of all these interventions is to protect and preserve as much of the heart as is possible, thus enabling it to continue functioning to the best of its ability.

Alleviation of Pain and Apprehension

Pain and apprehension stimulate sympathetic nervous innervation. Sympathetic innervation results in high production of *catecholamines* which increase the preload, contractility, afterload, and heart rate. *Consequently, the heart works harder to pump blood and increases its demand for oxygen, which is already in short supply.* The alleviation of pain and apprehension serve to decrease the level of circulating catecholamines and their detrimental effects on the ailing myocardium. Through a decrease in preload, contractility, afterload, and heart rate, the workload and oxygen consumption of the heart decrease, thus reducing potential ischemic damage and irreversible infarct.

Prevention and Management of Dysrhythmias

Electrical dysrhythmias must be evaluated and addressed. Warning dysrhythmias must be rectified before they degenerate into harder-to-manage potentially lethal dysrhythmias. Dysrhythmias represent aberrant conduction and abnormal stimulation of the heart that can promote an inadequate cardiac output.

Limiting the Size of the Infarction

Remember, rapid management of ischemic and injured tissue can halt the progression of a myocardial infarction. If successful, this prevents greater heart involvement and reduces the chances of detrimental complication. The concept of myocardial salvaging can significantly decrease the morbidity and mortality that may be inflicted by an acute MI.

Initiation of Thrombolytic Therapy

Thrombolytics have revolutionized the treatment of the acute MI. They dissolve blood clots and thus serve to reopen occluded arteries and reoxygenate the ischemic and injured tissue. As the injured myocardium is reperfused, there is an improvement in left ventricular function resulting in higher perfusion pressures. As coronary perfusion is improved, the overall size of the infarct is limited and the remaining myocardium protected. *Early initiation is paramount to the overall success of the treatment, as thrombolysis is extremely time dependent.*

Management of Specific AMI Presentations

Because the myocardial infarction can present in a variety of ways, treatment of the acute MI is quite variable. Therefore, management of the AMI will be discussed in terms of the following presentations:

- The AMI without complication
- The AMI with dysrhythmias
- The AMI with hemodynamic alteration

The following guidelines are recommended for those health care providers (paramedics, nurses, physicians, and others) who care for patients presenting with an actual or suspected myocardial infarction. The guidelines have been developed by a consortium of professional entities that include the American College of Cardiology and the American Heart Association, based on the best currently available medical information, research, and technology. These recommendations have been endorsed by the American Society of Echocardiography, the American College of Emergency Physicians, and the American Association of Critical-Care Nurses. The recommendations are incorporated into the discussion in this chapter. They are briefly summarized in Table 8-2 and presented in a more complete summary in the Appendix.[1]

The management of the acute MI begins with a brief, targeted history and thorough assessment that is geared toward the cardiovascular and associated systems. If an MI is suspected, management must be decisive and expedient. The acute myocardial infarction algorithm (Figure 8-7) outlines the treatment of the uncomplicated myocardial infarction and represents a basis on which all other presentations of a heart attack are managed. Keep in

[1]The guidelines for management of patients with myocardial infarction recommended by the American College of Cardiology and the American Heart Association—discussed in this chapter—have been published in: Ryan TJ, Anderon JL, Antman EM, Braniff BA, Brooks NH, Califf RM, Hillis LD, Hiratzka LF, Rapaport E, Riegel BJ, Russell RO, Smith EE III, Weaver WD. ACC/AHA guidelines for the management of patients with acute myocardial infarction: a report of the American College of Cardiology/American Heart Association Task Force on Practice Guidelines (Committee on Management of Acute Myocardial Infarction). *J Am Coll Cardiol.* 1996: 28; 1328-1428.

TABLE 8-2 SUMMARY OF RECOMMENDED GUIDELINES FOR THE MANAGEMENT OF MYOCARDIAL INFARCTION

Prehospital Issues	
Class I	1. 911 access 2. EMS service education on identifying, triaging, and initiating treatment for ischemic-chest-pain patients
Class IIa	1. First responder defibrillation 2. Community education on MI recognition, EMS access, and medications
Class IIb	1. 12-lead telemetry 2. Prehospital thrombolysis with >90 minutes transport time
Emergency Department Management	
Class I	1. MI protocol designed to identify the MI patient and obtain a 12-lead ECG within 10 minutes of arrival and deliver thrombolytics within 30 minutes of arrival 2. Routine measures to include: oxygen, intravenous nitroglycerin, thrombolysis, eligibility for primary PTCA, and specific pharmacological management of concurrent dysrhythmias
Hospital Management	
Class I	1. Continual ECG monitoring for reocclusion 2. Management of recurrent chest discomfort 3. Avoidance of Valsalva, bed rest 4. Hemodynamic monitoring as appropriate 5. Intra-aortic balloon counterpulsation as needed 6. Continued management of concurrent rhythm disturbances 7. Consideration for surgical interventions
Class IIb	1. Routine use of anxiolytics
Class III	1. Prolonged bed rest in uncomplicated MI patients

mind that not every intervention in the algorithm may be applicable to the particular MI at hand; therefore, each AMI must be considered individually.

Management of the Uncomplicated AMI
An uncomplicated AMI is one that presents without any electrical dysrhythmias or hemodynamic alteration. The following section discusses components of the AHA guidelines for management of the acute myocardial infarction as outlined in the AMI algorithm (Figure 8-7).

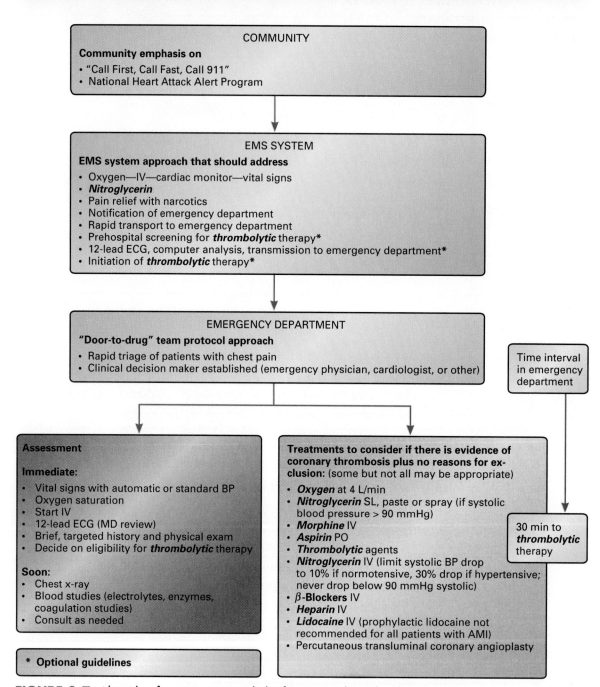

ALGORITHM: ACUTE MYOCARDIAL INFARCTION

COMMUNITY

Community emphasis on
- "Call First, Call Fast, Call 911"
- National Heart Attack Alert Program

EMS SYSTEM

EMS system approach that should address
- Oxygen—IV—cardiac monitor—vital signs
- *Nitroglycerin*
- Pain relief with narcotics
- Notification of emergency department
- Rapid transport to emergency department
- Prehospital screening for *thrombolytic* therapy*
- 12-lead ECG, computer analysis, transmission to emergency department*
- Initiation of *thrombolytic* therapy*

EMERGENCY DEPARTMENT

"Door-to-drug" team protocol approach
- Rapid triage of patients with chest pain
- Clinical decision maker established (emergency physician, cardiologist, or other)

Time interval in emergency department

Assessment

Immediate:
- Vital signs with automatic or standard BP
- Oxygen saturation
- Start IV
- 12-lead ECG (MD review)
- Brief, targeted history and physical exam
- Decide on eligibility for *thrombolytic* therapy

Soon:
- Chest x-ray
- Blood studies (electrolytes, enzymes, coagulation studies)
- Consult as needed

Treatments to consider if there is evidence of coronary thrombosis plus no reasons for exclusion: (some but not all may be appropriate)
- *Oxygen* at 4 L/min
- *Nitroglycerin* SL, paste or spray (if systolic blood pressure > 90 mmHg)
- *Morphine* IV
- *Aspirin* PO
- *Thrombolytic* agents
- *Nitroglycerin* IV (limit systolic BP drop to 10% if normotensive, 30% drop if hypertensive; never drop below 90 mmHg systolic)
- *β-Blockers* IV
- *Heparin* IV
- *Lidocaine* IV (prophylactic lidocaine not recommended for all patients with AMI)
- Percutaneous transluminal coronary angioplasty

30 min to *thrombolytic* therapy

* Optional guidelines

FIGURE 8-7 Algorithm for acute myocardial infarction. Adapted with permission. Journal of the American Medical Association, October 28, 1992, Volume 268, No. 16, *Guidelines for Cardiopulmonary Resuscitation and Emergency Cardiac Care*, p. 2230. ©1992 American Medical Association.

Oxygen

Oxygen is the most important and most effective drug in the treatment of the acute myocardial infarction! As such, it is considered to be a Class I intervention for symptomatic chest pain, and IIa with an uncomplicated MI during the first 2 to 3 hours. Because the infarcting myocardium is starving for oxygen, the administration of supplemental oxygen helps to relieve the discomfort of ischemic pain and limit the progression of the infarction.

Simply stated, oxygen must be given to any patient in whom an AMI is suspected. Even in the absence of dysrhythmias or other complications, supplemental oxygen must be provided.

Oxygen is administered in enough quantity to maintain an arterial saturation of >97%. This may be possible via a low-flow volume of 4–6 liters per minute through a nasal cannula, or by way of a nonrebreathing face mask utilizing a volume of 10–15 liters per minute. Any existing hypoxemia must be reversed. In the setting of an AMI, there are no immediate dangers in the utilization of oxygen.

A pulse oximeter provides invaluable feedback on the effectiveness of oxygen therapy and avoids arterial puncture, which may be contraindicated with the use of thrombolytics.

Intravenous Access

Due to the potential need for pharmacologic and fluid therapy, intravenous access in the myocardial infarction patient must be promptly established. Optimally, a large bore catheter should be placed in an arm/vein.

Concerning IV access in the AMI patient, several points are worthy of discussion. First, intravenous cannulation is painful and can promote anxiety and the release of catecholamines. Recall that catecholamines can induce a heart to work harder, thus encouraging the process of infarction. This is exactly the process that you are trying to prevent! So IV access must be established quickly and without multiple attempts.

Because of the anticoagulatory effects of drugs such as aspirin, heparin, and thrombolytics, any injury to the vein, which can cause hematoma or infiltration, must be avoided. Along the same lines, central access into noncompressible veins such as the subclavian is frowned on due to the potential complication of vascular bleeding and difficulty in controlling possible hemorrhage in this area.

While obtaining IV access, it is prudent to obtain blood samples for electrolyte, enzyme, and coagulation studies. However, do not delay further treatment while awaiting the results of these studies.

Electrocardiograph Monitoring

Since most early deaths associated with an acute myocardial infarction occur secondary to electrical disturbance, rapid application of the cardiac monitor is necessary. Dysrhythmias can present at any time and must be promptly evaluated. Even if they are not immediately life threatening, remember that such electrical disturbances can quickly degenerate into lethal dysrhythmias. Additionally, keep in mind that an individual suffering an acute MI is most prone to ventricular fibrillation during the first hour following the onset of cardiac symptoms. Successful conversion of ventricular fibrillation into a viable rhythm is time dependent. If the cardiac monitor/defibrillator is already in place, delays in identification and defibrillation are avoided. So as

IV initiation is considered standard treatment, so is ECG monitoring. It should be initiated early in the prehospital environment (if possible) and continued during the patient's movement through the Emergency Department and subsequent CCU and step down units.

As discussed earlier, a 12-lead cardiac monitor is optimal for the identification and location of ischemia, injury, and infarct. If a 12-lead machine is unavailable, a 3-lead monitor can supply the basic rate and rhythm information. *Remember, however, that a normal ECG tracing by itself does not preclude the presence of an AMI!* 12-lead ECG monitoring is recommended as a IIb intervention in the out-of-hospital environment; however upon arrival at the Emergency Department, acquisition of a 12-lead ECG is of paramount importance in the process of identifying the MI patient with acute ischemic-type chest pain.

Chest X-ray

As soon as is possible, a chest x-ray should be obtained. The chest x-ray may help to rule out other causes of chest pain that may mimic a myocardial infarction. Such conditions include cardiac tamponade, aortic dissection, and pulmonary embolism.

Nitroglycerin

Nitroglycerin is an effective drug in the management of an acute myocardial infarction. Nitroglycerin works to promote *venous dilation*. As a result, the veins retain a greater volume of blood and decrease preload. The decrease in arterial wall tension also lowers afterload. *These outcomes effectively decrease the myocardial workload and oxygen utilization.* Additionally, nitroglycerin may dilate coronary arteries and promote collateral circulation. This action allows for *the flow of blood into regions of the heart originally deprived of oxygen.* In accomplishing all this, *nitroglycerin assists in the alleviation of ischemic pain, stabilization of an electrically unstable myocardium, and limitation of infarct extension.*

Nitroglycerin should be given as a Class I intervention to any patient with ischemic-type chest pain. Caution should be exercised when considering nitroglycerin for a patient with a systolic pressure under 90 mmHg or a heart rate less than 50 or greater than 100 beats per minute. Nitroglycerin can be administered through a variety of routes in a variety of dosages, as outlined in Table 8-3.

TABLE 8-3 NITROGLYCERIN ADMINISTRATION	
Routes	**Dosages**
Sublingual pill	0.3–0.4 mg every 5 minutes
Sublingual spray	1 spray every 5 minutes
Topical paste	1–2 inches
IV infusion	10–20 µg per minute. Increase 5–10 µg per minute every 5-10 minutes.

Because it causes vasodilation, nitroglycerin must be used with extreme caution in any patient who actively exhibits hypotension. In this situation, a single tablet of nitroglycerin may be tried with caution if IV access for judicious fluid administration has been established. Since right ventricular infarcts typically present with hypotension, the administration of nitroglycerin must be used with particular caution in the presence of suspected right ventricular infarction. Nitroglycerin administration should be avoided if the patient declares sensitivity to the drug.

As stated, nitroglycerin can significantly lower the overall blood pressure. While in many cases this is beneficial, it must be emphasized that too drastic a pressure decrease can be detrimental. A sudden drop in blood pressure can induce syncope, bradycardia, reflex tachycardia, or even cardiac arrest as coronary artery perfusion bottoms out in relation to a decreasing diastolic pressure. IV infusion allows for the most control of the drug. An IV line should be initiated prior to oral administration, ready for prompt measures to counteract side effects.

If any of the above occur, volume expansion should accompany the normal ACLS procedures for any dysrhythmia. Furthermore, the patient must be placed supine with the legs elevated to enhance blood return to the heart and increase coronary artery perfusion. Pressor therapy (which acts to relieve the symptom of hypotension) should be avoided unless and until fluid volume expansion (which addresses the underlying problem) proves ineffective.

For the above reasons, remember that nitroglycerin should be used with extreme caution in the hypotensive patient. Additionally, after the blood pressure of a normotensive patient has sustained a mean drop of 10%, or a hypertensive patient has sustained a mean drop of 30%, continued administration should be carefully scrutinized.

Morphine Sulfate

Morphine sulfate is another agent that can be used in the management of the acute myocardial infarction. Similar to nitroglycerin, morphine sulfate decreases preload and afterload through the *dilation of the venous and arterial systems*, thus decreasing myocardial workload, alleviating ischemic chest pain, and limiting the overall progression of the infarct. In addition to the hemodynamic alterations, morphine also acts on the brain to produce an *analgesic effect*. Pain perception is decreased, in turn reducing the stress and anxiety that promote the release of harmful endogenous catecholamines.

Like nitroglycerin, morphine can be considered for the anxious acute MI patient complaining of continuing chest pain. Morphine should be discontinued if hypotension ensues and the systolic blood pressure drops below 90 mmHg. If hypersensitivity exists, morphine should be avoided.

Morphine is administered via IV in dosage increments of 1–3 mg. These dosages can be repeated as often as every 5 minutes until total pain alleviation has been accomplished. The total dosage of morphine must be evaluated in reference to a stable blood pressure. Additionally, since morphine can depress the respiratory center in the medulla, the patient's breathing must be monitored continuously.

A drastic reduction in preload and afterload can precipitate a decrease in cardiac output and dangerous hypotension, as with nitroglycerin. Again, the provider must be observant for a sudden drop in blood pressure and the dangerous manifestations of this drop. Should such a decrease bring about syncope, shock, bradycardia, reflex tachycardia, or cardiac arrest, judicious fluid therapy should accompany the normal ACLS protocol for the presenting dysrhythmias. The supine position with elevated legs should be implemented. Pressor agents should be avoided until it is obvious that the fluid challenge is ineffective.

If the administration of morphine sulfate results in dangerous hypoventilation, positive pressure ventilation is necessary. In severe cases of respiratory depression, *naloxone* (Narcan) can be given in 0.4–0.8 mg dosages.

It is important to remember that morphine sulfate should not be used by itself, but in conjunction with nitroglycerin, oxygen, and other appropriate interventions in the acute myocardial infarction.

Aspirin

Aspirin is becoming a prominent agent in emergent and long-term management of the acute myocardial infarction and is considered a Class I therapeutic intervention for known acute MI or suspected ischemic-type chest pain. Studies indicate the administration of aspirin in the setting of an AMI has achieved significant reduction in mortality comparable to some thrombolytic agents. Economically, aspirin is the most cost-effective therapy available.

Through a complex series of actions, aspirin functions as an antiplatelet factor that decreases the coagulation potential of the blood. This makes thrombus formation less likely in arteries with pre-existing occlusion. Even though the arteries are compromised, delivery of oxygenated blood to the myocardium can continue and help to limit ischemic pain and infarct size.

Aspirin should be given as soon as possible! Any patient with a presentation suggestive of an acute MI should receive aspirin, barring a declared hypersensitivity. Relative contraindications to the application of aspirin are actively bleeding ulcers or asthmatic conditions.

Aspirin should be given by mouth at a suggested dosage range of 160–325 mg. As always, avoid any oral tablet administration in the patient with a severely decreased level of consciousness to prevent possible airway occlusion and/or aspiration.

Platelet inhibition can lead to bleeding complications. As discussed earlier, carefully weigh the potential benefits against potential complications of administering aspirin to a patient with actively bleeding ulcers or a history of asthma.

Thrombolytic Therapy

Thrombolytic therapy has revolutionized the effective treatment of acute myocardial infarction occurring secondary to a thrombus-blocked artery.

Thrombolytic agents act to quickly dissolve an occluding blood clot and reopen a pathway through which the myocardium can receive vitally needed oxygenated blood. Subsequent reperfusion delivers oxygen to ischemic tissues and halts the infarction process. As a result, the overall size of the infarction can be limited and portions of the susceptible myocardium salvaged.

Thrombolytic eligibility determination and administration should occur as soon as possible! As "time is muscle," the maximum thrombolytic benefit appears to be achieved if the thrombolytic is administered within 6 hours of onset of symptoms (optimally within 30–60 minutes), although definite benefit is still seen in patients who receive the therapy within the first 12 hours of infarction. Thrombolysis is now known to be beneficial to most patients, irrespective of the individual's age, past medical history, or gender. However, some increased risks (e.g., intracranial hemorrhage) have been identified in those patients who are over 65 years of age, weigh less than 70 kg, display systolic hypertension, or receive tissue plasminogen activator.

Thrombolytics should be administered to a patient with objective evidence that indicates infarction, especially those suffering a transmural MI. Definitive diagnosis of an AMI is dependent on characteristic enzyme changes and the development of pathologic Q waves. As discussed earlier, the development of pathologic Q waves can lag hours to days behind the actual death of cardiac tissue. Additionally, ascertainment of laboratory results may require time. The progression of infarction is not considerate of such delays and continues right along at a rapid pace. Therefore, *thrombolytics may be administered as a Class I intervention on the presumption of infarction.* This presumption can be made upon ECG changes indicating injury (ST elevation) with a compatible history. The presumption of an MI can also be made if the patient displays evidence of a new bundle branch block (common to left anterior descending arterial occlusion) with a compatible history.

Several contraindications exist to the administration of thrombolytics. These contraindications all revolve around the potential for serious hemorrhage, as the human body's compensatory clotting mechanism is temporarily disabled by the thrombolytic. As listed by the AHA, absolute contraindications to thrombolytic therapy are:

- Active internal bleeding
- Suspected aortic aneurysm
- Known CPR trauma such as rib fractures or pneumothorax or a traumatic endotracheal intubation
- Severe persistent hypertension despite pain relief and initial drugs:
  systolic >180 mmHg
  diastolic >110 mmHg
- Recent head trauma or known intracranial tumor (neoplasm)
- History of CVA in past 6 months
- Pregnancy

Relative contraindications, in which the practitioner must use extreme discretion in the administration of thrombolytics, are:

- Recent trauma or major surgery in the past 2 months
- Initial blood pressure of >180 mmHg systolic and/or >110 mmHg diastolic that is controlled via medical treatment
- Active bleeding ulcers
- History of CVA, tumor, injury, or brain surgery
- Known bleeding disorder or use of wafarin (Coumadin)
- Significant liver or kidney dysfunction
- Previous use of the thrombolytic agents streptokinase or anistreplase within the past 12 months
- Known cancer or illness with possible thoracic, abdominal, or intracranial abnormalities
- Prolonged CPR efforts

TABLE 8-4 THROMBOLYTICS ADMINISTRATION

Thrombolytic Agent	Regimen
anistreplase	30 U IV over 2–5 minutes
alteplase	100 mg IV (60 mg in first hour—6–10 mg IV push initially—then 20 mg/hour over the next 2 hours) Note: An accelerated regimen* is used by some clinicians, as follows: • Give 15 mg IV bolus • Then 0.75 mg/kg over next 30 minutes (not to exceed 50 mg) • Then 0.50 mg/kg over next 60 minutes (not to exceed 35 mg) Total dose < 100 mg
streptokinase	1.5 million U in a 1-hour infusion
urokinase	1.5 million U IV over 2 minutes, then 1.5 million U IV over 90 minutes*

* FDA approval pending

Currently, several thrombolytic agents exist and are given intravenously. These agents and their dosage regimens are listed in Table 8-4.

It is important to remember that ventricular fibrillation can occur during the administration of thrombolytics! Refer to Chapter 7 for a detailed discussion of thrombolytics.

Heparin

Heparin is an anticoagulant that has no lytic effect on existing clots. Often heparin is used in conjunction with certain thrombolytic agents or by itself after thrombolysis has occurred.

Even after thrombolytics effectively dissolve an occlusive clot, a rough atherosclerotic surface remains. This surface provides an opportunity for the reformation of a thrombus with subsequent reocclusion. Through its anticoagulant properties, heparin works to prevent the recurrence of thrombus formation and provides for the maintenance of a patent coronary artery.

Also, in the setting of post-thrombolytic therapy, pieces of the thrombus may break off and be transported by the blood, only to lodge (as emboli) elsewhere in the body. Consequently, complications such as CVA and/or further infarct can arise. Heparin appears to decrease the incidence of such complications.

Among clinicians, there appears to be some controversy concerning the administration of heparin. However, heparin is considered a Class I indication for patients undergoing percutaneous or surgical revascularization, and a Class II intervention when administered with thrombolytics. Finally, it is a Class III intervention for routine IV use within 6 hours to patients receiving a nonselective fibrinolytic agent, who are not at a high risk for systemic embolism.

In the presence of active bleeding, severe hypotension, recent intracranial surgery, or bleeding tendencies, heparin is contraindicated for the same

TABLE 8-5 HEPARIN ADMINISTRATION	
AHA-Recommended Options	**Dosing Regimen**
Option 1: Administer heparin simultaneously with the thrombolytic agent. Option 2: Administer heparin on completion of a thrombolytic infusion. Option 3: Administer heparin empirically in patients with large anterior AMIs without thrombolytics.	• Bolus IV: 5000 U (Other regimens such as 100-150 U/kg are also acceptable.) • Continue: 1000 U/hour for 24-48 hours.

reason as are thrombolytics. The administration and dosing regimen for heparin are summarized in Table 8-5.

Beta Blockers

Beta blockers inhibit the uptake of catecholamines at the myocardial beta receptors. As a consequence, circulating catecholamines are prevented from increasing the heart's rate, contractility, and electrical excitability, in turn preventing adverse effects on workload and myocardial consumption of oxygen, ischemic pain, and ultimately infarct size. For these reasons, the administration of beta blockers can be considered a Class I intervention for the management of recurrent chest discomfort unresponsive to initial therapy.

Despite thrombolytic therapy, ischemic and injured tissues can continue to degenerate into dead tissue because of ongoing myocardial work. The administration of long-term beta blockers attempts to stop this process by chronically inhibiting the workload of the heart. In the presence of an MI, beta blockers also appear to decrease the incidence and mortality of ventricular fibrillation.

Beta blockers should be considered for any patient suffering an acute MI with excessive adrenergic activity. This activity includes an elevated heart rate or hypertension.

Because of their ability to reduce the activity of the heart, beta blockers are contraindicated in hypotension, congestive heart failure, and bradycardia. Recall that the bronchi and bronchioles are susceptible to beta stimulation and rely on this influence for relaxation. For this reason, beta blockers are contraindicated with any asthmatic or bronchospasmodic disposition.

Although many approaches are acceptable, the regimens of beta blockers commonly used are summarized in Table 8-6.

The administration of beta blockers in the setting of an AMI can be dangerous and must be used with judicious caution. By nature, beta blockers induce myocardial depression and therefore require constant observation. Always monitor for symptomatic bradycardic dysrhythmias.

The reduction in electrical excitability, heart rate, and contractility can adversely affect the stroke volume and cardiac output. Consequently,

TABLE 8-6 BETA BLOCKERS ADMINISTRATION

Beta Blocker	Regimen
metoprolol	5 mg IV infusion every 5 minutes to a total of 15 mg
atenolol	5 mg infusion over 5 minutes. Wait 10 minutes and give second dose of 5 mg over the course of 5 minutes.
propranolol	1 mg IV every 5 minutes to a total dose of 5 mg

a balance between decreased cardiac workload and optimal cardiac output must be found. Beta blockers are often continued 1 to 2 years after infarct.

Magnesium Sulfate

There is increased interest in a prominent role for magnesium sulfate in the management of the acute myocardial infarction. Magnesium deficiency has been associated with dysrhythmias and sudden death in the infarcting patient. Although the exact mechanisms are unknown, magnesium has been found to deter dysrhythmias and stabilize electrical activity in the myocardium. Additionally, magnesium sulfate exhibits vasodilatory properties, thus reducing preload and afterload and decreasing myocardial workloads.

Magnesium sulfate should be administered as a Class IIa intervention to any AMI patient with a known or suspected deficiency in magnesium. Magnesium deficiencies commonly occur in alcoholics, in patients on diuretics, or in those with poor dietary intake. Routine prophylactic administration of magnesium may possibly be helpful but has not yet been proven effective and, therefore, remains controversial (Class IIb). The regimen for magnesium sulfate is summarized in Table 8-7.

Even though magnesium sulfate is a generally safe drug that can be given quickly in a large quantity, some side effects may present. These include hypotension, drowsiness, and diaphoresis.

Percutaneous Transluminal Coronary Angioplasty (PTCA)

PTCA is a method of clearing an atherosclerotic-narrowed artery by mechanical means. A long catheter is inserted through a peripheral artery (usually brachial or femoral) and threaded through the aorta into the involved coronary artery. A balloon at the distal end of the catheter is inflated and deflated many times to flatten the atherosclerotic accumulation against

TABLE 8-7 MAGNESIUM SULFATE ADMINISTRATION

Indications	Regimen
Acute myocardial infarction	1–2 g diluted in 100 ml of normal saline. Infusion over 5–60 minutes, followed by maintenance infusion of 0.5–1.0 g/hour for up to the next 24 hours

the vessel wall. The net result is an opened coronary artery and reperfusion of an oxygen-deprived myocardial region.

PTCA addresses the underlying cause of the myocardial infarction, the atherosclerotic-narrowed coronary artery. Where thrombolytics will rectify a thrombogenic occlusion by dissolving the clot, PTCA opens the occluded artery by mechanically widening the lumen.

Individuals suffering an AMI for which thrombolytic therapy is contraindicated, or who don't respond to thrombolytic agents, are candidates for PTCA. Also, PTCA has shown positive results for those afflicted with cardiogenic shock or acute pump failure. Further, PTCA is indicated for those with occluded vein grafts from coronary artery bypass graft surgery.

PTCA must be performed by a specialist in the catheterization laboratory and is a Class I intervention when an alternative to thrombolytic therapy is needed. It assumes a class IIa rating when a patient is a candidate for reperfusion but has a risk of bleeding.

Individual Considerations

The ACLS algorithm as described earlier (and shown in Figure 8-7) stands as a general outline of interventions that should be considered in the emergent management of the acute myocardial infarction. Keep in mind, however, that consideration for the listed items should be done on an individual basis, with application tailored to the individual suffering the acute myocardial infarction.

Management of AMI Complicated by Dysrhythmia

Short of unstable dysrhythmias or cardiac arrest, the algorithm for acute myocardial infarction, as described above, also finds application to the acute myocardial infarction complicated by electrical dysrhythmia. Often, an electrical disturbance secondary to an acute MI serves to warn of extensive ischemia or serious underlying abnormalities such as acid-base imbalance, hypocalcemia, hypokalemia, or hypomagnesemia. Hence, these dysrhythmias are termed *warning dysrhythmias* and warrant immediate attention.

Frequently, warning dysrhythmias are rectified through application of the guidelines as described earlier. Among others, this includes the administration of oxygen, nitroglycerin, morphine, thrombolytics, and beta blockers. Therefore, prior to pharmacologic therapy specific to the dysrhythmia, these and other standard AMI treatment measures should be attempted with their effectiveness constantly evaluated. If the dysrhythmias persist despite these measures, standard therapy specific to the dysrhythmia should be considered.

An unstable rhythm or cardiac arrest requires immediate intervention —*regardless of the presence of an acute myocardial infarction*. The following section contains information that pertains to the management of the common dysrhythmias that occur secondary to an acute MI. As always, *treat the patient, not the monitor!*

The ACLS standard treatment algorithms for all of the dysrhythmias discussed below will be examined in detail in Chapter 10.

AMI and PVCs

When PVCs occur during an active infarction, it is essential to determine the cause. Often, PVCs in the setting of an acute MI occur secondary to an underlying abnormality. Underlying causes may include poor oxygenation, hypotension, electrolyte abnormalities, acid-base imbalances, high state of catecholamine stimulation, and others. It is up to the clinician to identify the cause and correct it, which should correct the PVCs as well.

In the presence of PVCs, examine the status of adequate oxygenation, efforts at pain relief, and the administration of nitroglycerin, morphine, and beta blockers. If PVCs are associated with a bradycardic rhythm, it is likely that the premature ventricular beats are escape beats and can be corrected by addressing the bradycardic rhythm itself.

Treatment with lidocaine (see Chapter 7 for the dosing regimen) should be considered if the PVCs persist despite the above measures or if they satisfy one or more of the following criteria:

- Six or more PVCs per minute
- PVCs that are closely coupled
- PVCs that fall on the preceding T wave (R-on-T phenomenon)
- PVCs that occur in couplets or runs of three
- PVCs that are multiform

AMI and Ventricular Dysrhythmias

Ventricular fibrillation must be promptly defibrillated. If ventricular fibrillation occurs in the presence of an acute MI, defibrillation should be conducted immediately. The incidence of ventricular fibrillation is highest during the first hour following the onset of myocardial infarction and continues over the next 48 hours. Ventricular fibrillation can be described as one of two types:

- *Primary ventricular fibrillation* occurs as a result of a problem with the heart itself. An example is aberrant conduction related to the ischemic and injured myocardial tissues.
- *Secondary ventricular fibrillation* typically occurs because of a problem elsewhere in the body. Among others, hypovolemia and pH disturbances are possible causes of secondary ventricular fibrillation. Because the underlying cause is external to the heart, secondary ventricular fibrillation is more difficult to correct. Successful treatment often relies on addressing the underlying abnormality.

Ventricular fibrillation is a potentially convertable rhythm, and prompt defibrillation carries a high incidence of conversion. Ventricular tachycardia often deteriorates into ventricular fibrillation and, therefore, must also be treated promptly. The clinician must first determine whether the ventricular tachycardia is stable, unstable, or pulseless and manage it accordingly.

AMI and Bradycardia

Bradycardia commonly accompanies an acute MI and is quite prevalent during the first hour of infarct. This slow rhythm often occurs in response to an increased parasympathetic influence and is frequently associated with an inferior- or posterior-wall MI. Bradycardia can present with a variety of underlying rhythms, including sinus bradycardia, junctional escape rhythms, and an assortment of different heart blocks.

Management of sinus bradycardia in the presence of an AMI represents a tricky issue. A slow rate can cause a decrease in cardiac output and produce insufficient peripheral and coronary artery perfusion. Consequently, the infarct can be worsened and cardiac arrest may result.

Conversely, a slow heart rate may exert a protective effect by slowing down the heart. From this perspective, the heart is intrinsically limiting ischemia and injury through a self-initiated decrease in workload and oxygen demand.

Any bradycardia that occurs secondary to an AMI should not be treated with pharmacologic therapy unless it is symptomatic and produces signs of hypoperfusion. As always, the provider should assure adequate oxygenation and pain relief in the attempt to limit the infarct progression.

AMI and Tachycardia

An acute MI with associated tachycardia is a signal that something else is occurring! Often, tachycardia is the physiologic response to stress, anxiety, heart failure, or hypovolemia. Tachycardia is a dangerous rhythm that must be immediately addressed, for the accelerated rhythm stands to worsen an overall infarct by *increasing the myocardial workload and overall oxygen consumption, leading to extensive myocardial damage.* Additionally, it is thought that excessive tachycardia lowers the threshold for the occurrence of ventricular fibrillation. As with PVCs, the key lies in the identification and treatment of the causal mechanism.

If sinus tachycardia, atrial flutter, atrial fibrillation, or atrial tachycardia is present, the clinician must ensure that effective oxygenation, pain control, and all other appropriate interventions of the myocardial algorithm have been correctly and adequately initiated. The use of beta blockers and morphine sulfate have special application with tachycardia.

Excessive tachycardia can lead to unstable conditions such as shortness of breath, pulmonary congestion, hypotension, increased chest pain, and shock. Tachycardias of this nature must be terminated immediately and are managed with synchronized electrical shock therapy and medications.

AMI and Conduction Blocks

An acute MI can present with a variety of conduction blocks. While some of these blocks require no more than careful observation, others are an ominous sign of extensive damage and require immediate and extensive intervention.

First Degree Conduction Block   A first degree conduction block requires little more than observation. The concern with a first degree block is the progression to a more serious block. If a first degree block is encountered, *careful observation* is necessary.

Second Degree Conduction Blocks   There are two types of second degree blocks. Second degree Type I block usually signifies an AV node block that is frequently caused by an enhanced vagal discharge. In the absence of symptomatic bradycardia and other symptoms, this block only requires *observation* for progression to a more serious block. If *symptomatic*, this block can be treated with a trial of atropine and the placement of a temporary pacemaker.

Second degree Type II block represents a very serious situation. This block signifies ischemia and damage to the myocardial conduction system. *With this block, there is significant risk for the transformation into a full heart block.* If encountered, a transvenous or transcutaneous pacemaker must be applied in anticipation of the progression to a third degree block.

Third Degree Conduction Block   A third degree heart block in an acute MI indicates extensive damage from the infarction. The only means of cardiac output comes from the ventricular escape rhythm. *Because this pacemaker is very unstable, a temporary pacemaker must be implemented as soon as possible.*

Intraventricular Block   If the intraventricular block is clinically significant, pacing and therapeutic management should be aggressively initiated. Pacing is a must in a right bundle branch block; however, authorities are unsure of its effectiveness in a left bundle branch block.

Management of AMI with Hemodynamic Alteration

Depending on the nervous system response or the contractile damage to the heart as a pump, variable hemodynamic states can accompany the acute myocardial infarction. The following section discusses the acute MI with hypertension and the acute MI with hypotension. As emphasized earlier, all interventions listed in the algorithm need to be evaluated for implementation on a one-by-one basis.

Keep in mind that hemodynamic alteration can occur in response to mechanisms that are not related to the MI. Such causes include massive pulmonary embolism, hypovolemic shock, septic shock, cardiac tamponade, and a dissecting aortic aneurysm.

AMI and Hypertension

During the process of myocardial infarction, a patient may present with hypertension, which can be typical for the patient or may signify an increased circulation of catecholamines secondary to pain and anxiety. *Regardless of its origin, hypertension (systolic >140 mmHg and/or diastolic > 90 mmHg) in the setting of an acute MI needs to be addressed.*

Because the heart must work harder to eject blood against an increased afterload, hypertension can produce an *increase in myocardial oxygen demand and result in an extension of the infarct.* For the same reasons, persistent hypertension can also harm the recovery of a weak heart. Further, hypertension in the setting of an acute infarction can precipitate wall rupture as the weakened tissue is subject to heightened stress from an increased effort to eject blood.

Many times, hypertension is transient; rest and reassurance along with the administration of supplemental oxygen, nitroglycerin, and morphine are enough to alleviate the release of catecholamines. If these measures prove ineffective in reducing the hypertension, or if the hypertension is severe, IV nitroglycerin (10–20 mg/min.) and beta blockers may be effective. If all of these measures fail, nitroprusside (0.1–5.0 µg/kg/min) can be administered.

AMI and Hypotension

Symptomatic hypotension in the presence of an acute myocardial infarction is an ominous sign. Hypotension indicates a decrease in cardiac output due to a decrease in stroke volume or a heart rate that is too slow or too rapid to permit adequate ventricular filling. *Symptomatic hypotension can result in hypoperfusion of the body tissues, including the heart itself. Without intervention, further damage or cardiac arrest can ensue.*

Hypotension associated with an acute MI can be of several origins. The etiology must be identified and corrected as is appropriate. (The algorithm in Figure 8-8 represents the current guidelines for treatment of acute pulmonary edema, hypotension, and shock.)

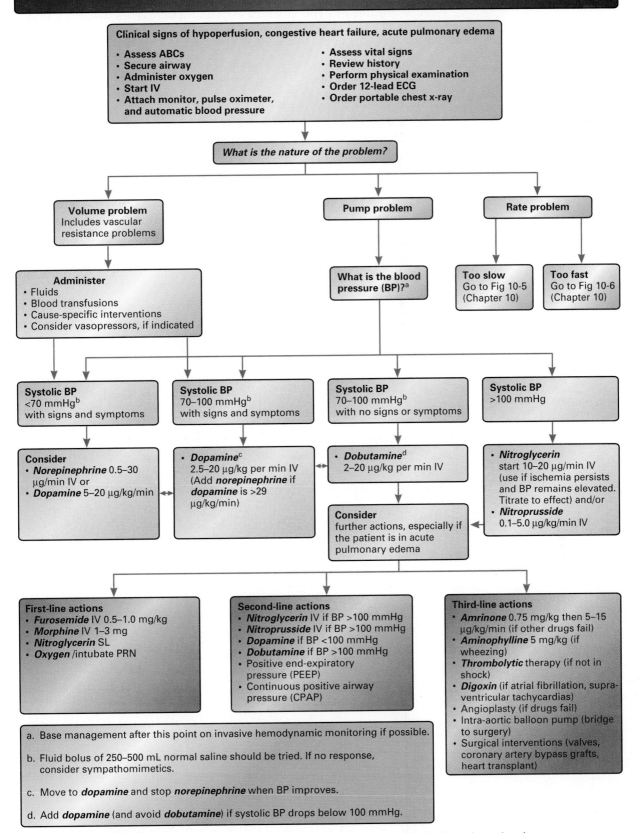

ALGORITHM: HYPOTENSION/SHOCK/ACUTE PULMONARY EDEMA

Clinical signs of hypoperfusion, congestive heart failure, acute pulmonary edema

- Assess ABCs
- Secure airway
- Administer oxygen
- Start IV
- Attach monitor, pulse oximeter, and automatic blood pressure

- Assess vital signs
- Review history
- Perform physical examination
- Order 12-lead ECG
- Order portable chest x-ray

What is the nature of the problem?

Volume problem
Includes vascular resistance problems

Pump problem

Rate problem

Administer
- Fluids
- Blood transfusions
- Cause-specific interventions
- Consider vasopressors, if indicated

What is the blood pressure (BP)?[a]

Too slow
Go to Fig 10-5 (Chapter 10)

Too fast
Go to Fig 10-6 (Chapter 10)

Systolic BP
<70 mmHg[b]
with signs and symptoms

Systolic BP
70–100 mmHg[b]
with signs and symptoms

Systolic BP
70–100 mmHg[b]
with no signs or symptoms

Systolic BP
>100 mmHg

Consider
- *Norepinephrine* 0.5–30 µg/min IV or
- *Dopamine* 5–20 µg/kg/min

- *Dopamine*[c] 2.5–20 µg/kg per min IV (Add *norepinephrine* if *dopamine* is >29 µg/kg/min)

- *Dobutamine*[d] 2–20 µg/kg per min IV

- *Nitroglycerin* start 10–20 µg/min IV (use if ischemia persists and BP remains elevated. Titrate to effect) and/or
- *Nitroprusside* 0.1–5.0 µg/kg/min IV

Consider
further actions, especially if the patient is in acute pulmonary edema

First-line actions
- *Furosemide* IV 0.5–1.0 mg/kg
- *Morphine* IV 1–3 mg
- *Nitroglycerin* SL
- *Oxygen* /intubate PRN

Second-line actions
- *Nitroglycerin* IV if BP >100 mmHg
- *Nitroprusside* IV if BP >100 mmHg
- *Dopamine* if BP <100 mmHg
- *Dobutamine* if BP >100 mmHg
- Positive end-expiratory pressure (PEEP)
- Continuous positive airway pressure (CPAP)

Third-line actions
- *Amrinone* 0.75 mg/kg then 5–15 µg/kg/min (if other drugs fail)
- *Aminophylline* 5 mg/kg (if wheezing)
- *Thrombolytic* therapy (if not in shock)
- *Digoxin* (if atrial fibrillation, supra-ventricular tachycardias)
- Angioplasty (if drugs fail)
- Intra-aortic balloon pump (bridge to surgery)
- Surgical interventions (valves, coronary artery bypass grafts, heart transplant)

a. Base management after this point on invasive hemodynamic monitoring if possible.

b. Fluid bolus of 250–500 mL normal saline should be tried. If no response, consider sympathomimetics.

c. Move to *dopamine* and stop *norepinephrine* when BP improves.

d. Add *dopamine* (and avoid *dobutamine*) if systolic BP drops below 100 mmHg.

FIGURE 8-8 Algorithm for acute pulmonary edema, hypotension, and shock. Adapted with permission. *Journal of the American Medical Association*, October 28, 1992, Volume 268, No. 16, *Guidelines for Cardiopulmonary Resuscitation and Emergency Cardiac Care*, p.2227. ©1992 American Medical Association.

Possible origins of hypotension associated with MI are discussed below.

Bradycardia As the heart rate is slow, the cardiac output has fallen. See the earlier section of this chapter, "AMI and Bradycardia," for the proper management of this condition.

Tachycardia As the heart rate is too rapid, adequate ventricular filling is discouraged. Consequently the cardiac output falls. See the earlier section of this chapter, "AMI and Tachycardia," for the proper management of this condition.

Left Ventricular Pump Failure Left ventricular pump failure occurs when a significant-sized infarct decreases the effective wall motion necessary for contraction. Through this complication, the heart is unable to eject an acceptable stroke volume. When left ventricular pump failure occurs, a decrease in cardiac output and/or pulmonary congestion ensue. Even though the patient is hypotensive, the cardiac output may still be able to meet the immediate demands of the body; but be aware of the potential for deterioration into cardiogenic shock, as discussed below.

Initial treatment of left ventricular failure focuses on aggressive airway control and oxygenation. If the heart rate is not the cause, treatment should center on enhancing systemic vascular resistance to increase the blood pressure. The suggested guidelines are outlined in Table 8-8. These approaches are dictated by blood pressure readings. The possible use of vasodilators and beta blockers must be carefully weighed in light of the patient's hypotensive state.

Cardiogenic Shock *When cardiac output is no longer adequate to perfuse the tissues of the body and the heart, cardiogenic shock must be suspected.* Cardiogenic shock will manifest itself with systemic hypotension and pulmonary edema. Cardiogenic shock results when more than 35% of the left ventricle has been destroyed by an infarct. The prognosis is poor, and the majority of patients do not survive.

Treatment originates with aggressive airway management and oxygenation. The treatment of cardiogenic shock is similar to the treatment of left ventricular failure. Dopamine and/or norepinephrine at the lowest effec-

---

TABLE 8-8 TREATMENT FOR AMI WITH HYPOTENSION (PUMP OR VOLUME PROBLEM)

Initial treatment for symptomatic hypotension in the presence of an AMI focuses on aggressive airway control and oxygenation. If there is a pump or volume problem (if heart rate is not the causal mechanism), treatment should center on vasoconstriction to increase the blood pressure, as follows:

Systolic Blood Pressure	Agent/Dosage	
<70 mmHg with signs of shock	Norepinephrine	0.5–30 µg/min
	Dopamine	5–20 µg/kg/min
70–100 mmHg with signs of shock	Dopamine	2.5–20 µg/kg/min
	Add norepinephrine if > 20 µg/kg/min	

tive dose is advised. Pulmonary edema secondary to cardiogenic shock should be treated as described under "AMI and Pulmonary Edema," below. Cardiogenic shock is an indication for advanced procedures such as PTCA and intra-aortic balloon pump catheterization.

Right Ventricular Pump Failure   In right ventricular failure, the right ventricle cannot eject blood into the pulmonary circulation. This results in a decreased volume available for the left ventricle to pump to the remainder of the body. Consequently, profound hypotension ensues with the associated danger of decreased systemic and coronary artery perfusion.

The key to treatment lies in the administration of fluids. Under *Starling's Law* of contractility, the more the ventricle is stretched, the more forceful the contraction will be. Therefore, if a greater preload is available to the right ventricle, the ventricle will eject more volume into the lungs, thus delivering a greater amount of blood to the left ventricle for systemic dispersement. Vasodilators should be strictly avoided, in that these will only serve to decrease preload and worsen the entire situation.

AMI and Pulmonary Edema
If the pumping ability of the left ventricle has been seriously impaired and blood backs up into the pulmonary vessels, as described earlier, the pressure increase can force serum and other fluids from within these vessels into the interstitial spaces and even into the alveoli. This series of events not only compromises cardiac output but also impairs the ability of the lungs to adequately oxygenate blood for delivery to the entire body.

In pulmonary edema, respiratory distress is accompanied by adventitious lung sounds (rales). Depending on how seriously the left ventricle has been damaged, and the degree to which the adrenergic nervous system has been stimulated, the clinician may note profound hypotension or adrenergically induced hypertension as the body attempts to compensate for this deficit. In severe cases, blood and other frothy material from the lungs can be seen at the patient's mouth and/or nose.

Emergency treatment of acute pulmonary edema revolves around decreasing the amount of blood that the impaired left ventricle must eject and the resistance against which it must pump. This will reduce the buildup in the pulmonary vessels and, in turn, reduce the pressure that forces the blood from the pulmonary vessels into the interstitial spaces and/or alveoli.

After sitting the patient upright and administering high flow oxygen, nitroglycerin is useful in increasing the venous capacitance and decreasing the amount of preload presented to the heart for pumping. Because of its similar action, morphine sulfate may also find application in this situation. Finally, if an increase in venous capacitance does not rectify the situation, the diuretic furosemide (Lasix) can be given at a dosage of 0.5–1.0 mg/kg via IV bolus to reduce pressure by stimulating the kidneys to excrete water. IV nitroglycerin, nitroprusside, or dopamine can be administered if the blood pressure is greater than 100 mmHg.

If the patient is hypotensive and vasodilators are not applicable, dobutamine can be utilized in an attempt to raise the overall blood pressure. Dobutamine administered at a dosage of 2–20 µg/kg/minute functions to increase the contractility of the heart with reflex decreases in systemic vascular resistance.

CASE STUDY FOLLOW-UP

You are working a lonely holiday-night shift at an urgent care center when Kathy Miller brings in her husband Steve who has been suffering chest pain for more than 24 hours and, as you talk with him, is becoming somewhat combative.

Assessment

Your initial assessment of Steve reveals a lethargic male patient with a cardiac history experiencing a possible myocardial infarction. Upon further investigation, you note obvious distention of the jugular veins accompanied by edema to the abdomen and feet. While the lung sounds are clear of any crepitance, you obtain a pulse oximetry reading of only 68%. Knowing that decisive action must be taken quickly, you prepare to treat the patient for a possible infarct of the right ventricle.

Treatment

Because of the important role oxygen plays in the treatment of chest pain, you quickly place Steve on 100% oxygen through a nonrebreather. While applying the cardiac monitor, you instruct your helper to initiate an IV of normal saline.

Once Steve is on the 12-lead cardiac monitor, you note a bradycardic rhythm at a rate of 48 beats per minute that includes unifocal PVCs at a rate of 12 per minute. The 12-lead ECG reveals ST segment elevation and Q wave changes to the right precordial lead.

Your helper asks if you want him to administer nitroglycerin for the chest pain or lidocaine hydrochloride for the PVCs. You instruct him not to, as the patient is already hypotensive and the PVCs are most likely escape beats resulting from the slow rhythm. Rather, you order a complete set of lab tests and a fluid bolus of 500cc of normal saline in an attempt to increase cardiac

As always, remember that ventilatory effort may need assistance with positive pressure ventilation so as to force fluid from the alveoli and increase the delivery of oxygen into the pulmonary fields.

SUMMARY

Acute coronary syndromes, mainly acute myocardial infarctions, are devastating events that claim many lives each year. Many of these deaths are unnecessary because both preventive practices and rapid treatment have led to improved outcomes.

Successful management of the acute MI hinges on an application of procedures tailored to the particular presentation of the infarction. Consequently, a strong working knowledge of the heart as a pump and the overall cardiovascular system is a must.

The fact that treatments exist for the acute MI is only half the battle. Individuals suffering an acute MI tend to wait 2 to 4 hours before seeking medical attention. "Time is muscle," and the success of many management techniques is extremely time dependent. These delays result in unnecessary disability and death.

It is the responsibility of the community at large to become educated in the prevention and recognition of infarction symptoms. General awareness and avoidance of modifiable risk factors, recognition of a heart attack, and training in CPR are just a few examples of how the myocardial infarction can be challenged in the community. Most important of all may be an understanding of the need to seek help promptly.

(continued)

output by raising the left ventricular filling pressure.

Additionally, you administer 1 mg of atropine and apply the transcutaneous cardiac pacer as a precaution. Within a minute, Steve's heart rate increases to 68 beats per minute with a blood pressure reading of 88 over 50 mm Hg. There is also a concomitant increase in his level of orientation and ability to respond. Quickly, you send the blood sample off for seratologic and enzyme analysis and notify a local ambulance for transport to a city hospital.

While waiting for the ambulance, you administer 325 mg of aspirin and complete a checklist for thrombolytic therapy. Steve appears eligible for thrombolytic therapy, and you include this information when you notify the receiving cardiologist over the telephone of the patient you are sending him. At this juncture, the ambulance arrives and quickly transports Steve to the awaiting facility.

The next evening, you get a call from Kathy Miller informing you that Steve successfully underwent thrombolytic therapy for a thrombus in the right coronary artery. She tells you that Steve is now on heparin and will be in the ICU for the next two weeks. The cardiologist has told them both that he expects Steve to make a full recovery but that he will have to modify his lifestyle if he is going to live to see his grandchildren get married!

Knowing that your actions were integral to Steve's successful outcome, you proceed into the break room with a large grin on your face. You are about to eat a large jelly-filled donut when it occurs to you that this may be part of the lifestyle that landed Steve in the hospital. You decide on an unbuttered bagel instead—and are just about to take the first bite when your coworker yells for you to come and assess a gentleman who has sustained a severe laceration to his left forearm.

Your work is never done....

Here the phrase *"dial first, dial fast, dial 911"* finds poignant application.

REVIEW QUESTIONS

1. Of the following situations, which would serve most to diminish the cardiac output?
   a. increased afterload with a decrease in preload
   b. increase in heart rate while stroke volume remains the same
   c. decrease in heart rate with an increase in stroke volume
   d. decrease in stroke volume with an increase in heart rate

2. A patient suffering an acute MI presents with systemic hypotension and lung sounds that are clear of any adventitious noises. Which of the following should be suspected by the health care professional?
   a. possible left ventricular failure
   b. possible right ventricular failure
   c. a left ventricular MI with right ventricular involvement
   d. an acute MI with no ventricular involvement

3. In which of the following situations will the myocardial oxygen demand be decreased the most?
   a. increase in afterload
   b. increase in preload
   c. decrease in afterload
   d. increase in contractility

4. You are administering oxygen to a patient with an acute MI. Which of the following is most likely to occur as a result?
   a. increase of activity in the infarct region
   b. restoration of function to all injured cells
   c. increase in myocardial workload
   d. improvement of function to ischemic tissue

5. Of the following patients, which could be said to be suffering the greatest infarct in terms of size?
   a. patient with occlusion in the left coronary artery
   b. patient with occlusion in the left descending coronary artery
   c. patient with blockage in the left circumflex artery
   d. patient with blockage of the left subclavian artery

6. In the acute MI, which of the following pathophysiological processes is responsible for the majority of deaths?
   a. myocardial wall rupture
   b. electrical instability in the infarcted tissue
   c. aberrant conduction through ischemic and injured tissue
   d. the formation of aneurysms on the left ventricle

7. When assessing a patient with a possible acute myocardial infarction, which of the following would most support the evaluation that an acute MI is occurring?
   a. the presence of chest pain
   b. ST elevation in leads V_4 and V_5
   c. a blood pressure of 90/66
   d. ST elevation in leads V_2 and V_5

8. A 53-year-old female patient has the chief complaint of shortness of breath. Upon questioning, she denies the presence of chest pain. On the cardiac monitor, you note a sinus rhythm of 88 beats per minute with ST elevation in leads V_3 and V_4. You would suspect
   a. the patient has COPD.
   b. the patient has an occlusion of the right coronary artery.
   c. no infarction is occurring because of the absence of chest pain.
   d. a possible anterior-wall infarction is occurring.

9. Of the following choices, which **definitively** indicates an acute myocardial infarction?
   a. patient with serum enzyme changes and pathologic Q waves
   b. patient with ST elevation in leads V_3 and V_5
   c. patient with shortness of breath and chest pain
   d. patient with symmetrically inverted T waves in leads V_5 and V_6

10. A 67-year-old male presents with crushing chest pain and is diaphoretic. Upon inspection, you note sinus bradycardia with ST elevation in lead V_{4R}, blood pressure of 94/70, and engorgement of the neck veins. Which of the following represents the **best** course of treatment for this patient?
    a. oxygen
    b. oxygen with nitroglycerin and morphine
    c. oxygen with a bolus of normal saline
    d. oxygen with nitroglycerin and beta blockers

11. A physician orders a bolus of heparin to a patient after thrombolytic therapy has been completed. The rationale for such a move is to
    a. keep opened artery patent.
    b. lower the returning preload.
    c. decrease myocardial workload.
    d. prevent active bleeding elsewhere in the body.

12. Which of the following choices represents the **most** prudent order of treatment for a hemodynamically stable MI patient presenting with 10 multifocal
PVCs per minute?
    a. lidocaine, oxygen, beta blockers
    b. oxygen, lidocaine, nitroglycerin
    c. lidocaine, oxygen, morphine
    d. oxygen, nitroglycerin, lidocaine if needed

13. A COPD patient is incurring a left ventricular infarction. The patient is
confused, diaphoretic, and displays a pulse oximeter reading of 87%.
Which of the following treatments would be most beneficial for the
patient?
    a. high flow oxygen delivered by a nonrebreather
    b. oxygen at 4 liters per minute delivered through a simple face mask
    c. low flow oxygen delivered through a nasal cannula
    d. withhold oxygen so as not to depress respiratory drive

14. After administering nitroglycerin to a chest pain patient, the patient's blood
pressure drops drastically, and she goes into pulseless electrical activity
(PEA). Your best course of action would be to
    a. place the patient supine with legs elevated and defibrillate.
    b. give large amounts of fluid while administering CPR.
    c. administer dopamine at 10 µg/kg/min.
    d. administer CPR only.

15. Of the following patients, which would be **most** eligible for thrombolytic
therapy?
    a. male with transmural infarct and BP 150/120
    b. female with transmural infarct and CVA 11 months ago
    c. male involved in car crash with right ventricular infarct and head injury
    d. female with left ventricular infarction and pregnant

16. Which of the following electrical disturbances represents the greatest life
threat to occur within the first hour post infarct?
    a. PEA   c. asystole
    b. ventricular tachycardia d. ventricular fibrillation

17. You are treating a severely lethargic patient in cardiogenic shock from a
massive left ventricular MI. Which of the following regimens best describes
the appropriate treatment of this patient?
    a. oxygen, dopamine, norepinephrine
    b. intubation, oxygen, nitroglycerin, dopamine
    c. oxygen, IV, cardiac monitor, nitroglycerin
    d. intubation, oxygen, dopamine, norepinephrine

18. Of the following cardiac drugs, which is the most important in the management of the acute myocardial infarction?
    a. nitroglycerin
    b. oxygen
    c. morphine sulfate
    d. beta blockers

19. You are treating a patient who complains of chest pain and exhibits respiratory distress with adventitious lung sounds heard on auscultation. As you examine the patient, you note a pink froth beginning to appear at the corners of her mouth. You note a systolic blood pressure of 140 mmHg. Which of the following represents the **best** choice for the initial treatment of this patient?
    a. oxygen at 15 lpm
    b. IV nitroglycerin
    c. furosemide
    d. nitroglycerin given by mouth

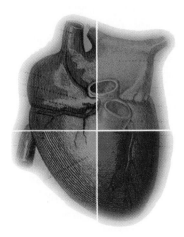

Acute Stroke

The emergency assessment and management of stroke has evolved drastically over the last several years. Previously, the stroke patient was basically provided supportive care and assessed for maximal neurologic deficit. However, management of the acute ischemic stroke, known today as a "brain attack," has taken on a new aggressive assessment approach and treatment plan in an attempt to reduce the neurologic deficit and disability associated with its incidence. Early and prompt recognition of the signs and symptoms of stroke, expeditious transport by EMS, and aggressive assessment and intervention by the emergency department physician and staff is paramount to reducing the morbidity and mortality of an acute ischemic stroke.

Topics to be covered in this chapter are:

- Acute Stroke and Transient Ischemic Attack (TIA)
- Initial Assessment of the Patient with an Acute Stroke or TIA
- Treatment Strategies for the Acute Stroke Patient

CASE STUDY

You are called to the scene for a 56-year-old male patient complaining of a sudden onset of weakness to one side of the body. As you arrive, you find the patient in the living room sitting in a recliner. His wife states that her husband, John, was relaxing and watching television when he began to complain that his right arm was getting numb. She noticed that his speech was slurred and his face appeared to be drooping. Having just recently read a pamphlet on the signs and symptoms of stroke, she recognized the urgency of his condition and immediately called 911 to access the EMS system.

You approach John as he explains, with slurred speech, that his arm is numb. You note a droop to the right side of the face. He is holding his right arm with his left hand while attempting to make gross motor movements. He is upset and frightened.

How would you proceed to assess and care for this patient? This chapter will describe the assessment and management of a patient suffering from an acute ischemic stroke. Later we will return to the case and apply the information learned.

Introduction

An acute stroke (or brain attack) is yet another cardiovascular emergency that, like a myocardial infarction (heart attack), can cause airway, breathing, and circulation compromises and, on occasion, cardiac arrest. It is the third leading cause of death behind cardiac disease and cancer, accounting for more than 150,000 deaths annually.

Acute Stroke and Transient Ischemic Attack (TIA)

The term *acute ischemic stroke* (sometimes called a cerebral vascular accident, or CVA) refers to an acute onset of signs and symptoms of stroke with evolving brain ischemia and injury. This is also termed a "brain attack" because, like a heart attack, it results in ischemia and injury that require immediate assessment and treatment in order to limit the amount of damage associated with the ischemic event—in this case damage to the brain. A *transient ischemic attack (TIA)*, has a similar etiology and presentation to a stroke, however, the signs and symptoms are temporary and the patient suffers no permanent neurologic dysfunction. It is, however, often the precursor to a full acute ischemic stroke.

Etiology of an Acute Stroke

Stroke is an emergency that arises when a blood vessel that perfuses the brain becomes occluded or ruptures. This disruption of blood flow results in ischemia and necrosis in the area of the brain perfused by that vessel. Ischemia of the brain tissue results in local edema as well as abnormal nerve function and transmission, which in turn causes characteristic signs and symptoms of a stroke. Ischemic strokes occur because of an occlusion, whereas, hemorrhagic strokes are due to a ruptured vessel. Thrombotic and embolic strokes are considered to be ischemic.

Causes of occlusive stroke include thrombus formation at the site of the infarct (usually at pre-existing atherosclerotic plaque), or thrombus formation in the heart or carotids which then embolizes into the cerebral vessels.

Emboli can also be formed from atherosclerotic plaques, cardiac valvular vegetations, air or other gases (e.g., nitrogen from diving accidents), amniotic fluid, tumors, or fat.

Hemorrhagic strokes result from subarachnoid hemorrhage (SAH) or intracerebral hemorrhage (ICH). SAH often occurs from a ruptured cerebral aneurysm, with the blood then filling the subarachnoid space and compressing adjacent brain tissue. ICH generally occurs from hypertensive bleeds (rupture of small vessels within the brain that have been damaged by long-standing hypertension), or from ruptured arteriovenous malformations (AVM).

Etiology of a Transient Ischemic Attack (TIA)

A transient ischemic attack (TIA) is thought to occur when there is a temporary disruption in cerebral blood flow. Once circulation is restored, symptoms resolve. The most common etiology is a small thromboembolus traveling through the cardiovascular system that becomes lodged in a cerebral blood vessel too small for it to pass through. A TIA is only temporary because the body is able to lyse, or dissolve, the clot causing the obstruction, or the thromboembolus will fragment into clinically insignificant microemboli and pass through to a more distal site, thereby returning normal perfusion and abating the signs and symptoms.

Although a TIA is a "temporary" emergency, it is extremely important for TIAs to be recognized. About one-third of all TIA patients experience a full acute ischemic stroke shortly after the initial event. Therefore, a TIA in the adult patient is considered to be a warning sign of an impending acute ischemic stroke.

Upon identification of a TIA, the patient should be carefully evaluated by a physician so that additional diagnostic tests can be completed to determine the likelihood of an acute ischemic stroke and preventive management initiated. If carotid atherosclerotic plaques are found to be the etiology of the TIA symptoms, there is also a strong possibility of coronary artery disease in the same patient, which also places that person at risk for future myocardial ischemic events.

Clinical Presentation of an Acute Stroke or TIA

Clinically, strokes of hemorrhagic etiology have some distinguishing characteristics from those of occlusive (ischemic) origins. A hemorrhagic stroke will typically be of abrupt onset (seconds), occur during stress or exertion, and rapidly progress to maximal deficit. Patients with severe hemorrhage may rapidly progress through a stuporous state to coma and death. If able to give a history, these patients will often describe a "pistol-shot headache," which is an abrupt-onset headache of maximal intensity. Other common symptoms include nausea and vomiting.

If subarachnoid hemorrhage (SAH) occurs, there may be no lateralizing features. The blood may distribute in the subarachnoid space leading to bilateral symptoms of compression and or herniation. These patients may have findings of nuchal rigidity (neck stiffness) or complain of neck pain. Conversely, intracerebral hemorrhage (ICH), which occurs in one of the cerebral hemispheres, does tend to show initial lateralizing findings. These findings persist until enough midline shift occurs to produce contralateral compression, coma, and herniation syndromes.

Acute ischemic strokes and TIAs may present as very insidious, nonspecific symptoms such as memory loss, auditory disturbances, vertigo, gait disturbances, or very focal weakness or paresthesias that go unreported or unrecognized by patients and their families. They may also present with more characteristic patterns of findings suggesting the vessel of origin.

Strokes or TIAs involving occlusion of the anterior circulation (carotid artery) typically present with weakness and numbness of the face and extremities on the opposite side of the body from the damaged cerebral cortex. If the dominant hemisphere is involved there may also be aphasia (speech impairment). If the posterior circulation (vertebro-basilar artery) is the occluded vessel, there may be bilateral findings such as facial numbness on one side of the body with contralateral weakness. Vertigo, bilateral blindness, ataxia (impaired muscular coordination) and general weakness are also possibilities as these vessels supply the cerebellum, occipital lobe, and brainstem (including cranial nerves). The Circle of Willis connects the two major blood supplies of the brain and, if intact, often limits the degree of damage done by the acute ischemic stroke.

Understanding what a stroke is, and knowing the common indicators, will help you identify the acute ischemic stroke or TIA early in its progression when treatment will be most beneficial. Early recognition is critical to successful management with minimal residual effects. There is a correlation between the length of time between onset of the acute ischemic stroke and successful treatment. The longer the stroke exists without proper management, the worse the prognosis and the overall severity of the emergency.

The signs and symptoms of an acute ischemic stroke and of a TIA are essentially the same, since both result from inadequate perfusion to an area of the brain. The difference is that the signs and symptoms seen during a TIA resolve spontaneously within 24 hours of onset. During the initial stages of a stroke or TIA, it is usually not feasible (nor absolutely necessary with regard to initial supportive management) to delineate between the two. Table 9-1 identifies some common signs and symptoms seen with an acute ischemic stroke or TIA.

An acute ischemic stroke or TIA should be suspected in any patient who has experienced a rapid onset of neurologic deficits or an alteration in mental status. The additional physical findings listed in Table 9-1 may exist alone or in combination with each other. As well, they may progressively worsen, wax and wane, or be maximally severe at onset.

Initial Assessment of the Patient with an Acute Stroke or TIA

As with any cardiovascular emergency, only a good patient assessment can lead to sound medical treatment. Even though acute cardiovascular decompensation is rare with strokes, oftentimes the health care provider will be faced with airway maintenance challenges, which do occur frequently in the acute ischemic stroke patient who is unresponsive.

Airway
In conjunction with initial airway management, remember to stabilize the spine if trauma is suspected. Remember, also, that the decreasing mental

TABLE 9-1 SIGNS AND SYMPTOMS OF ACUTE STROKE OR TIA

- Headache (possible severe, may be associated with neck pain/rigidity)

- Paralysis (usually hemiplegic)

- Paresis (weakness to one or more extremities)

- Ataxia (lack of coordinated muscle movement)

- Dysphagia (difficulty in swallowing)

- Aphasia (difficulty with speech due to brain impairment)

- Dysarthria (difficulty with speech due to impairment of the muscles of speech)

- Diplopia (double vision)

- Disturbances in sensory perception (in one or more parts of the body)

- Amaurosis fugax (temporary blindness due to thromboembolus in opthalmic artery)

- Vertigo (dizziness)

- Changes in cognition (anything from mild confusion to unresponsiveness)

- Loss of muscle tone to one side of the face, with paralysis to opposite extremities

- Possible seizures, incontinence, vomiting

status or unresponsiveness of the acute stroke patient may result in a loss of the patient's ability to protect his airway. The mandible will become relaxed and fall posteriorly while the person lies supine. As the mandible is displaced posteriorly, so are the muscles that support the tongue and epiglottis. This can lead to a partial or total obstruction as the tongue falls against the posterior wall of the hypopharynx and the epiglottis partially occludes the glottic opening. Another threat is the accumulation of saliva, blood, or vomitus in the hypopharynx. Thoroughly assess the airway and apply suction, if necessary, to remove any secretions, blood, vomitus, or foreign materials.

You may need to insert a simple mechanical device, such as an oropharyngeal airway in the absence of a gag reflex or a nasopharyngeal airway, to help keep the airway open while positive pressure ventilation is initiated. Eventually, any acute stroke patient in need of ventilatory support should be intubated, if necessary using a rapid sequence induction intubation technique (described later), and hyperventilated until proven not to have evidence of increased intracranial pressure (ICP) by CT scan.

Vital Signs
Vital sign changes are not usually very clear indicators of the presence of an acute stroke and depend on the severity and location of the stroke. Commonly,

an acute stroke will not cause hypotension or shock. If the patient shows signs of shock you should seek an alternative cause (for example, internal hemorrhage). An acute stroke more commonly causes hypertension, occasionally severe enough to require pharmacological therapy. This is one reason why the monitoring of vital signs is an integral part of emergency stroke management. Also be alert for dysrhythmias, as they are more likely to occur as the stroke progresses and involves more and more of the brain stem. Treat any life-threatening dysrhythmias with the appropriate pharmacological therapy.

Respiratory Effort

Abnormal breathing patterns are another possible finding in an acute ischemic stroke. They are one of the most useful indicators of brainstem function. *Cheyne-Stokes respiratory pattern* will occur when there is bilateral cerebral hemisphere damage resulting from a large hemorrhagic stroke. It indicates bilateral cerebral cortical injury, functionally disconnecting cerebral influence on the brainstem respiratory centers. This breathing pattern is characterized by a waxing and waning hyperpneic respiratory pattern, followed by a short period of apnea before repeating itself. The apneic period occurs after CO_2 levels decrease from the hyperpneic (full deep respiration) phase.

Central neurogenic hyperventilation is characterized by increased rate and depth of respiration resulting from early herniation or primary damage to the pons or lower midbrain. The respiratory control centers in the lower brainstem no longer inhibit respiration due to hypocapnea (low CO_2 levels), and this allows for continued hyperventilation and respiratory alkalosis.

Apneustic breathing is a pattern in which there is a 2-to-3-second pause after full inspiration that results from lower pontine lesions seen in basilar artery occlusion. Lastly, if the medulla is compressed or injured, *Biot's breathing* may be noted, characterized by chaotic irregular breathing regularly interrupted by apneic episodes. This progresses to irregular inspiratory gasps and then apnea.

Most patients who die of neurologic insult will die a respiratory death. So, just as you must maintain the airway when the patient cannot, you must also supplement any inadequate respiratory effort with positive pressure ventilation and oxygenation. Also consider hyperventilating the patient, since this will temporarily lower the $PaCO_2$ and cause cerebral vasoconstriction, lowering cerebral blood volume and reducing intracranial pressure.

Circulatory Status

As mentioned previously, cardiac arrest is an uncommon complication of an acute stroke. When it does occur, it is usually secondary to respiratory arrest associated with the stroke. While the need for chest compressions is rare, cardiac monitoring is imperative, since acute ischemic strokes often cause abnormalities in blood pressure and cardiac rhythms. Hypertension is more commonly caused by an acute stroke than hypotension. Hypertension is thought possibly to be a result of the body's response to the stroke, increasing blood flow to the ischemic areas by increasing its driving pressure. Hypertension may also be a stress response by the body to the cerebral insult, or more likely is one of the contributing factors to the acute stroke itself. (Hypertension is a major risk factor.)

If hypotension is seen in conjunction with an acute stroke, you should rapidly seek out other causes for the hypotension. Only with severe brain insults at the terminal stages will the pressure start to drop. Thus, hypotension is not usually an initial finding with an acute stroke.

Neurological Assessment

Constant monitoring of the acute stroke/TIA patient will help you to decide if the patient is improving or deteriorating. While the assessment techniques you use need not be exhaustive, they do need to be reliable, and the most reliable finding in the acute stroke patient is the level of consciousness. A depressed mental status, or a deteriorating mental status, indicates a major insult to the brain. Stroke patients who present or become unresponsive are at the greatest risk of death from the acute stroke.

The Glasgow Coma Scale (Figure 9-1) provides a standardized way to assess the severity of the neurological injury. A benefit of this scale is that it can be used by any health care provider with a high degree of objectivity and accuracy. Any numeric change upon reassessment indicates a general improvement, or worsening, in the patient's condition. The scale uses assessments of three parameters: eye opening, motor response, and verbal response. The total score can range from 3 to 15. In general, a score of 8 or less indicates a severe neurological insult with a poor prognosis.

Since responsiveness requires an intact brain stem, you can infer some type of dysfunction of the brain stem from altered mental status or unresponsiveness. Assess the following to gain an idea about the status of the brain stem:

- Reactivity of the pupils to light
- Size and equality of the pupils (inequality may indicate herniation of the temporal lobe)
- Corneal reflexes
- Gag reflex

Glasgow Coma Scale

Eye Opening	Spontaneous	4	
	To Voice	3	
	To Pain	2	
	None	1	
Verbal Response	Oriented	5	
	Confused	4	
	Inappropriate Words	3	
	Incomprehensible Words	2	
	None	1	
Motor Response	Obeys Commands	6	
	Localizes Pain	5	
	Withdraw (Pain)	4	
	Flexion (Pain)	3	
	Extension (Pain)	2	
	None	1	
Glasgow Coma Score Total			

FIGURE 9-1   Glasgow Coma Scale

TABLE 9-2 NIH STROKE SCALE	
Level of Consciousness (LOC)	0 = alert 1 = not alert, arousable 2 = not alert, obtunded 3 = nonresponsive
Questions	0 = answers two correctly 1 = answers one correctly 2 = answers neither correctly
Commands	0 = performs 2 tasks 1 = performs 1 task 2 = performs neither task
Gaze	0 = no visual loss 1 = partial gaze palsy 2 = forced deviation
Visual fields	0 = no visual loss 1 = partial hemianopia 2 = complete hemianopia 3 = bilateral hemianopia
Facial palsy	0 = normal 1 = minor paralysis 2 = partial paralysis 3 = complete paralysis
Motor Arm a - left b - right	0 = no drift 1 = drift before 10 sec. 2 = falls before 10 sec. 3 = no effort against gravity 4 = no movement

- Doll's eyes maneuver (in coma, eyes turning with the head like a doll's eyes indicate brain-stem damage; eyes remaining focused upward when the head is turned indicate an intact brain stem)

The NIH Stroke scale (Table 9-2) was developed by the National Institutes of Health and is used as a measure of severity of stroke. This scale was utilized by the National Institute of Neurologic Disorders and Stroke rt-PA Study.[1] This study demonstrated that the study-group patients receiving rt-PA were 30 percent more likely to have minimal or no deficit at 3 months than patients treated with a placebo. The incidence of symptomatic intracranial

[1]NEJM.12/95;333(24):1581-1587

TABLE 9-2 *(continued)*

Motor Leg **a - left** **b - right**	0 = no drift 1 = drift before 5 sec. 2 = falls before 10 sec. 3 = no effort against gravity 4 = no movement
Ataxia	0 = absent 1 = one limb 2 = two limbs
Sensory	0 = absent 1 = mid to moderate loss 2 = severe to total loss
Language	0 = normal 1 = mild to moderate aphasia 2 = severe aphasia 3 = mute
Dysarthria	0 = normal 1 = mild to moderate 2 = severe
Extinction/Inattention	0 = normal 1 = mild–one modality 2 = severe–more than one modality

Developed by the National Institute of Neurological Disorders and Stroke/National Institutes of Health, Bethesda, Maryland.

hemorrhage in the treatment group within 36 hours after onset of stroke was 6.4 percent.

The mnemonic *FAST* may be used as a quick assessment tool to help confirm the suspicion of an acute stroke in the conscious patient:

- **F**acial symmetry
- **A**ctive strength/coordination testing
- **S**ensation
- **T**alk/language

TABLE 9-3 DIFFERENTIAL DIAGNOSIS FOR ACUTE STROKE
• Hemorrhagic versus ischemic stroke
• Meningitis/encephalitis
• Drugs/narcotic overdose
• Intracranial mass (tumor, subdural hematoma)
• Craniocerebral trauma/cervical trauma
• Seizures (although seizures could be caused by a stroke)
• Hypertensive crisis
• Metabolic causes
• Glucose levels (hypoglycemia or hyperglycemia)
• Post-arrest cerebral ischemia
• Drug use/abuse

Differential Diagnosis for the Acute Ischemic Stroke/TIA Patient

Prior to administering any treatment, consider the variety of emergencies that may have precipitated the presenting signs and symptoms in order to avoid administering treatment that may be inappropriate or harmful. For example, a hypoglycemic patient and an acute ischemic stroke patient may both display an altered mental status, focal neurologic deficits such as aphasia (inability to speak) hemiparesis (partial paralysis), or unresponsiveness. But if dextrose (which is appropriate for a hypoglycemic patient) is administered to an unresponsive patient who is actually suffering an acute ischemic stroke, the neurological damage may be worsened by the dextrose.

Rapid bedside testing may be employed to help identify certain possible causes of the patient's neurological emergency. For example, a bedside glucose measurement will help identify hypoglycemia, and there are other bedside tests that can determine the presence or absence of drugs. There may also be specific physical findings that point toward certain other etiologies. For example, needle tracks may point to drug abuse and bites on the tongue or inner cheek are common to seizures. Table 9-3 presents the most common differential diagnoses for suspected acute ischemic strokes.

After you have properly assessed and treated threats to the airway, breathing, and circulation, attention must be turned to the underlying cause of the neurologic deficit. It is important for the physician to determine not only the presence or absence of a stroke but also the type of stroke. Since an acute ischemic stroke from a brain infarction (embolus or thrombus) is managed radically differently from a stroke from a cerebral hemorrhage, this determination is imperative.

To assist with this determination, the emergency department physician has advanced diagnostic capabilities at his disposal. While a complete discussion of

TABLE 9-4 DIAGNOSTIC EVALUATIONS FOR PATIENTS WITH ACUTE STROKE
• Computed tomography (CT)
• Magnetic resonance imaging (MRI)
• Electrocardiogram
• Serum electrolytes
• Other chemistries (osmolarity, renal, liver, calcium, toxicology screen)
• Glucose levels
• Arterial blood gas levels
• Hematologic studies
• Lateral cervical spine x-rays
• Skull x-rays

these alternative diagnostic exams is well beyond the scope of this text, we mention them to help you understand the additional studies the ED physician may be requesting. Table 9-4 identifies these additional diagnostic studies which will help isolate the presence or absence and type of acute stroke.

Treatment Strategies for the Acute Stroke Patient

Acute stroke, or brain attack as it is now called, is a true medical emergency. Care and treatment[2] depends on rapid evaluation and determination of the cause of the event. If the cause is determined to be a nonhemorrhagic occlusive acute ischemic stroke, then thrombolytic therapy may be appropriate in certain patient populations.[3] (Refer to Table 9-5 for contraindications for thrombolytic therapy.) These patients must:

- Be thoroughly evaluated
- Have a CT scan
- Be ready for treatment within 3 hours of symptom onset
- Be at least 18 years of age or older
- Have an NIH Stroke Scale score of >4 and <22

TIAs need further diagnostics to determine the need for surgical treatment if carotid stenosis is found to be the etiology. If the patient is not a surgical candidate, then anticoagulant therapy is considered in the high risk patient population (see Table 9-6), or antiplatelet therapy may be utilized if the patient is not a candidate for anticoagulants.

---

[2]National Stroke Consensus Statement. May 1993;4(1):1-12)

[3]NINDS. NEJM. DEC 1995;330: 1581-1587)

TABLE 9-5 CONTRAINDICATIONS TO THROMBOLYTIC THERAPY

- Intracranial hemorrhage diagnosed

- Recent acute ischemic stroke or head trauma, within 3 months

- Undergone major surgery within 14 days

- Uncontrolled Systolic BP >185, or diastolic BP >110 with initial treatment

- Rapidly improving symptoms

- GI or urinary tract hemorrhage within 21 days

- Arterial puncture of a noncompressible vessel within 7 days

- Seizure at onset of stroke

- Anticoagulant therapy within 48 hours with elevated PT or PTT

- Platelet count below 100,000

- Glucose <50 mg/dl or >400 mg/dl

Patients determined to have hemorrhagic strokes will require immediate neurosurgical consultation to determine the appropriateness of surgical intervention. SAH of grade 1-3 (see Table 9-7), may also benefit from the use of the calcium channel blocker nimodipine. Nimodipine 60 mg is suggested every 6 hours orally for 21 days to prevent arterial vasospasm that may further ischemia.

General Considerations in Initial Care of Acute Stroke

As emphasized earlier, initial management is geared toward supporting the ABCs. In the acute stroke patient this is of paramount concern, since vomiting with subsequent aspiration is common. The airway should initially be assessed for patency, while suctioning as appropriate. If the patient cannot maintain his

TABLE 9-6 HIGH-RISK PATIENTS WITH TIA SYNDROME

- Patients with high grade carotid stenosis (70-99%) anatomically related to symptoms

- Patients already on antiplatelet therapy

- Patients with chronic atrial fibrillation or other cardiac etiology to emboli

- TIAs occurring with increasing frequency

TABLE 9-7	CLINICAL GRADES OF SUBARACHNOID HEMORRHAGE (SAH)
Grade 1:	Asymptomatic or minimal headache or stiff neck
Grade 2:	More severe headache/stiff neck
Grade 3:	Drowsy or confused, may have mild hemiparesis
Grade 4:	Deeply stuporous, may have moderate to severe hemiparesis, early decerebrate signs
Grade 5:	Deeply comatose

J.Neurosurg 1968.28:1920-1968

airway, insert a nasopharyngeal or oropharyngeal airway initially, and consider endotracheal intubation. Positive pressure ventilation is appropriate for those patients who have a disturbance in their minute ventilation (by a decrease in the respiratory rate, inadequate tidal volume, or ataxic ventilations). Oxygenation should always accompany ventilations, and hyperventilation may be of benefit to the acute stroke patient since it can reduce intracranial pressure. Monitor oxygenation by applying a pulse oximeter. If the patient has been intubated, an end-tidal CO_2 monitor may be used.

Initiate intravenous access with an isotonic solution in a patent vein, and run it at 30 ml/h. Preferably, this should be done with 0.9% NaCl (normal saline), but lactated Ringer's may also be used. Dextrose-containing solutions should be avoided because the dextrose will be metabolized by the body, leaving free water which is hypo-osmolar (hypotonic) and will leave the vascular space which, in turn, will potentiate the cerebral edema. As well, large volumes of crystalloid solution (normal saline, lactated Ringer's) should also be avoided unless the patient is hypotensive. In conjunction with initiating the IV, draw blood samples so that a stat lab report may be obtained for the blood values.

The administration of the "rule-out" drugs (dextrose, Narcan®, and thiamine) early in the management regime should be guided by conscious assessments and interpretations, and not a "knee-jerk" reaction. Although relatively safe to use in the normal patient, dextrose administration may worsen neurologic outcome. The administration of 25 grams of D_{50} should be done only after a bedside glucose assessment demonstrates hypoglycemia. Thiamine (vitamin B_1) may be administered at 100 mg IM or IV push for any patient who demonstrates neurologic deficits in conjunction with suspected malnourishment, chronic alcoholism, or thiamine deficiency. Narcan® (naloxone, a narcotic antagonist) may also be considered at a 0.4 to 2.0 mg initial dose for those patients suspected to be under the influence of narcotics.

Prehospital Assessment and Management

The prehospital management of the acute stroke patient emphasizes quick recognition, supportive measures, expeditious transport, and notification of the emergency department. It is essential to provide airway control when the gag and cough reflexes are diminished or absent and to hyperventilate when an increased ICP is suspected. Prehospital management must include the following:

- Determination of time of onset of symptoms
- Oxygen therapy
- Immediate transport
- IV normal saline or lactated Ringers KVO (do en route; don't delay transport)
- Notification of emergency department to initiate acute ischemic stroke response team

Initial Emergency Department Treatment

A patient suffering from an acute stroke or TIA could potentially be a challenge, since acute strokes may present with neurological abnormalities anywhere on the continuum from alert and oriented to unresponsive with cardiovascular instability. The management of an acute stroke/TIA patient in the initial phases (until advanced diagnostic exams isolate the type of stroke) is geared toward maintaining the airway, breathing, and circulatory status. After that, there are additional interventions, discussed below, that can help limit the acute stroke progression and reduce the intracranial pressure.

After initial stabilization, the advanced diagnostic procedures are conducted to determine the nature of the acute stroke/TIA. If the health care facility is unable to perform these advanced procedures, the patient should be transferred to another facility capable of doing them after the initial stabilization is completed.

Emergency Department Acute Stroke Response Team

Patients determined by exam and CT to have an occlusive acute ischemic stroke, who present within 3 hours of onset of symptoms, may be candidates for thrombolytic therapy. This therapy has been approved by the FDA but is being implemented with caution due to the risk of intracranial hemorrhage.

The following is a suggested protocol for thrombolytics in occlusive/ischemic stroke:

- Team approach initiated, with immediate response of emergency nursing personnel and the emergency physician to the bedside for a rapid initial assessment (includes NIH stroke scale score >4/<22 and ruling out of contraindications to thrombolysis); CT Department notified of priority case
- ABCs appropriately stabilized; 2 peripheral IV lines placed with blood draw for CBC, PT, PTT, E-lytes, liver profile, type and screen, HCG (female of reproductive age), and urinalysis
- Blood pressure treated if systolic >185, diastolic >110 mmHg (consider labetalol, nitroprusside)
- If screening exam confirms suspected acute ischemic stroke, patient immediately sent to CT; neurologist/neurosurgeon and radiologist notified for consultation
- If all criteria are met and consultants are in agreement, initiation of rt-PA 0.9 mg/kg body weight, with 10% given as a bolus, and the remaining 90% given over 1 hour IV piggyback

- All anticoagulant therapy and antiplatelet therapy held for 24 hours
- Admission to ICU for intensive monitoring and serial examinations

If the patient is not a candidate for thrombolytics, antiplatelet aggregation therapy with aspirin or ticlodipine may provide some benefit to those patients with occlusive/ischemic stroke who have no contraindications to therapy with these agents in preventing recurrent acute ischemic stroke.

Special Considerations in the Management of the Acute Stroke Patient

Each stroke patient presents with a myriad of signs and symptoms and potential complications. Some of the conditions require special treatment considerations. Common complications and special considerations that may require specific management techniques are discussed in the following segments.

Management of Hypertension

Adequate cerebral blood flow (CBF) is necessary to maintain adequate cerebral functioning. And neurologic abnormalities seen in an acute stroke can be described according to changes in CBF. CBF is dependent upon a normal cerebral perfusion pressure (CPP). CPP is simply a relationship between arterial blood flow and the amount of resistance it meets as it passes through the brain. The relationship is as follows:

CPP = mean arterial pressure (MAP) – intracranial pressure (ICP)

As long as the MAP stays high enough to overcome the ICP, the cerebral blood flow remains adequate. Relating this to an acute stroke, a hemorrhagic stroke would cause an increase in ICP (due to extra blood volume in a closed cranial vault), thereby causing a resistance the MAP might be unable to overcome. Conversely, an MAP that is reduced (from poor cardiac output) will be insufficient to overcome even the normal ICP, which will also lead to inadequate cerebral blood flow.

Here is a quick-reference summary of these abbreviations:

CBF	cerebral blood flow
CPP	cerebral perfusion pressure
ICP	intracranial pressure
MAP	mean arterial pressure

It is important to understand this concept when treating hypertension in an acute stroke patient. If your patient is suffering a hemorrhagic stroke and is also hypertensive, that hypertension may be caused by a reflex response of the body to increase MAP in an attempt to overcome elevated ICP caused by the accumulation of blood in the cranium. In essence, this hypertension is present so the body can maintain a normal CBF. The problem is, the increases in mean arterial pressure can also add to, and worsen, the hemorrhage. So you will want to take actions to reduce the arterial pressure to limit the hemorrhage, but not so much that the MAP cannot overcome the ICP.

Experts still disagree about the specifics of hypertension management. However, there is agreement that hemorrhagic strokes (as identified by advanced diagnostic studies) should be treated with antihypertensives to premorbid (before the hemorrhage) levels if known, to limit the size of the bleed and opportunities for rebleeding. Ischemic thrombotic or embolic strokes do not require the aggressive management of hypertension, because the blood pressure typically decreases within a couple of hours. The only exception to this is if the hypertension is persistent at levels above 220/120 mmHg during serial evaluations every 15 minutes of at least 60–90 minutes duration, or is in association with AMI or left ventricular failure.

The administration of antihypertensives should be guided by a physician who is knowledgeable and experienced in neurologic emergencies. For your background information, however, Table 9-8 offers the general guidelines for the treatment of hypertension in conjunction with an acute stroke.

Constant monitoring of the blood pressure is important in titrating the drugs listed in Table 9-8 to achieve the effective response. Labetalol essentially works by dropping cardiac output through its beta-blocking effects (hence causing a drop in MAP), while sodium nitroprusside is a rapid-acting vasodilator which will also decrease the MAP, but may actually increase ICP by cerebral vasodilation. Intravenous administration of nitrates, other beta blockers, or calcium channel blockers may be considered as alternatives or adjuncts to therapy.

TABLE 9-8 ANTIHYPERTENSIVE ADMINISTRATION FOR THE HEMORRHAGIC STROKE

Blood Pressure Measurements	Appropriate Antihypertensive Therapy
If the systolic B/P is <160 torr with a diastolic pressure <105 torr in conjunction with a *prehemorrhage* B/P that was significantly lower . . .	Consider administration of hypertensives to achieve premorbid pressures.
If the systolic B/P is > 160 torr or diastolic B/P is >105 torr on consecutive assessments . . .	Consider administration of labetalol (a beta-blocker) at 10 mg IV over 1-2 min. You may repeat doses of the same or doubled amount every 20 min to a maximum of 300 mg or until desired effect is achieved. If unsuccessful, consider sodium nitroprusside. Avoid labetalol in any patient who should not receive beta-blocking drugs.
If the systolic B/P is >220 torr or a diastolic pressure is >120 torr on consecutive assessments . . .	Initiate labetalol therapy and, if unsuccessful, use an infusion of sodium nitroprusside at 0.5 to 10 µg/kg/min, or nitroglycerin infusion at 10–20 µg/min with the understanding that this may increase ICP.

Management of Increased Intracranial Pressure

As a result of an acute stroke, there may be dramatic increases in the ICP by either a space-occupying hematoma, with a hemorrhagic stroke, or edema that may be seen with ischemic strokes. Getting back to the concept of normal CBF, any increase in ICP without a change in MAP will result in inadequate CPP and a drop in CBF. Or, simply put, an increase in the pressure within the skull, without a reflexive increase in the blood pressure to force the blood through, will cause an inadequate amount of blood flow through the brain.

Common sense would dictate that in an acute stroke, it would not be a desirable intervention to purposely make the systolic pressure rise with sympathomimetic drugs. This could actually complicate matters as well as increase myocardial workload. As an alternative, however, certain interventions can be used that will help reduce the excessively high ICP, thereby allowing whatever the systolic pressure is to be more effective in maintaining normal blood flow. These measures can include simple maneuvers like semi-Fowler's positioning, limitation of IV fluids, and hyperventilation following endotracheal intubation with rapid sequence induction intubation, to more aggressive interventions including specific drug administration.

Rapid Sequence Induction Intubation   *Rapid sequence induction intubation (RSI)* allows for the patient to be sedated and paralyzed for endotracheal intubation with specific pharmacologic agents chosen to lower ICP and blunt the increased ICP response to laryngoscopy. A suggested regimen includes:

- Preoxygenation with 100% oxygen, cardiac monitoring, and continuous pulse oximetry
- Lidocaine IVP 1.0–1.5 mg/kg
- Pancuronium 0.01 mg/kg IVP as a defasiculating agent
- Let above medications circulate 3 minutes with careful monitoring to ensure the quality of rate and depth of respirations
- Sodium pentothal 3.0–5.0 mg/kg IVP (not to be used in patients at risk for hypotension)
- Sellick's maneuver (cricoid pressure to prevent aspiration of gastric contents)
- Succinylcholine 1.5 mg/kg IVP (rapid)
- Intubate trachea and inflate cuff
- Assess breath sounds bilaterally and, if correct placement confirmed, may release cricoid pressure and begin hyperventilation therapy
- Consider administration of a longer-acting nondepolarizing muscle relaxant such as Norcuron ® 0.10-0.15 mg/kg to keep the patient paralyzed for 30–45 minutes while diagnostics are being obtained with consideration for further sedation using a barbiturate or benzodiazepine.

Hyperventilation   Hyperventilation of the acute stroke patient will not only assure normal PaO_2 values, it will also eliminate excessive levels of CO_2. The drop in CO_2 causes a temporary drop in ICP by promoting cerebral vasoconstriction. Lowering the $PaCO_2$ to 25–30 mmHg is probably safe; lower reductions may be detrimental by causing profound cerebral vasoconstriction and an inadvertent reduction in cerebral blood flow. But remember, this is only a temporary measure.

Mannitol   Mannitol is a hyperosmolar agent which will draw interstitial fluid into the vasculature, to eventually be eliminated by the kidneys. This elimination of excessive interstitial fluid in the brain will reduce the ICP and allow the MAP to be more effective in maintaining CBF. Mannitol can be administered at 0.5 g/kg of a 20% solution over a 20-minute period. Its onset is about 20 minutes with a 4–6 hour duration. Repeat dosage can be administered at 0.25 g/kg every 4–6 hours. Caution should be exercised in those patients who may not tolerate an increase in intravascular volume well (e.g., those with CHF or renal disease).

Management of Seizures   Seizures are a relatively infrequent, but potentially life-threatening, complication of a stroke. About 1% of thrombotic, 5%–10% of embolic, and 15% of hemorrhagic strokes present with seizures. The reason they are detrimental is that they increase metabolic activity in the brain, increase core temperature, increase waste production, and consume large amounts of energy and oxygen due to the constant muscular contractions. These effects only worsen the ICP, which in turn will reduce the CPP and hence reduce the CBF. The following is an outline of management principles for the acute stroke patient with concurrent seizures:

- Protect the airway and provide positive pressure ventilation with supplemental oxygen
- Maintain a normal temperature
- Administer diazepam 5–10 mg IV push
    [or]
  Administer lorezapam 1–4 mg IV push over 10 minutes

It may be necessary to administer a long-acting anticonvulsant to control seizures in acute stroke patients. Since almost all anticonvulsants depress respirations, attention must be paid to the respiratory status. Intubation with positive pressure ventilation may be necessary. The following therapies have a longer duration of action in controlling seizures:

- Administer phenytoin at 50 mg/min until a maximum dose of 16 mg/kg is achieved
    [or]
  Administer IV phenobarbital to a maximum of 20 mg/kg, followed by 30–60 mg every 6–8 hours
- If the patient is experiencing intractable seizures that are not terminated by phenytoin or phenobarbital, consider the administration of pentobarbital. Pentobarbital is a very potent drug and should only be administered within intensive care environments.

Anticoagulant and Thrombolytic Therapy

Heparin administration has been considered under the premise that its anticoagulation properties may help prevent the recurrence or propagation of a thrombus. Likewise, thrombolytic therapy has proved to be an effective strategy in the management of an acute stroke due to its thrombolytic actions in selected patients. However, neither heparin nor thrombolytic therapy has been proven (or disproven) as a universally safe and effective treatment for an acute stroke patient. Therefore, it is still not recommended as a routine treatment for the stroke patient, and its administration, if any, should be under the strict guidance of the patient's neurologist.

Overall Goals of Acute Stroke/TIA Management

During the acute management phase of a patient experiencing either an acute ischemic stroke or TIA, the goals are to support any lost or diminished functions of the airway, breathing, and circulation. Additionally, the care provider should treat any cardiac emergencies according to the appropriate algorithms presented elsewhere in this text, and initiate ICP reduction measures. There should be expedited transfer of the patient to initiate advanced diagnostic studies so that additional treatment, potentially including thrombolytics, may be appropriately rendered. Figure 9-2 identifies the treatment algorithm for the patient with an acute ischemic stroke.

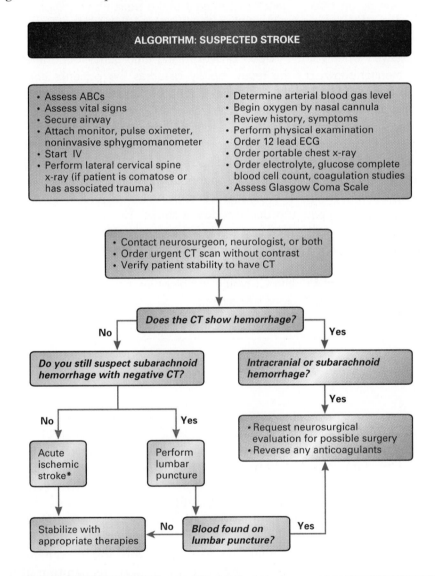

ALGORITHM: SUSPECTED STROKE

- Assess ABCs
- Assess vital signs
- Secure airway
- Attach monitor, pulse oximeter, noninvasive sphygmomanometer
- Start IV
- Perform lateral cervical spine x-ray (if patient is comatose or has associated trauma)

- Determine arterial blood gas level
- Begin oxygen by nasal cannula
- Review history, symptoms
- Perform physical examination
- Order 12 lead ECG
- Order portable chest x-ray
- Order electrolyte, glucose complete blood cell count, coagulation studies
- Assess Glasgow Coma Scale

- Contact neurosurgeon, neurologist, or both
- Order urgent CT scan without contrast
- Verify patient stability to have CT

Does the CT show hemorrhage?

No — *Do you still suspect subarachnoid hemorrhage with negative CT?*

Yes — *Intracranial or subarachnoid hemorrhage?*

Yes — • Request neurosurgical evaluation for possible surgery
• Reverse any anticoagulants

No — Acute ischemic stroke*

Yes — Perform lumbar puncture

Stabilize with appropriate therapies ← No — *Blood found on lumbar puncture?* — Yes

* The detailed management of acute stroke is beyond the scope of the ACLS program. Management of cardiovascular emergencies in stroke victims is similar to the management in other patients. Never forget, however, that acute stroke can coexist with acute cardiovascular problems.

FIGURE 9-2 Algorithm for initial evaluation of suspected stroke. Adapted with permission. Journal of the American Medical Association, October 28, 1992, Volume 268, No. 16, *Guidelines for Cardiopulmonary Resuscitation and Emergency Cardiac Care,* p.2243. ©1992 American Medical Association.

CASE STUDY FOLLOW-UP

You are called to the scene for a 56-year-old male patient who is complaining of a sudden onset of weakness to the right side of his body. Noting his slurred speech and facial droop, John's wife recognized the signs of a stroke and called 911.

Assessment

Your initial assessment of John reveals an open airway, adequate ventilation, and good peripheral pulses. His skin is warm and dry. However, the right side of his face droops excessively when you ask John to make a smile. The monitor shows a normal sinus rhythm at 86 beats per minute. His blood pressure is 178/96 and respiratory rate is 19/minute. His pulse oximeter reading is 97%.

You find severe weakness to the left extremities while performing a motor examination by testing grip strength in the upper extremities and plantar and dorsal flexion in the lower extremities. In addition, his response to sensory stimuli by pin prick and light touch is not accurate. His pupils are equal and reactive to light. Initially, John is alert and oriented to person, place, and time; however, as time progresses, his speech becomes more garbled and less comprehensible as his mental status continues to deteriorate.

Treatment

You immediately place John on a nonrebreather at 15 lpm while constantly monitoring his ventilation status for inadequacy. You initiate an intravenous line of normal saline and draw blood. You continue to monitor the patient and prepare him for transport. En route, you notify the emergency department of the patient's condition and request that they activate the stroke response team.

Upon arrival to the emergency department, the team rapidly assesses the patient's condition. The physician conducts an initial assessment and derives an NIH stroke score. He notifies the CT team that they may need to scan a stroke patient. He orders laboratory studies and establishes a second IV line. The blood pressure remains unchanged. Based on his assessment, the emergency department physician suspects an acute occlusive stroke. He sends the patient to CT scan. He immediately calls for a neurologist and radiologist for a consultation to consider thrombolytic therapy. The physicians wait for the CT results to determine how to proceed with John's treatment.

SUMMARY

The acute stroke, similar to the acute myocardial infarction, is a devastating cardiovascular event that claims thousands of lives each year. It results from ischemic damage to the brain caused by the occlusion or rupture of a blood vessel that perfuses the brain. A transient ischemic attack (TIA) has a similar etiology with similar signs and symptoms, but resolves itself within 24 hours. However, a TIA is often the precursor of a full acute ischemic stroke.

The initial management goals are to support any lost or diminished functions in the airway, breathing, and circulation. Early recognition of the signs and symptoms of stroke, expeditious transport by EMS, and aggressive assessment and intervention by the emergency department physician and staff are paramount to reducing the morbidity and mortality of an acute ischemic stroke.

Review Questions

1. While an acute stroke and a TIA may both produce focal neurologic deficits, only an acute ischemic stroke
   a. will have an abatement of signs and symptoms within 24 hours.
   b. is caused by a hemorrhage only, while a TIA is from a thrombus.
   c. will not cause cardiac arrest.
   d. will result in death of brain cells.
   e. none of the above

2. Why is the identification of a TIA so important?
   a. because it may foretell an impending acute ischemic stroke
   b. so anticonvulsant medications can be administered early
   c. to limit the extent of residual damage
   d. so that the patient can be put on a healthy diet and exercise plan

3. Essentially any neurologic abnormality can occur with an acute stroke or a TIA.
   a. true
   b. false

4. Upon noxious stimuli application to a patient suffering an acute stroke, he opens his eyes and tries to push your hand away while making incomprehensible sounds. Based on this limited information, his Glasgow Coma Scale score would be
   a. 3.
   b. 5.
   c. 7.
   d. 9.
   e. 11.

5. Which of the following treatments may be beneficial in reducing ICP early in the management of an acute stroke or TIA patient?
   a. hyperventilation
   b. IV therapy
   c. Trendelenburg positioning
   d. administration of anticonvulsants to prevent seizures

6. Which of the following is a common distinguishing sign or symptom of a hemorrhagic stroke?
   a. hemiparesis and hemiplegia
   b. abrupt onset of a severe headache
   c. pupillary fixation and dilation
   d. nausea and vomiting

7. When bilateral cerebral hemisphere damage has occurred due to a large acute stroke, which respiratory pattern will most likely occur?
   a. central neurogenic hyperventilation
   b. Biot's
   c. Cheyne-Stokes
   d. apneustic

8. The doll's eyes maneuver in the comatose patient provides an indication of
   a. the integrity of the brainstem.
   b. encroachment on the third cranial nerve.
   c. herniation through the tentorial incisura.
   d. cerebellar function.

9. For thrombolytic therapy to be considered in the acute ischemic stroke patient, the drug must be administered within how many hours from onset of symptoms?
   a. 1
   b. 3
   c. 6
   d. 36

10. Aggressive management of hypertension should be considered in which of the following types of stroke etiology?
    a. embolic
    b. thrombotic
    c. hemorrhagic
    d. none of the above

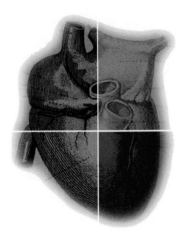

Putting It All Together: The Algorithms

An algorithm is a simplified method to illustrate a systematic approach to emergency cardiac care management. The series of steps is used as a guideline to stimulate thought and clinical action and should not be used as a legal standard of care. Critical interventions that are based on scientific evidence or standard practice are identified as a recommended course of treatment for the various types of cardiac arrest and cardiovascular and cardiopulmonary conditions.

Topics to be covered in this chapter are:

- Classification of Therapeutic Interventions
- Key Considerations in the Algorithm Approach to Emergency Cardiac Care
- Algorithms for Patients in Cardiac Arrest
- Postresuscitation Patient Management
- Algorithms for Patients Not in Cardiac Arrest

CASE STUDY

You are on call at a local community hospital emergency department when you finally get to sit down and sip your cold, 2-hour-old coffee after a grueling night of constant patient flow.

Suddenly, the doors of the emergency department slam open and an older man comes running frantically up to the triage desk. He is out of breath and screaming, "My wife, my wife! Please help her!" You proceed out to his car, which is parked under the canopy, and find an elderly woman who is slumped over on the front seat. She is ashen gray and motionless. You yell, "I need help out here right now! Bring a gurney and get the cardiac resuscitation room ready!"

How would you proceed to assess and care for this patient? This chapter will describe the systematic algorithm approach to managing a patient in cardiac arrest or one who is suffering from a cardiovascular or cardiopulmonary compromise. Later we will return to the case and apply the procedures learned.

Introduction

The algorithm approach to managing a patient in cardiac arrest or one who is suffering from cardiovascular or cardiopulmonary compromise is an oversimplified guideline that is used mainly as an educational tool to illustrate and summarize important emergency care steps. These are not rigid and inflexible steps that set a legal standard of care; instead, they are designed to provide a systematic approach to consider when managing these types of patients. The steps should stimulate thought that is based on clinical understanding.

Classification of Therapeutic Interventions

The American Heart Association uses a classification system for the efficacy of interventions adopted from the 1992 National Conference on Cardiopulmonary Resuscitation and Emergency Cardiac Care. The classification assigned to an intervention is based on the experts' evaluation of available scientific information about the specific intervention.

The classification system assigns a range of therapeutic benefit or detriment to the clinical interventions identified in the algorithms. The classification is based on the amount of supporting scientific evidence for that particular intervention. The classification identifies the potential benefit of using a particular medication or nonpharmacologic intervention in each algorithm. Likewise, possible harmful effects of interventions or those interventions that lack supporting scientific evidence are also identified. You should take into consideration the assigned classification when you make a clinical decision regarding the potential benefit or harm of a medication or a nonpharmacologic intervention you are considering administering or initiating.

The classifications listed here are from the American Heart Association "Guidelines for Cardiopulmonary Resuscitation and Emergency Cardiac Care," *Journal of the American Medical Association* 1992; 268:2171-2302.

Class I.—An intervention that is usually indicated, always acceptable, and considered useful and effective. (Typically, this is the treatment of choice.)

Class II.—An intervention that is acceptable, however is of uncertain effectiveness, and may be controversial.

Class IIa.—An intervention in which the evidence supports its use and effectiveness.

Class IIb.—An intervention that is not well supported by scientific evidence but is considered possibly helpful and not harmful.

Class III.—An intervention that is not supported by scientific evidence and is considered inappropriate and possibly harmful.

Key Considerations in the Algorithm Approach to Emergency Cardiac Care

When applying the algorithms to patient management, it is necessary to consider the following clinical recommendations:

- Treat the patient, not a rhythm. It is necessary to consider the etiology of a rhythm when providing care. Likewise, you must attempt to determine the reason why a patient may be in a persistent rhythm. This is accomplished by managing the "whole" patient and not developing tunnel vision while performing specific skills.
- Proceed through the algorithm until the rhythm is changed or the patient is no longer in cardiac arrest.
- CPR is continued throughout the algorithm as long as the patient remains in cardiac arrest.
- Perform alternative interventions when the appropriate indications exist.
- The guidelines in the algorithms represent primarily Class I interventions. Other interventions may be noted for consideration.
- Airway management, effective ventilation, oxygenation, chest compressions, and defibrillation are key basic components in patient management. These interventions take precedence over more advanced care such as intravenous therapy and medication administration.
- Lidocaine, atropine, and epinephrine can be administered down the endotracheal tube at 2 to 2.5 times the intravenous dose.
- Intravenous medications should be administered by a rapid bolus, with a few exceptions. The administration should be followed by a 20 to 30 ml bolus of intravenous fluid in conjunction with elevation of the extremity. This expedites delivery of the medication to the core circulation, which may take 1 to 2 minutes.

The following are general considerations for medication administration applied to the cardiac arrest algorithms.

- **Epinephrine**—1 mg of epinephrine should be administered IV push every 3 to 5 minutes. If this does not produce favorable results, the following doses are recommended as a Class IIb consideration:

– Intermediate dose is 2 to 5 mg IV push repeated every 3 to 5 minutes.
– Escalating dose is 1 mg, 3 mg, 5 mg IV push administered 3 minutes apart.
– High dose is 0.1 mg/kg IV push repeated every 3 to 5 minutes.

- **Sodium Bicarbonate**—is administered at a dose of 1 mEq/kg repeated at 0.5 mEq/kg every ten minutes.

It is a Class I recommendation if the patient is known to be hyperkalemic. It is a Class IIa recommendation in the following conditions:
– Known preexisting acidosis that is responsive to sodium bicarbonate.
– An overdose of tricyclic antidepressants.
– Alkalinizing urine agent in drug overdose.

It is considered a Class IIb recommendation in the following conditions:
– Prolonged cardiac arrest in an intubated patient.
– Following return of spontaneous circulation after prolonged cardiac arrest.

It is a Class III recommendation in hypoxic lactic acidosis.

- **Atropine**—A 3-minute interval for repeat administration of atropine is a Class IIb recommendation in cardiac arrest.

Algorithms for Patients in Cardiac Arrest

Universal Algorithm
Any resuscitation efforts must begin with the universal algorithm (Figure 10-1). This algorithm follows the primary ABCD survey and secondary ABCD survey. It is a systematic approach that allows you to make a quick initial assessment and develop a management plan based on the presenting rhythm, precipitating events that led to the cardiac arrest, and any other information that is pertinent to the differential diagnosis of the patient.

Universal Algorithm: Key Points
- Establishing unresponsiveness is the first action that must be performed. Immediately call for additional resources to get a defibrillator to the patient. Early recognition and defibrillation of ventricular fibrillation or ventricular tachycardia is imperative to successful resuscitation.
- Open the airway and assess for breathing. If the patient is breathing, assess for adequacy and the need for ventilation. Place the patient in the recovery position if there is no suspicion of a spinal injury. Provide positive pressure ventilation if necessary, oxygen therapy, initiate intravenous therapy, and assess vital signs. If necessary, intubate the patient. Gather a history, perform a physical examination, and attach a continuous ECG monitor. Acquire a 12-lead ECG if necessary.
- If no breathing is present, administer two slow breaths and check for a pulse. Assess for a carotid pulse. If the patient is pulseless, begin chest compressions and ventilation.
- Defibrillation is the most important intervention that can be performed. As soon as the defibrillator is available and ventricular fibrillation or pulseless ventricular tachycardia is verified, defibrillate the patient.
- If defibrillation is not indicated, proceed to the secondary ABCD survey. Intubate the patient, confirm tube placement, assess effective ventilation, and attempt to determine the etiology of the cardiac arrest and rhythm.

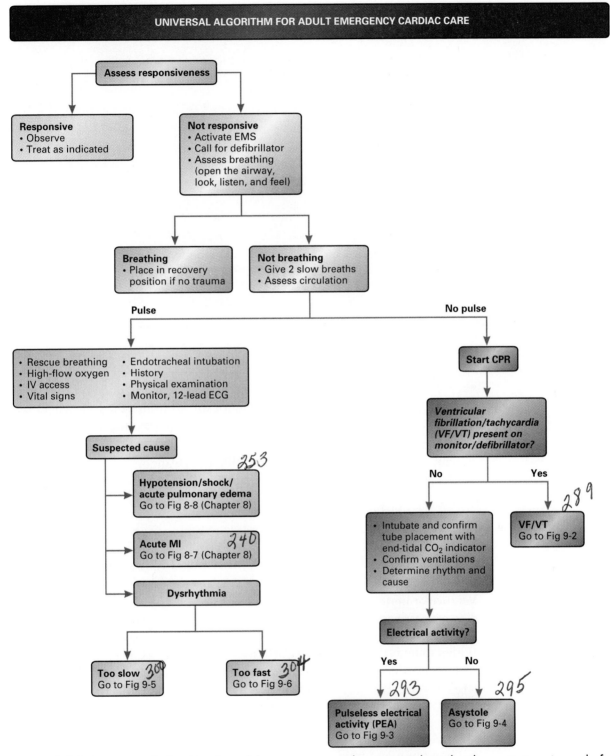

FIGURE 10-1 Universal algorithm for adult emergency cardiac care. Adapted with permission. Journal of the American Medical Association, October 28, 1992, Volume 268, No. 16, *Guidelines for Cardiopulmonary Resuscitation and Emergency Cardiac Care*, p.2216. ©1992 American Medical Association.

- If the patient is pulseless and electrical activity is present, with the exception of ventricular fibrillation and ventricular tachycardia, proceed to the pulseless electrical activity (PEA) algorithm.

Universal Algorithm: Summary

1. Assess for responsiveness.
   - If unresponsive, call for additional help, activate EMS system, call for defibrillator.
2. Open the airway, assess for breathing.
   - If the patient is breathless, administer two slow breaths over 2 to 4 seconds.
3. Assess for a carotid pulse.
   - If pulseless, initiate CPR.
4. Attach monitor/defibrillator and assess for ventricular fibrillation and pulseless ventricular tachycardia.
5. Defibrillate ventricular fibrillation or pulseless ventricular tachycardia by delivering three stacked shocks at 200 J, 300 J, and 360 J.
   - If VF/VT persists, proceed to VF/VT algorithm.
   - If the patient remains pulseless and electrical activity is present, proceed to the PEA algorithm.
   - If the patient remains pulseless and no electrical activity is present, proceed to the asystole algorithm.
   - If the patient regains a pulse, assess breathing, rhythm, and vital signs.

- If the patient is pulseless and no electrical activity is noted on the oscilloscope, proceed to the asystole algorithm. Consider the following possibilities when confronted with a flat line on the monitor:
  - The leads are loose.
  - The leads are not connected to the patient.
  - The leads are not connected to the monitor/defibrillator
  - The power to the monitor/defibrillator is not turned on.
  - The ECG gain is set too low.
  - Isoelectric VF/VT or true asystole exist.

Ventricular Fibrillation/Pulseless Ventricular Tachycardia (VF/FT) Algorithm

Ventricular fibrillation or pulseless ventricular tachycardia is the most viable cardiac arrest rhythm that a patient can be in. Approximately 80% to 90% of patients in nontraumatic sudden cardiac arrest initially present with VF or VT. Within minutes, the rhythm will deteriorate into a nonviable rhythm. The earlier defibrillation is done, the better the chance of converting the patient's rhythm into a perfusing rhythm. That is why early defibrillation is imperative in increasing the survival rate of patients both in and out of the hospital (Figure 10-2).

VF/VT Algorithm: Key Points

- In a witnessed cardiac arrest when a defibrillator is not immediately available, a precordial thump can be delivered. It is considered a Class IIb intervention. It can convert a patient from VF/VT to a perfusing rhythm. Conversely, it can convert a patient with organized cardiac electrical activity into VF/VT or asystole. If the defibrillator is immediately available, **do not delay defibrillation to deliver the precordial thump; go immediately to defibrillation.**

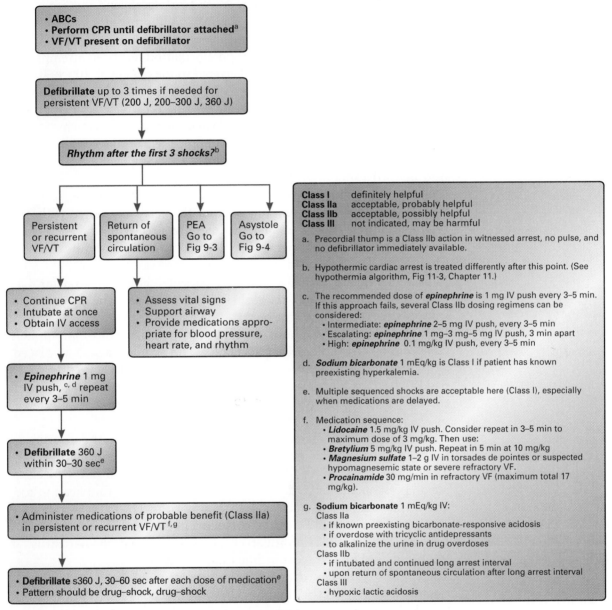

FIGURE 10-2 Ventricular Fibrillation/Pulseless Ventricular Tachycardia (VF/VT) algorithm. Adapted with permission. Journal of the American Medical Association, October 28, 1992, Volume 268, No. 16, *Guidelines for Cardiopulmonary Resuscitation and Emergency Cardiac Care*, p.2217. ©1992 American Medical Association.

- Ventricular fibrillation is the most common rhythm that patients will be in immediately following collapse from cardiac arrest. The majority of patients who will survive will be converted from ventricular fibrillation or pulseless ventricular tachycardia. Once the patient has deteriorated from VF/VT to asystole, the chance of survival is drastically decreased.
- Remember: With each passing minute, the chance of the rhythm deteriorating into a nonviable rhythm increases significantly.

- The treatment for ventricular fibrillation and pulseless ventricular tachycardia is defibrillation. It is imperative to maintain a patent airway and provide adequate ventilation and chest compressions. However, the method to terminate VF/VT to a perfusing rhythm is defibrillation and not endotracheal intubation, intravenous therapy, or drug administration. Those are considered only adjuncts to defibrillation and should be performed after defibrillation has been attempted.

- Initially, three stacked shocks are delivered to the patient at 200 J, 300 J, and 360 J. These should be delivered in as rapid a sequence as possible, with safety to the resuscitation team a key consideration. A pulse check is done following the third defibrillation and not between shock 1, shock 2, and shock 3. The paddles should be left on the chest and the rhythm reanalyzed quickly as the paddles are being charged for the next defibrillation.

- Quick-look paddles can be used to quickly assess the rhythm for VF/VT and deliver defibrillation without the delay associated with connecting monitor lead cables. The paddles are already on the chest and can be immediately charged if VF/VT is identified. Be careful of artifact associated with use of paddles.

- Remove nitroglycerin patches from the patient's chest prior to defibrillation. The patch may cause the electrical current to arc. The nitroglycerin substrate will not explode or burn.

- Do not place the defibrillator paddles over the generator of an implanted automatic defibrillator or pacemaker. The paddles should be placed approximately 5 inches from the generator. Energy discharged from paddles over an implanted device can damage, disable, or misprogram the implanted device. Also, the defibrillation current may be blocked by the implanted device.

- If an implanted automatic defibrillator is in place and not delivering a shock to the patient in VF/VT, proceed with normal defibrillation.

- The person delivering the defibrillation must ensure team safety by clearing all personnel prior to defibrillation. You must look from head to toe and say aloud, "One, I'm clear. Two, you're clear. Three, everybody's clear," assessing for and clearing personnel in contact with the patient.

- Following the stacked defibrillations, CPR is initiated, the patient is intubated, and an intravenous line established.

- Epinephrine is the first drug of choice administered after the defibrillation at 1 mg every 3 to 5 minutes. If an intravenous line is not established, the epinephrine can be administered down the endotracheal tube at 2 to 2.5 times the normal dose. If the standard dose of epinephrine is not effective, consider using the intermediate, escalating, or high dose regimens.

- You should defibrillate at 360 J within 30 to 60 seconds following the administration of each drug. The sequence is drug–shock, drug–shock.

- Antidysrhythmic medications that can be used in VF/VT are:
  - *Lidocaine*: 1.0 to 1.5 mg/kg IV push initial dose repeated in 3 to 5 minutes at 1.0 to 1.5 mg/kg to a maximum dose of 3 mg/kg. A single dose of 1.5 mg/kg can be administered, followed by bretylium.
  - *Bretylium*: 5 mg/kg IV push repeated in 5 minutes at 10 mg/kg to a total dose of 30 mg/kg.

- *Magnesium sulfate*: 1 to 2 grams IV for torsades de pointes, suspected hypomagnesemia, or refractory VF.
- *Procainamide*: 30 mg/minute to a total dose of 17 mg/kg for refractory VF.
- Lower loading doses of lidocaine should be used in patients of advanced age and those with liver dysfunction. A single loading dose of 1 mg/kg is administered.
- Lidocaine is only administered as a bolus during cardiac arrest. Once circulation has been restored, an infusion is started at 2 to 4 mg/minute.
- Bretylium is used when lidocaine fails to convert VF following defibrillation or the patient reverts back to VF with lidocaine administration.
- Once the circulation has been restored, an infusion of the antidysrhythmic agent that was effective in aiding in the conversion of the rhythm should be initiated. If the patient was converted by defibrillation alone or without any antidysrhythmic medication administration, an IV bolus loading dose of lidocaine at 1.0 to 1.5 mg/kg should be administered. The infusion medications are:
  - *Lidocaine*: 2 to 4 mg/minute
  - *Bretylium*: 1 to 2 mg/minute
  - *Procainamide*: 1 to 4 mg/minute
- Human clinical evidence does not suggest that the administration of lidocaine is superior to bretylium.

VF/VT Algorithm: Summary

1. Perform CPR.
2. Defibrillate at 200 J, 300 J, 360 J.
   - If no pulse, continue CPR
3. Intubate the patient, establish an IV line, and connect the continuous ECG monitor.
4. Epinephrine 1.0 mg IV push or endotracheally at 2 to 2.5 mg and repeated every 3 to 5 minutes throughout the entire resuscitation.
   - Wait 30 to 60 seconds following epinephrine and defibrillate at 360 J.
5. Lidocaine 1.0 to 1.5 mg/kg IV push or endotracheally at 2 to 3 mg/kg. Repeat every 3 to 5 minutes to a total cumulative dose of 3 mg/kg.
   - Wait 30 to 60 seconds and defibrillate at 360 J.
6. Bretylium at 5 mg/kg IV push. Repeat every 5 minutes at 10 mg/kg to a total cumulative dose of 30 mg/kg.
   - Wait 30 to 60 seconds and defibrillate at 360 J.
7. Consider Class IIb dosing regimens for epinephrine.
8. Consider magnesium sulfate at 1 to 2 grams IV push.
   - Wait 30 to 60 seconds and defibrillate at 360 J.
9. Consider sodium bicarbonate at 1 mEq/kg repeated every 10 minutes at 0.5 mEq/kg.
10. The sequence is drug–shock, drug–shock, with a 30-to-60-second wait to defibrillate after the administration of each medication.

Pulseless Electrical Activity (PEA) Algorithm

When electrical activity is identified on the monitor, other than VF or VT, in the absence of a pulse, it is termed pulseless electrical activity (Figure 10-3). There are myriad conditions that may cause PEA.

PEA Algorithm: Key Points

- PEA is comprised of a group of rhythms that include:
  - electro-mechanical dissociation (EMD)
  - pseudo-EMD
  - idioventricular rhythms
  - ventricular escape rhythms
  - post-defibrillation idioventricular rhythms
  - bradyasystolic rhythms
- EMD is characterized by a condition in which electrical depolarization occurs without shortening of the myocardial fibers and no mechanical contraction.
- Pseudo-EMD is associated with electrical depolarization with subsequent mechanical contraction that does not produce a measurable or detectable pulse. The most common cause is severe hypovolemia.
- The major key to PEA management is to find the possible cause. Etiologies of PEA include:
  - hypovolemia
  - hypoxia and hypoventilation
  - cardiac tamponade
  - tension pneumothorax
  - hypothermia
  - massive pulmonary embolism
  - drug overdose
  - hyperkalemia
  - acidosis
  - massive myocardial infarction
- Fluid challenges are used to manage or rule out hypovolemia.
- Aggressive hyperventilation is used to combat hypoventilation and hypoxia.
- Drug overdoses of tricyclic antidepressants, beta blockers, calcium channel blockers, and digitalis are only a few of the drugs that may precipitate PEA.
- A Doppler ultrasound should be used to detect possible blood flow not obtainable by regular palpation. If a pulse is detected by Doppler in PEA, proceed to the severe hypotension algorithm.
- Atropine is used in PEA rhythms that have underlying rates of less than 60 complexes per minute, assuming that the undetectable BP may be rate dependent and reversible. If the rate is greater than 60 complexes per minute, atropine is not administered.
- Pericardiocentesis is the treatment of choice for suspected pericardial tamponade.
- If a tension pneumothorax is suspected, perform a needle decompression by inserting an angiocath in the second intercostal space at the midclavicular line on the affected side.

FIGURE 10-3 Pulseless Electrical Activity (PEA) algorithm. Adapted with permission. Journal of the American Medical Association, October 28, 1992, Volume 268, No. 16, *Guidelines for Cardiopulmonary Resuscitation and Emergency Cardiac Care*, p.2219. ©1992 American Medical Association.

ALGORITHM: PULSELESS ELECTRICAL ACTIVITY (PEA)

Includes
• Electromechanical Dissociation (EMD)
• Pseudo-EMD
• Idioventricular rhythms
• Ventricular escape rhythms
• Bradyasystolic rhythms
• Postdefibrillation idioventricular rhythms

• **Continue CPR**   • **Obtain IV access**
• **Intubate at once**   • **Assess blood flow using Doppler ultrasound**

Consider possible causes
(Parentheses = possible therapies and treatments)

• Hypovolemia (volume infusion)
• Hypoxia (ventilation)
• Cardiac tamponade (pericardiocentesis)
• Tension pneumothorax (needle decompression)
• Hypothermia (see hypothermia algorithm, Fig 11-3, Chapter 11)
• Massive pulmonary embolism (surgery, *thrombolytics*)
• Drug overdoses such as tricyclics, digitalis, β-blockers, calcium channel blockers
• Hyperkalemia[a]
• Metabolic acidosis[b]
• Massive acute myocardial infarction (Go to Fig 8-7, Chapter 8)

• *Epinephrine* 1 mg IV push, [a, c] repeat every 3–5 min

• If absolute bradycardia (<60 BPM) or relative bradycardia, give *atropine* 1 mg IV
• Repeat every 3–5 min to a total of 0.04 mg/kg[d]

Class I   definitely helpful
Class IIa   acceptable, probably helpful
Class IIb   acceptable, possibly helpful
Class III   not indicated, may be harmful

a. *Sodium bicarbonate* 1 mEq/kg is Class I if patient has known preexisting hyperkalemia.

b. *Sodium bicarbonate* 1 mEq/kg

  Class IIa
  • if known preexisting bicarbonate-response acidosis
  • if overdose with tricyclic antidepressants
  • to alkalinize the urine in drug overdoses

  Class IIb
  • if intubated and continued long arrest interval
  • upon return of spontaneous circulation after long arrest interval

  Class III
  • hypoxic lactic acidosis

c. The recommended dose of *epinephrine* is 1 mg IV push every 3–5 min. If this approach fails, several Class IIb dosing regimens can be considered:

  • Intermediate: *epinephrine* 2–5 mg IV push, every 3–5 min
  • Escalating: *epinephrine* 1 mg–3 mg–5 mg IV push, 3–5 min apart
  • High: *epinephrine* 0.1 mg/kg IV push, every 3–5 min

d. Shorter *atropine* dosing intervals are possibly helpful in cardiac arrest (Class IIb)

PEA Algorithm: Summary

1. Initiate CPR.

2. Intubate and establish intravenous access.

3. Assess for arterial blood flow by Doppler ultrasound, end-tidal CO_2, echocardiography, or arterial line.

4. Consider possible causes:
    - hypoxia
    - hypothermia
    - acidosis
    - hypovolemia
    - drug overdose
    - tension pneumothorax
    - cardiac tamponade
    - hyperkalemia
    - acute MI
    - massive pulmonary embolism

5. Epinephrine 1 mg IV push repeated every 3 to 5 minutes.
    - Consider Class IIb dosing regimens for epinephrine
    - Consider sodium bicarbonate at 1 mEq/kg repeated every 10 minutes at 0.5 mEq/kg

6. If the complex rate is less than 60 per minute, Atropine 1 mg IV push repeated every 3 to 5 minutes to a total dose of 0.04 mg/kg.

Asystole Algorithm

Asystole is associated with no electrical activity. The prognosis of survival is very poor when a patient presents in this rhythm (Figure 10-4). Management of asystole is very similar to PEA.

Asystole Algorithm: Key Points

- Determining the etiology of the cardiac arrest and possible causes of the rhythm must be aggressively pursued during the differential diagnosis phase of the secondary ABCD survey.

- Asystole should be confirmed in more than one lead to ensure that the patient is not truly in a fine or medium ventricular fibrillation.

- Atropine is administered as a routine medication in asystole. A strong parasympathetic tone may eliminate ventricular and supraventricular pacemaker activity and lead to asystole. Since atropine is a parasympatholytic, also known as a vagolytic, it will block the parasympathetic tone and may restore pacemaker activity.

- Defibrillation of asystole produces parasympathetic discharge and may prevent any spontaneous pacemaker activity. Routine defibrillation of asystole is strongly discouraged.

- Studies have found that the asystolic heart almost never responds to cardiac pacing. It is considered a Class IIb intervention. To be effective, pacing must be initiated immediately after the cardiac arrest. If pacing is to be initiated, it should be done early along with CPR and the administration of medications.

- When endotracheal intubation, intravenous access, CPR, and medication have been successfully performed or administered, but there has been no response, cessation of resuscitation should be considered. Exceptions include hypothermia, electrocution, and drug overdose.

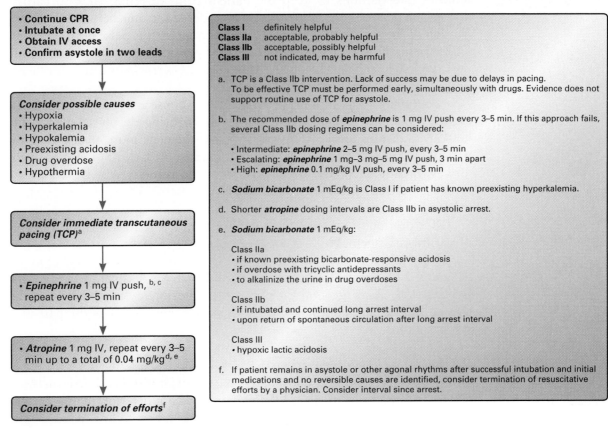

FIGURE 10-4 Asystole algorithm. Adapted with permission. Journal of the American Medical Association, October 28, 1992, Volume 268, No. 16, *Guidelines for Cardiopulmonary Resuscitation and Emergency Cardiac Care*, p.2220. ©1992 American Medical Association.

Asystole Algorithm: Summary

1. Continue CPR.

2. Confirm asystole in more than one lead.

3. Intubate and initiate intravenous access.

4. Consider possible causes to include:
   - hypoxia
   - hyperkalemia
   - hypokalemia
   - acidosis
   - drug overdose
   - hypothermia

5. Consider early transcutaneous pacing.

6. Epinephrine 1 mg IV push repeated every 3 to 5 minutes.

7. Atropine 1 mg IV push repeated every 3 minutes to a total cumulative dose of 0.04 mg/kg.

8. Consider Class IIb dosing regimens for epinephrine.

9. Consider sodium bicarbonate at 1 mEq/kg repeated every 10 minutes at 0.5 mEq/kg.

10. Consider termination of resuscitation efforts.

Postresuscitation Patient Management

The time following post cardiac arrest is critical to patient survival and requires interventions to keep the patient from reverting back to cardiac arrest. The postresuscitation period is considered the time between the resuscitation of the patient and restoration of a spontaneous pulse until the transfer to the intensive care unit. Generally, this period is approximately 30 minutes. Patient management during this period is critical and may influence patient survival and neurological outcome.

Following resuscitation, the patient's response may range from being alert, awake, and hemodynamically stable to being deeply comatose and hemodynamically unstable. Aggressive management must ensure that the patient's condition does not deteriorate because of lack of attention to the airway, breathing, or circulation. Perform the primary ABCD survey and secondary ABCD survey (as discussed in Chapter 2) to allow for a systematic and organized evaluation of the patient.

Restoration of circulation to the brain and other tissue is the key goal of patient management.

The tachycardia, bradycardia, and hypotension algorithms should not be applied to the postresuscitation period tachycardias, bradycardia, and hypotension. As a general rule, postresuscitation dysrhythmias are not treated during the immediate postresuscitation period unless the patient is symptomatic.

Postresuscitation Interventions

Following successful resuscitation of the patient, it is imperative to perform certain interventions to ensure the patient does not deteriorate into cardiac arrest. The following critical actions must be taken following successful cardiac arrest.

Airway

Reassess the airway to ensure it is patent. Reverify endotracheal tube placement by reassessment of breath sounds and use of an end-tidal CO_2 detector, endotracheal tube aspirator, and chest x-ray.

Breathing

Administer supplemental oxygen. Continue to provide positive pressure ventilation as necessary by bag-valve or other ventilation device. Assess bilateral breath sounds and chest wall movement during ventilation. Monitor oxygen saturation by pulse oximetry and arterial blood gas analysis.

If spontaneous respirations do not return, it will be necessary to mechanically ventilate the patient. You may need to sedate and paralyze the patient to accomplish this effectively. The ventilatory support is guided by blood gas analysis, respiratory rate and volume, and the patient's breathing effort.

Assess the patient closely for potential complications that may have resulted from the resuscitation. Pneumothorax, fractured ribs, sternal fracture, and a misplaced endotracheal tube are all possible complications.

Circulation

It is necessary to assess vital signs. Establish an intravenous line if one is not present. Continuously monitor the ECG rhythm, blood pressure, and pulse oximeter reading. Also, it is necessary to monitor urine output.

If the patient was in VF or VT during the cardiac arrest and no anti-dysrhythmic agent was administered during the course of the resuscitation, usually because of a short resuscitation time, a lidocaine bolus must be administered and an infusion started. This would be contraindicated in patients with ventricular escape rhythms since the lidocaine would tend to abolish the only perfusing beat.

If an antidysrhythmic agent was administered during the resuscitation, then initiate an infusion of the agent that was successful in converting the VF or VT to a perfusing rhythm. Lidocaine, bretylium, or procainamide are acceptable medications for maintenance infusion.

Thrombolytic therapy may be considered for patients suffering an acute myocardial infarction. This may be evident by a postresuscitation 12-lead ECG. Be aware of contraindications such as prolonged resuscitation, trauma, and central line placement.

Differential Diagnosis
Attempt to determine the etiology of the cardiac arrest. Identify any potential complications that may have occurred secondary to the cardiac arrest. Perform a detailed physical examination and gather and review the history. Order appropriate lab studies, such as magnesium and calcium levels, cardiac enzymes, and serum electrolytes.

Other Interventions and Considerations
Intravenous lines that were started hastily and without precise aseptic technique should be changed. Ensure that all intravenous lines are patent and running appropriately. Insert a nasogastric tube and a Foley catheter. Treat any identified abnormalities in the electrolytes. Continuously monitor the patient during transport to an appropriate facility or critical care unit.

Special Considerations in Postresuscitation Care
The postresuscitation period presents a very delicate time for patient management. Special considerations must be taken for certain conditions that may arise. The following are special considerations that may be encountered in the postresuscitation care of the patient.

Cerebral Perfusion   The whole goal of resuscitation is to restore the patient to as nearly the normal neurologic prearrest state as possible. Protect cerebral function by ensuring a patent airway, adequate ventilation, and effective perfusion. Normothermia should be maintained since hyperthermia increases oxygen requirements. Seizures also increase cerebral oxygen requirements; therefore, they must be controlled. Elevate the head to 30 degrees to decrease intracranial pressure and increase cerebral venous drainage.

Hypotension   Consider the etiology of the low blood pressure to be associated with either a volume, a rate, or a pump problem. A fluid bolus of 250 to 500 ml of normal saline is appropriate to administer, unless fluid overload or pump failure is suspected. Hypotension that persists following fluid administration may need to be treated with inotropic and vasopressor agents. The goal is to maintain adequate cerebral perfusion.

Recurrent VF/VT   Following successful resuscitation, an antidysrhythmic agent should be administered to reduce the likelihood that the patient will revert back to VF/VT. If VF/VT does recur, it is considered to be refractory. Whatever original therapy was successful in converting the rhythm initially, it should be reinstituted. Consider magnesium sulfate at 1 to 2 grams intravenously for refractory VF/VT. Reassess the airway and ventilation status. Poor ventilation, acid-base disturbances, hypovolemia, and electrolyte imbalances are often the reason for refractory or recurrent VF/VT.

Tachycardia in Postresuscitation Supraventricular tachycardias in the postresuscitation period should be left untreated unless the patient becomes hypotensive. High amounts of circulating catecholamines are usually the cause of tachycardia.

Bradycardia in Postresuscitation Atropine, pacing, and catecholamine infusions should be considered only in profound bradycardia with hypotension and evidence of hypoperfusion. Otherwise, reevaluate the airway, breathing, and circulation status and do not immediately administer atropine.

Premature Ventricular Contractions in Postresuscitation Most often, PVCs are an indication that there is an existing problem in the secondary ABCDs. Increase oxygenation if possible. Monitor the patient closely as the acid-base and catecholamine levels normalize. An infusion of lidocaine, procainamide, or bretylium is acceptable and probably helpful. If the patient did not receive an IV bolus or antidysrhythmic agent, consider a bolus and infusion at this time.

Algorithms for Patients Not in Cardiac Arrest

It is just as critical to be able to manage the patient who is not in cardiac arrest but has the potential to deteriorate to cardiac arrest. The following conditions must be managed to prevent cardiac arrest from occurring:

- Serious nonlethal dysrhythmias that are too fast or too slow
- Acute MI
- Hypotension, cardiogenic shock, and acute pulmonary edema

The universal algorithm, introduced earlier in this chapter for patients in cardiac arrest, also applies to the patient who is not in cardiac arrest. Reassessment of the airway and ventilation is a critical consideration in this particular patient. Management of the patient should include the following critical actions:

- Administer supplemental oxygen.
- Initiate intravenous access.
- Maintain continuous ECG monitoring.
- Continuously evaluate and reassess the airway and ventilation.
- Perform endotracheal intubation as necessary.
- Assess vital signs.
- Obtain and evaluate the patient's medical history.
- Perform a primary and secondary survey.
- Acquire a 12-lead ECG, especially if the patient is complaining of chest pain.

Like the patient in cardiac arrest, it is necessary to concentrate on the whole patient and not the rhythm, blood pressure, or findings of the 12-lead ECG. The following conditions are most likely to lead to cardiac arrest if not rapidly diagnosed and managed:

* Acute MI
* Acute pulmonary edema
* Dysrhythmias
* Hypotension and shock

Rhythms can be simply classified into two broad categories. Cardiac arrest (lethal) rhythms and non-cardiac arrest (nonlethal) rhythms. The cardiac arrest rhythms are segregated into four basic types (which have been discussed earlier in this chapter):

* Ventricular fibrillation
* Ventricular tachycardia
* Asystole
* Pulseless electrical activity

The non-cardiac arrest (nonlethal) rhythms are separated into two broad categories:

* Too slow (less than 60 beats per minute)
* Too fast (greater than 100 beats per minute)

When evaluating these rhythms it is necessary to concentrate on the patient and not the ECG rhythm. Look for evidence of physiologic instability such as hypotension, decreased mental status, chest pain, and other signs and symptoms. Use the primary and secondary ABCD survey to identify clinical compromise.

The algorithms for AED use and synchronized cardioversion were discussed in Chapter 6. The algorithms for acute myocardial infarction and for acute pulmonary edema, hypotension, and shock were discussed in Chapter 8.

Bradycardia Algorithm

This algorithm is used for patients who are not in cardiac arrest (Figure 10-5). The bradycardia is categorized into either absolute or relative bradycardia. It is important to determine if the patient is symptomatic, that is, displaying signs and symptoms of physiologic instability.

Signs and symptoms of physiologic instability associated with bradycardia are:

* Chest pain
* Shortness of breath
* Decreased level of consciousness
* Hypotension
* Evidence of poor perfusion and shock
* Pulmonary congestion
* Congestive heart failure
* Acute myocardial infarction

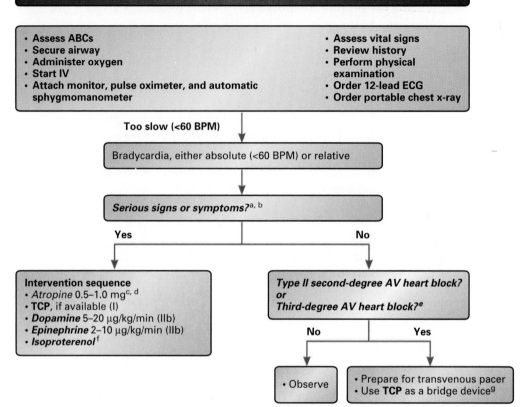

FIGURE 10-5 Bradycardia algorithm. Adapted with permission. Journal of the American Medical Association, October 28, 1992, Volume 268, No. 16, *Guidelines for Cardiopulmonary Resuscitation and Emergency Cardiac Care*, p.2221. ©1992 American Medical Association.

Bradycardia Algorithm: Key Points

- As with all other rhythms, treat the patient and not the rhythm. Continue to assess the patient for evidence of physiologic instability. Concentrate on treating the symptomatic patient.

- Absolute bradycardia is referred to as a heart rate less than 60 beats per minute. Relative bradycardia is a low rate, 68 for example, in a patient who is symptomatic.

- Assess for signs and symptoms of physiologic instability in bradycardia. This determines the need and extent of the patient management. You must determine if the slow rate is the actual etiology of the signs and symptoms or if the signs and symptoms are due to some other cause.

- Heart transplant patients have denervated hearts that will not respond to atropine. Thus, proceed directly to pacing or catecholamine infusion in the intervention sequence.

- Atropine is administered at 0.5 mg to 1 mg every 3 to 5 minutes to a total dose of 0.03 to 0.04 mg/kg. If the patient is severely symptomatic, use the 3 minute dosing interval. Use atropine with caution in the patient suffering from a Type II AV block and third degree block with wide QRS complexes (Class IIb).

- Never use lidocaine to treat a third degree heart block or any other ventricular rhythm.

- Isoproterenol should be used with extreme caution at low doses (Class IIb). At higher doses, it is considered harmful (Class III).

- Atropine will rarely accelerate the atrial rate in a second degree Mobitz Type II block and may increase the AV nodal block. This will decrease the ventricular rate and blood pressure and worsen the patient's condition.

- If the signs and symptoms associated with bradycardia are only mild, atropine should be considered the first-line drug of choice. The dose is 0.5 mg to 1.0 mg IV every 3 to 5 minutes up to a total dose of 0.03 mg/kg. The maximum vagolytic dose when used in asystolic cardiac arrest is 0.04 mg/kg.

- Dopamine, at a rate of 5 µg/kg/minute, should be used if hypotension is associated with the bradycardia. You can proceed directly to an epinephrine infusion if the signs and symptoms are severe. Infuse epinephrine at an initial rate of 1 to 2 µg/minute.

- Transcutaneous pacing is a Class I intervention in the symptomatic bradycardia patient. In a severely unstable patient, you should move immediately to transcutaneous pacing. A trial of atropine may be administered while the transcutaneous pacer is prepared.

- Patients with right ventricular infarction may present with bradycardia and hypotension. The hypotension is due to reduction in preload and not the bradycardia. A judicial fluid challenge may increase the right ventricular filling pressure with a subsequent increase in the force of right ventricular contractions, based on Starling's law.

- The Type II second degree AV block can rapidly convert to a third degree AV block. The patient needs to be prepared for transvenous pacing while the transcutaneous pacer is used as an immediate intervention.

- Atropine is relatively contraindicated in the third degree AV block patient. Transcutaneous pacing, dopamine, and an epinephrine infusion should be considered while awaiting a transvenous pacer.

Bradycardia Algorithm: Summary

Asymptomatic bradycardia:

1. Oxygen therapy
2. IV access
3. Continuous ECG monitoring
4. Reassess and monitor for development of signs and symptoms of hemodynamic instability.

Symptomatic bradycardia:

1. Oxygen therapy
2. IV access
3. Continuous ECG monitoring
4. Assess vital signs
5. Initiate transcutaneous pacing if immediately available. *
6. Atropine 0.5 mg to 1.0 mg IV push every 3 to 5 minutes to a total dose of 0.03 mg/kg [†, ‡]
7. Dopamine infusion beginning at 5 μg/kg/minute (titrate to acceptable heart rate and blood pressure up to 20 μg/kg/min)
8. Epinephrine infusion at 2 to 10 μg/minute
9. Isoproterenol at 2 to 10 μg/minute (Class IIb)

*Pacing is always a Class I intervention.
†A trial of atropine can be used in second degree Type II and third degree blocks as infusions and transcutaneous pacing is being prepared.
‡Go to pacing, dopamine, and epinephrine infusion in denervated hearts.

Tachycardia Algorithm

Tachydysrhythmias can be broken into two basic categories based on the morphology (wave form) of the ECG tracing: narrow complex and wide complex. Each of these types can be further categorized, as shown below.

Tachydysrhythmia Categories Based on Morphology of ECG Tracing	
Narrow Complex Tachycardias:	Wide Complex Tachycardias:
• Atrial fibrillation or atrial flutter	• Ventricular tachycardia
• Supraventricular tachycardia	• Wide complex tachycardia of an uncertain type (unknown whether the impulse origin is supraventricular or ventricular)

Tachydysrhythmias are also categorized based on hemodynamic stability, which is primarily determined by signs and symptoms exhibited by the patient. Patients who are exhibiting signs and symptoms of hemodynamic instability are categorized as "unstable," whereas the patient who has no complaints or who is not showing any signs or symptoms is considered to be "stable." Thus, all of the tachydysrhythmias, whether narrow or wide complex, can be clinically categorized as either stable or unstable.

Tachydysrhythmia Categories Based on Patient's Hemodynamic Status	
Stable: • Patient has no complaints, signs, or symptoms.	Unstable: • Patient has signs and symptoms of hemodynamic instability

You must not only determine the rhythm but also the hemodynamic status of the patient, since the management is significantly different for the stable vs. the unstable patient. This requires you to assess and treat the "whole" patient and not just the rhythm. Whether the rhythm is wide complex, narrow complex, atrial flutter/fibrillation, supraventricular, ventricular, or uncertain, the urgency of management is based on the patient's hemodynamic status and ability to compensate while in the rhythm. Symptomatic, unstable patients require immediate intervention.

The signs and symptoms of hemodynamic instability are the same for tachycardias as for bradycardias. Signs and symptoms of an unstable tachycardia requiring immediate intervention are:

- Hypotension
- Congestive heart failure
- Decreased level of consciousness
- Chest pain
- Acute MI
- Shortness of breath
- Evidence of poor perfusion and shock
- Pulmonary congestion

When treating a patient with an unstable (symptomatic) tachydysrhythmia, it is important to determine whether the tachycardia is a result of an underlying condition that is also producing the signs and symptoms (for example, both tachycardia and chest pain resulting from an MI) or if the signs and symptoms are a result of the tachycardia (for example, chest pain resulting from tachycardia).

When considering management of the patient based on the algorithm approach (Figure 10-6), it is best to categorize the patient and rhythm into one of the following:

- Stable supraventricular tachycardia (narrow complex)
- Unstable supraventricular tachycardia (narrow complex)
- Stable ventricular tachycardia (wide complex)
- Unstable ventricular tachycardia (wide complex)
- Stable wide-complex tachycardia of an uncertain type
- Unstable wide-complex tachycardia of an uncertain type

Tachycardia Algorithm: Key Points
Atrial Fibrillation/Flutter

- Cardioversion is the treatment of choice for an unstable tachycardia. This is performed prior to the use of antidysrhythmic agents.
- Do not do carotid sinus massage in patients with carotid bruits. Likewise, do not use the ice water immersion vagal technique if the patient has ischemic heart disease.

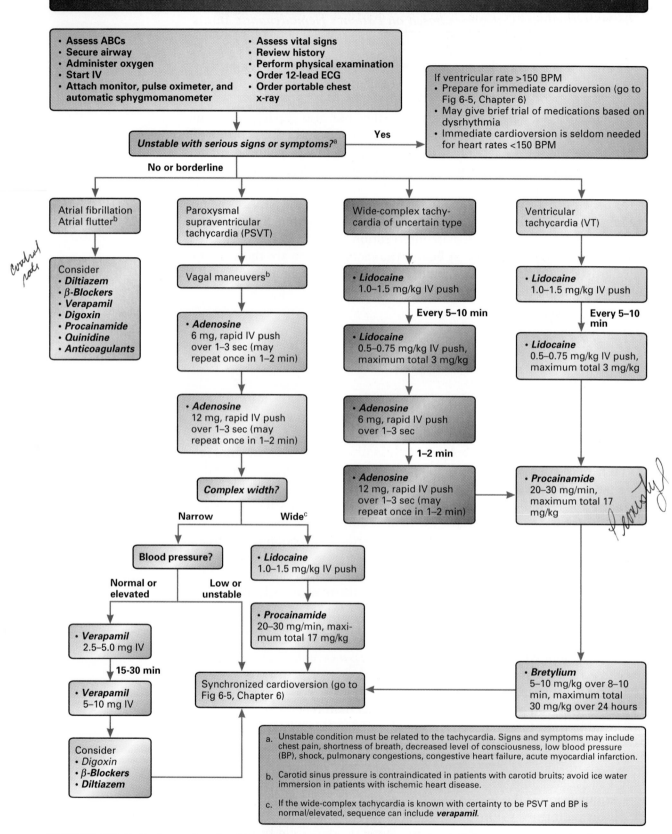

ALGORITHM: TACHYCARDIA

- Assess ABCs
- Secure airway
- Administer oxygen
- Start IV
- Attach monitor, pulse oximeter, and automatic sphygmomanometer

- Assess vital signs
- Review history
- Perform physical examination
- Order 12-lead ECG
- Order portable chest x-ray

If ventricular rate >150 BPM
- Prepare for immediate cardioversion (go to Fig 6-5, Chapter 6)
- May give brief trial of medications based on dysrhythmia
- Immediate cardioversion is seldom needed for heart rates <150 BPM

Unstable with serious signs or symptoms?[a] → **Yes**

No or borderline

Atrial fibrillation Atrial flutter[b]

Consider
- *Diltiazem*
- *β-Blockers*
- *Verapamil*
- *Digoxin*
- *Procainamide*
- *Quinidine*
- *Anticoagulants*

Paroxysmal supraventricular tachycardia (PSVT)

Vagal maneuvers[b]

- *Adenosine* 6 mg, rapid IV push over 1–3 sec (may repeat once in 1–2 min)

- *Adenosine* 12 mg, rapid IV push over 1–3 sec (may repeat once in 1–2 min)

Complex width?

Narrow / **Wide**[c]

Blood pressure?

- *Lidocaine* 1.0–1.5 mg/kg IV push

- *Procainamide* 20–30 mg/min, maximum total 17 mg/kg

Normal or elevated / **Low or unstable**

- *Verapamil* 2.5–5.0 mg IV

15-30 min

- *Verapamil* 5–10 mg IV

Consider
- *Digoxin*
- *β-Blockers*
- *Diltiazem*

Wide-complex tachy-cardia of uncertain type

- *Lidocaine* 1.0–1.5 mg/kg IV push

Every 5–10 min

- *Lidocaine* 0.5–0.75 mg/kg IV push, maximum total 3 mg/kg

- *Adenosine* 6 mg, rapid IV push over 1–3 sec

1–2 min

- *Adenosine* 12 mg, rapid IV push over 1–3 sec (may repeat once in 1–2 min)

Ventricular tachycardia (VT)

- *Lidocaine* 1.0–1.5 mg/kg IV push

Every 5–10 min

- *Lidocaine* 0.5–0.75 mg/kg IV push, maximum total 3 mg/kg

- *Procainamide* 20–30 mg/min, maximum total 17 mg/kg

- *Bretylium* 5–10 mg/kg over 8–10 min, maximum total 30 mg/kg over 24 hours

Synchronized cardioversion (go to Fig 6-5, Chapter 6)

a. Unstable condition must be related to the tachycardia. Signs and symptoms may include chest pain, shortness of breath, decreased level of consciousness, low blood pressure (BP), shock, pulmonary congestions, congestive heart failure, acute myocardial infarction.

b. Carotid sinus pressure is contraindicated in patients with carotid bruits; avoid ice water immersion in patients with ischemic heart disease.

c. If the wide-complex tachycardia is known with certainty to be PSVT and BP is normal/elevated, sequence can include *verapamil*.

FIGURE 10-6 Tachycardia algorithm. Adapted with permission. Journal of the American Medical Association, October 28, 1992, Volume 268, No. 16, *Guidelines for Cardiopulmonary Resuscitation and Emergency Cardiac Care*, p.2223. ©1992 American Medical Association.

- Atrial fibrillation and atrial flutter may not require any intervention unless the patient develops signs and symptoms of hemodynamic instability. This usually occurs as the result of a rapid ventricular response. The management is geared toward slowing the ventricular response and not converting the rhythm to normal sinus.
- Atrial flutter is a less stable rhythm than atrial fibrillation.
- Calcium channel blockers and beta blockers are used as medications to control the rate in atrial fibrillation and flutter.
- Vagal maneuvers may slow the rhythm enough to allow for diagnosis of atrial fibrillation or flutter versus other supraventricular tachydysrhythmias.
- Cardioversion should be performed if the patient develops hemodynamic instability.

Paroxysmal Supraventricular Tachycardia (PSVT)
- Immediate cardioversion is needed if serious signs and symptoms of hemodynamic instability are evident.
- If the complexes are wide, treat the tachycardia like ventricular tachycardia.
- Vagal maneuvers should be performed prior to medications in the stable patient. Pressure on the eyeball as a vagal maneuver should be discouraged because of the chance of causing retinal detachment.
- Adenosine is an effective agent in the conversion of PSVT. It produces less hypotension and has a much shorter half-life than verapamil. Adenosine, at a dose of 6 mg, must be administered as a rapid IV push followed by a 20 ml fluid bolus as a flush and elevation of the arm. It can be repeated after 1 to 2 minutes at 12 mg.
- Verapamil is administered at 5 mg IV push over a two minute period. A significant side effect is hypotension. A repeat bolus at 10 mg can be administered after 15 to 30 minutes.
- Hypotension secondary to verapamil administration can be controlled by placing the patient in the Trendelenburg position, administration of fluids, or the administration of 0.5 to 1.0 grams of calcium chloride.
- Beta blockers, digoxin, sedation and rest, overdrive pacing, cardioversion, and other antidysrhythmics may be considered following failure of adenosine or verapamil to convert the rhythm in the stable PSVT patient.

Wide-Complex PSVT and Wide-Complex Tachycardias of Uncertain Type
- Verapamil should never be given to a patient with a wide-complex tachycardia of an uncertain type. Administration of verapamil to a patient in ventricular tachycardia can be lethal.
- Lidocaine is the first-line drug of choice in the wide-complex tachycardia of an uncertain type. This is a Class I intervention.
- Adenosine does not produce any harm in this situation and should follow lidocaine if unsuccessful. This is a Class IIa intervention.
- If lidocaine and adenosine are unsuccessful, procainamide can be administered. Hypotension is a concern following the administration of procainamide. It is also a Class I intervention.
- Verapamil should only be used if the wide-complex tachycardia is certainly supraventricular and hypotension is not present.

Ventricular Tachycardia

- Ventricular tachycardia is classified as:
  - pulseless ventricular tachycardia
  - unstable ventricular tachycardia
  - stable ventricular tachycardia
- Pulseless ventricular tachycardia is managed exactly the same as ventricular fibrillation.
- A patient in ventricular tachycardia with hypotension, shortness of breath, chest pain, altered level of consciousness, or pulmonary edema is considered to be unstable. Immediate cardioversion is the treatment of choice.
- The stable ventricular tachycardia patient is treated with antidysrhythmic agents. Lidocaine is the first-line drug of choice. An initial loading dose of 1.0 to 1.5 mg/kg is administered with repeat doses of 0.5 to 0.75 mg/kg after 5 to 10 minutes. A total maximum cumulative dose is 3 mg/kg. If lidocaine was successful in converting the rhythm, a maintenance infusion of 2 to 4 mg/minute should be initiated. The correct bolus/infusion ratios are shown below.

Total Cumulative Lidocaine Bolus Dose	Lidocaine Maintenance Infusion Dose
1.0–1.75 mg/kg	2 mg/minute
2.0–2.75 mg/kg	3 mg/minute
3.0 mg/kg	4 mg/minute

- Procainamide is the second-line drug of choice in the stable VT patient. It is administered as an infusion at 20 to 30 mg/minute. A total loading dose is 17 mg/kg.
  The end points for administration of procainamide are:
  - hypotension ensues
  - the QRS complex widens by 50% the original width
  - the maximum dose of 17 mg/kg is administered
  - the rhythm is abolished
- If procainamide is effective in abolishing the rhythm, a maintenance infusion of 1 to 4 mg/minute should be initiated.
- Bretylium is used as the third-line drug of choice in stable VT. It is administered by mixing 5 mg/kg of the drug in 50 to 100 ml of normal saline and infusing it over an 8 to 10 minute period. If bretylium is effective in eliminating the VT, initiate a maintenance infusion at 1 to 2 mg/minute.

Synchronous vs. Unsynchronized Cardioversion

- Synchronized cardioversion should be performed in a patient who is unstable or who has not responded adequately to medication. Because of a potential delay in complex recognition, unsynchronous cardioversion may be performed in severely unstable tachycardias.

Torsades de Pointes

- The amplitude and direction of the electrical activity continuously changes. Consider torsades when traditional VT therapy does not convert patients not in cardiac arrest.

- Electrical pacing is the treatment of choice.
- Magnesium sulfate at 1 to 2 grams over a 1 to 2 minute period is the drug of choice following an infusion of 1 to 2 grams over 1 hour.
- Isoproterenol can be used to overdrive the ventricular rate and abolish the dysrhythmia. It is administered at 2 to 8 µg/minute.
- Torsades is commonly due to tricyclic antidepressant, other drug overdose, or hypokalemia.

Stable PSVT (Narrow Complex Tachycardia): Summary

1. Initiate oxygen therapy.
2. Establish intravenous access.
3. Initiate continuous ECG monitoring.
4. Assess vital signs.
5. Perform vagal maneuvers.
6. Administer adenosine at 6 mg rapid IV push.
7. Repeat adenosine at 12 mg rapid IV push after 1 to 2 minutes.
8. Repeat adenosine at 12 mg after 1 to 2 minutes.
9. Administer verapamil at 2.5 to 5 mg slow IV push repeated after 15 to 30 minutes at 5 to 10 mg slow IV push.
   - Consider digoxin, beta blockers, and diltiazem.
   - Consider synchronized cardioversion.
10. If the patient becomes unstable, proceed directly to cardioversion.
11. Assess BP prior to verapamil administration.

Unstable PSVT (Narrow Complex Tachycardia): Summary

1. Initiate oxygen therapy.
2. Establish intravenous access.
3. Provide continuous ECG monitoring.
4. Assess vital signs.
5. Consider a brief trial of adenosine at 6 mg.
6. Premedicate with 2 to 5 mg of diazepam if patient condition and time permits.
7. Deliver synchronized cardioversion at: [*],[†]
   50 J
   100 J
   200 J
   300 J
   360 J
8. Administer adenosine or verapamil.

[*]Deliver asynchronous cardioversion if tachydysrhythmia is greater than 160 beats per minute or the circuit does not capture.
[†]If successful conversion occurs but PSVT recurs, do not continue with cardioversion.

Stable Ventricular (Wide Complex) Tachycardia: Summary

1. Initiate oxygen therapy.

2. Establish intravenous access.

3. Provide continuous ECG monitoring.

4. Assess vital signs.

5. Administer lidocaine at 1 to 1.5 mg/kg IV push repeated every 5 to 10 minutes at 0.5 to 0.75 mg/kg to a total cumulative maximum dose of 3 mg/kg.

6. Administer procainamide at 20 to 30 mg/minute IV infusion to a total dose of 17 mg/kg.

7. Administer bretylium at 5 to 10 mg/kg diluted in 50 to 100 ml of normal saline as an IV infusion over an 8 to 10 minute period. Repeat every 15 to 30 minutes to a total dose of 30 mg/kg.

8. Consider synchronized cardioversion if drug therapy is ineffective.

9. Initiate a maintenance infusion of the medication that converted the rhythm:
   – lidocaine at 2 to 4 mg/minute
   – procainamide at 1 to 4 mg/minute
   – bretylium at 1 to 2 mg/minute

10. If at any time the patient becomes unstable, proceed to cardioversion.

Unstable Ventricular (Wide Complex) Tachycardia: Summary

1. Initiate oxygen therapy.

2. Establish intravenous access.

3. Provide continuous ECG monitoring.

4. Assess vital signs.

5. Consider brief trial of lidocaine.

6. Consider sedation.

7. Provide cardioversion at:
   100 J
   200 J
   300 J
   360 J
   Note: Polymorphic ventricular tachycardia—begin at 200 J

8. Administer lidocaine at 1 to 1.5 mg/kg.

9. Cardiovert at 360 J.

10. Continue with sequence of drug–shock to include the administration of procainamide and bretylium.

11. If the patient is severely unstable, bretylium should follow the administration of lidocaine.

Stable Wide-Complex Tachycardia of Uncertain Type: Summary

1. Initiate oxygen therapy.
2. Establish intravenous access.
3. Provide continuous ECG monitoring.
4. Assess vital signs.
5. Administer lidocaine at 1.0 to 1.5 mg/kg IV push.
6. Repeat lidocaine at 0.5 to 0.75 mg/kg every 5 to 10 minutes to a total maximum cumulative dose of 3 mg/kg.
7. Administer adenosine at 6 mg rapid IV push.
8. Repeat adenosine after 1 to 2 minutes at 12 mg rapid IV push. Adenosine could be repeated once more in 1 to 2 minutes at 12 mg rapid IV push.
9. Administer procainamide at 20 to 30 mg/minute to a total maximum dose of 17 mg/kg.
10. Administer bretylium at 5 mg/kg over an 8 to 10 minute period.
11. Repeat bretylium every 15 to 30 minutes at 5 to 10 mg/kg to a total maximum cumulative dose of 30 to 35 mg/kg.
12. Consider synchronized cardioversion at:
    100 J
    200 J
    300 J
    360 J

Unstable Wide-Complex Tachycardia of Uncertain Type: Summary

1. Initiate oxygen therapy.
2. Establish intravenous access.
3. Provide continuous ECG monitoring.
4. Assess vital signs.
5. Consider a brief trial of lidocaine.
6. Consider sedation.
7. Provide cardioversion at:
    100 J
    200 J
    300 J
    360 J
8. Administer lidocaine at 1 to 1.5 mg/kg IV push.
9. Cardiovert at 360 J.
10. Repeat lidocaine every 5 to 10 minutes at 0.5 to 0.75 mg/kg until a total maximum cumulative dose of 3 mg/kg is reached. Cardiovert at 360 J after each lidocaine bolus.
11. Administer adenosine at 6 mg rapid IV push.
12. Repeat adenosine after 1 to 2 minutes at 12 mg rapid IV push. Adenosine could be repeated once more in 1 to 2 minutes at 12 mg rapid IV push.
13. Administer procainamide at 20 to 30 mg/minute to a total maximum dose of 17 mg/kg. Continue the sequence of drug–shock with the administration of procainamide and bretylium.
14. Administer bretylium at 5 mg/kg over an 8 to 10 minute period. Bretylium can be repeated at 5 to 10 mg/kg every 15 to 30 minutes to a total maximum cumulative dose of 30 to 35 mg/kg.

CASE STUDY FOLLOW-UP

You are frantically summoned by an elderly man to attend to his wife who is found slumped in the front seat of his car. The elderly woman is ashen gray and motionless. You immediately call for help and direct the others to get the cardiac resuscitation room ready.

Basic-Life-Support

You open the car door and shout at the woman, "Hey, ma'am, can you hear me?!" You shake her shoulder and get no response. You open her airway and assess for breathing. The patient is breathless. You deliver two quick ventilations with a pocket mask. You assess for a carotid pulse and find none. You and two others immediately remove the woman from the car, place her on the gurney, and begin CPR as she is quickly wheeled into the cardiac resuscitation room.

Advanced Life Support

You immediately perform a quick look with the defibrillation paddles and identify ventricular fibrillation on the oscilloscope. You place defibrillation pads on the chest and scan the patient while shouting, "I'm clear, you're clear, everyone's clear," as you begin to charge the defibrillator to 200 J. You deliver the first shock and hold the paddles firmly on the chest as you wait for the rhythm to return to the isoelectric line on the oscilloscope. The monitor shows V-fib. You charge to 300 J as you again shout to clear the patient. You deliver the shock and reassess the rhythm. It remains V-fib. You charge to 360 J and deliver the third shock in the stacked shock sequence. You check for the carotid pulse and do not find one.

By this time, your resuscitation team has assembled in the room. You instruct Mike to continue chest compressions. Heather is at the airway and resumes bag-valve-mask ventilation. You instruct her to hyperventilate the patient and perform endotracheal intubation. George is establishing intravenous access in an antecubital vein in the right arm. You hook up the continuous monitoring ECG cable.

Heather yells, "Tubes in." You check for chest rise and fall while you listen to the epigastrium. No sounds are heard in the stomach, so you pro-

SUMMARY

In this chapter we have provided algorithms for managing patients who are in cardiac arrest or suffering from other common dysrhythmias. The algorithms are to be used only as guidelines and not as a legal standard of care. You must use your clinical judgment and expertise when making patient management decisions, since all patients are different and require individual consideration.

When managing the patient in cardiac arrest or one who is suffering from a dysrhythmia, it is imperative that you treat the whole patient and not just the rhythm. Developing tunnel vision and managing rhythms will only lead to unsuccessful resuscitation attempts. Assess your patient and consider conditions that may have led to the cardiac arrest or conditions that are preventing you from successfully converting the rhythm. Get to the etiology of the problem, save the heart, and most importantly save the head!

REVIEW QUESTIONS

1. A drug that is not well supported by scientific evidence but is considered possibly helpful and not harmful, is classified as
   a. I.
   b. IIa.
   c. IIb.
   d. III.

(continued)

ceed to assess breath sounds over the lungs. You indicate, "Breath sounds are equal and clear bilaterally. Secure the tube."

You ask, "George, where's my IV line?" George states, "This lady has bad veins. The IV just blew." You instruct Heather to administer 2 mg of epinephrine down the endotracheal tube and aggressively hyperventilate for 30 to 60 seconds. After the 30 to 60 seconds, you clear the patient and defibrillate at 360 J. You check for a carotid pulse and find none.

You order, "Continue compressions and ventilations." George has now established a patent IV line. You estimate the patient's weight at 80 kg. You instruct him to administer 120 mg of lidocaine IV push. You wait 60 seconds following the drug administration, clear the patient, and defibrillate at 360 J. No pulse is found. The monitor now shows asystole. You switch to Leads I and III to be sure the patient is not still in V-fib in another lead. The monitor shows asystole in each lead.

You order continuation of the compressions and ventilations while you administer 1 mg of atropine IV push. After 2 minutes you stop and assess the rhythm. You find V-fib on the oscilloscope. You immediately defibrillate at 360 J. No pulse is found, so CPR is continued. You administer another bolus of 1 mg of epinephrine, followed by another 120 mg of lidocaine. After 30 seconds, you defibrillate at 360 J. No pulse is found, and you instruct the team to continue CPR. You administer 400 mg of bretylium IV push. After 60 seconds you defibrillate at 360 J.

Transfer
You find a faint pulse upon assessment, and the monitor shows a sinus rhythm at a rate of 82. The blood pressure is 102/64. You instruct George to mix a bretylium infusion and run it at 2 mg/minute. The patient remains unresponsive with no spontaneous ventilation. You reassess the endotracheal tube and IV line and ensure that the bretylium infusion is running properly. You contact the critical care unit and prepare the patient for transfer. The patient is transferred to the unit without further incident.

You learn the next day that the patient coded later that night and died.

2. Which of the following medications **cannot** be administered endotracheally?
   a. bretylium
   b. naloxone
   c. lidocaine
   d. epinephrine

3. Which of the following would be considered an acceptable alternative dose regimen for epinephrine?
   a. 1 mg/kg IV push repeated every 3 to 5 minutes
   b. 5 mg IV push repeated every 10 minutes
   c. 0.5 mg, 1 mg, 3 mg IV push repeated every 3 to 5 minutes
   d. 0.1 mg/kg IV push repeated every 3 to 5 minutes

4. In which of the following conditions is sodium bicarbonate a class III intervention?
   a. prolonged cardiac arrest in an intubated patient
   b. a patient with suspected hypoxic lactic acidosis
   c. a tricyclic antidepressant overdose
   d. a patient found to be hyperkalemic

5. Immediately upon identifying ventricular fibrillation on the monitor, you should
   a. defibrillate at 200 joules.
   b. begin chest compression and ventilation.
   c. establish an intravenous line and intubate the patient.
   d. attach the continuous ECG monitor and check a second lead.

6. During the resuscitation, the rhythm converts to asystole. You should immediately
   a. defibrillate at 200 joules, since it may be a fine ventricular fibrillation.
   b. check a second lead to ensure that it is not ventricular fibrillation.
   c. stop chest compression and decompress the chest.
   d. administer a bolus of sodium bicarbonate.

7. You have provided the initial three stacked defibrillations to a patient in ventricular fibrillation. The patient regains a pulse for a few minutes, then suddenly reverts back into ventricular fibrillation. You should immediately
   a. administer a bolus of lidocaine at 1 mg/kg.
   b. defibrillate at 200 joules.
   c. defibrillate at 360 joules.
   d. hyperventilate and perform endotracheal intubation.

8. The appropriate dose of bretylium, when used for a patient in ventricular fibrillation, is
   a. 5 mg/kg repeated in 5 minutes at 10 mg/kg to a total dose of 30 mg/kg.
   b. 10 mg/kg repeated in 5 minutes at 5 mg/kg to a total dose of 30 mg/kg.
   c. 30 mg/kg repeated in 10 minutes at 30 mg/kg.
   d. 5 mg/kg mixed in 50 ml of normal saline repeated every 8 minutes.

9. Following the administration of a drug in the patient in ventricular fibrillation, you should
   a. immediately defibrillate at 360 joules.
   b. perform CPR for 30 to 60 seconds, then defibrillate at 360 joules.
   c. perform CPR for 1 to 2 minutes, then defibrillate at 360 joules.
   d. repeat the defibrillation sequence at 200 J, 300 J, and 360 J.

10. Hypovolemia, hypoxemia, tension pneumothorax, and pericardial tamponade are all possible etiologies of
    a. ventricular fibrillation.
    b. symptomatic bradycardia.
    c. unstable ventricular tachycardia.
    d. pulseless electrical activity.

11. The treatment of choice for a patient in PEA from a tension pneumothorax is
    a. 250 ml fluid bolus of normal saline.
    b. needle thoracentesis.
    c. administration of 1 mg of epinephrine.
    d. transcutaneous pacing.

12. The total cumulative dose of atropine in a 70 kg patient in asystole is
    a. 1.0 mg.   c. 2.8 mg.
    b. 2.1 mg.   d. 4.0 mg.

13. Following successful resuscitation, the patient's blood pressure remains hypotensive. Your **first** consideration in management of the blood pressure would be to
    a. administer a fluid bolus of 250 to 500 ml if fluid overload is not suspected.
    b. initiate a norepinephrine infusion at 20 µg/minute.
    c. initiate a dopamine infusion starting at 1 to 2µg/kg/minute.
    d. begin transcutaneous pacing at a rate of 80 and 100 milliamp.

14. The patient you have just successfully resuscitated is in a supraventricular tachycardia. He is normotensive and perfusing well. The treatment of choice for the supraventricular tachycardia in this case is
    a. administration of adenosine at 6 mg rapid IV bolus.
    b. to leave the rhythm untreated unless the patient becomes hypotensive.
    c. synchronized cardioversion starting at 50 joules.
    d. administration of verapamil at 5 mg, then repeated in 15 minutes at 10 mg.

15. You encounter a patient who is in a third-degree heart block at a ventricular rate of 30 beats/minute. The monitor shows couplets of premature ventricular contractions. Your treatment of choice is
    a. administration of a lidocaine bolus of 1 to 1.5 mg/kg.
    b. administration of atropine at 1.0 mg.
    c. initiation of transcutaneous pacing.
    d. initiation of an epinephrine infusion at 2 to 10 µg/minute.

16. You are treating a symptomatic patient in a second-degree Mobitz Type I heart block. You have attached the external pacer, adjusted the milliamps, and there is still no capture occurring. Your next intervention should be
    a. continue with external pacing.
    b. administer a bolus of epinephrine at 1 mg.
    c. initiate an infusion of dopamine at 5 µg/kg/minute.
    d. initiate an epinephrine infusion at 2 µg/minute.

17. A patient comes into the emergency department complaining of palpitations. The patient denies any chest pain, weakness, dyspnea, or any other complaints. He is alert and oriented to person, place, and time. His skin is warm and dry. His vital signs are: blood pressure 142/66, respirations 16, and pulse 196/minute. You attach the monitor and it reveals a narrow complex supraventricular tachycardia at a rate of 196. The treatment of choice is
    a. administer 6 mg of adenosine IV push.
    b. perform a vagal maneuver.
    c. administer 5 mg of verapamil IV push.
    d. perform synchronized cardioversion at 50 joules.

18. While treating a stable supraventricular tachycardia patient, he suddenly becomes weak, lightheaded, and pale and complains of chest discomfort. Your next immediate action should be
    a. perform synchronized cardioversion at 50 joules.
    b. defibrillate at 200 joules.
    c. try another vagal maneuver.
    d. administer verapamil at 5 mg slow IV push.

19. The treatment of choice for the patient in torsades de pointes is
    a. administration of lidocaine at 1.0 to 1.5 mg/kg IV push.
    b. initiation of electrical pacing.
    c. administration of magnesium sulfate at 1 to 2 grams IV.
    d. perform vagal maneuvers.

20. You have just administered a third bolus of 0.5 mg/kg of lidocaine to a patient having PVCs. You have administered a total cumulative bolus dose of 2.0 mg/kg when the ectopy is abolished. You initiate a lidocaine infusion. The infusion should be run at
    a. 1 mg/minute.   c. 3 mg/minute.
    b. 2 mg/minute.   d. 4 mg/minute.

Chapter**Eleven**

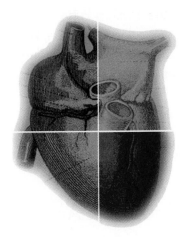

Case Studies: Application Exercises

It has no doubt occurred to you that you can learn all about a variety of advanced-cardiac-life-support topics—how to perform an intubation, how to gain IV access, how to read an ECG, and so on—and yet have no idea how, or if, you will be able to apply it all when a real patient is turning blue in front of you, lights are flashing, the noise level is rising, people are running around, and panic threatens to destroy your thinking processes.

During your ACLS course, you will work through a set of case studies that provide a framework to practice functioning as part of an ACLS team in simulated cardiac emergencies. This chapter presents the core case studies from the ACLS course to help you preview them and practice applying the advanced-cardiac-life-support concepts and skills you have studied in the preceding chapters.

The topics that will be covered are:

- Some Questions and Answers about the ACLS Course
- The Core Cases
- Respiratory Arrest with a Pulse
- Witnessed Ventricular Fibrillation, Adult Cardiac Arrest
- Adult Ventricular Fibrillation/Pulseless Ventricular Tachycardia
- Pulseless Electrical Activity
- Asystole
- Adult Myocardial Infarction
- Bradycardia
- Unstable Tachycardia
- Stable Tachycardia

Some Questions and Answers about the ACLS Course

Why did you come to the course?

The ACLS course can be one of the most valuable and rewarding classes that you will ever take. Many clinicians have received extensive professional training, but the training may fall short in practical, applicable instruction on what to do in the most critical patient situations. The ACLS course will provide this kind of practical instruction and significantly increase your confidence in managing cardiac emergencies.

What should you get out of the course?

The major goal of the American Heart Association's Advanced Cardiac Life Support course is for you to master the knowledge, skills, and attitudes you will need to assume the role as team member during the first 10 minutes of a cardiac arrest. Your specific role will depend on your clinical background, work environment, and experience. The challenge of the ACLS course is to be sensitive to your individual background and the role that you will assume in cardiac arrest management as part of your clinical practice. It is difficult to be all things to all people; but the Heart Association's course uses an interdisciplinary approach to emphasize the importance of the team concept to cardiac emergencies.

The team concept is ideal for managing a cardiac arrest. Each member is vitally important in a successful resuscitation. Each member must take his role seriously and work with the team in a synchronized fashion.

The typical arrest team includes the following roles:

- **Team leader**—the individual who leads the arrest, performs the patient assessment, interprets ECGs, uses the monitor/defibrillator, and directs and oversees the actions of the team members. The team leader makes all of the clinical decisions *with input and suggestions from the team.* It is *not* necessary for the team leader to be the most highly certified, senior, or experienced member of the team. In fact, it is beneficial for less-experienced individuals to serve as the team leader to gain experience and become better team members.

- **Airway and ventilation**—one individual to manage the airway and ventilate the patient, as directed by the team leader. This usually includes intubating the patient.
- **IV and medications**—one individual to gain IV access and administer medications, as directed by the team leader
- **External chest compressions**—one individual to perform external chest compressions, as directed by the team leader
- **Record keeper**—one individual to record the times and all pertinent assessment findings, patient status, interventions performed, medications given, and events of the resuscitation

There will be circumstances where there are initially not enough individuals to form a complete team. If fact, it is generally true that you have *either* too few *or* too many people on the arrest team. In the case of too few people, some members of the team will assume multiple roles. If too many people become distracting, the team leader should take control and ask those not directly involved in the treatment of the patient to leave.

But, I will NEVER have to run a code where I work!

The ACLS course is designed to make you more effective as an arrest team member. In order to accomplish this objective, you will be expected to serve as the team leader during the course. Regardless of the role you assume in actual clinical situations, the experience of working as team leader will help you to be able to

- anticipate the actions of the team leader
- offer valuable suggestions and input to the team leader
- appreciate the priorities in managing problems
- anticipate and manage problems and inform the team leader of your actions

It is always easier to be a "Monday morning quarterback" or comment from the bleachers. In the ACLS course you will be the quarterback. This will help you appreciate how difficult it can be to serve as team leader and, therefore, help you be a better team member. This should not be an intimidating or frightening experience. This is an opportunity to practice and increase your cardiac arrest management skills in a non-threatening, supportive environment, when no patient's well-being is on the line.

So what is case-based teaching?

The revised ACLS class uses a number of standardized cases to illustrate common cardiac emergency situations. You will have an opportunity to work through these cases during the course, but this text will present them in writing to prepare you for the course. All of the cases integrate knowledge, skills, and attitudes, but each has been designed to address specific facets of emergency cardiac care. If you pay careful attention to the key points and unacceptable actions, you will be well prepared for the ACLS class, and you will find that you have much greater confidence when treating cardiac emergencies.

An instructional difficulty in the course is that significant teaching that is done during a case study can become distracting to the flow of the case.

It is easy to become sidetracked in how to use the defibrillator or the characteristics of various ECGs and "get lost" in the scenario. This book resolves this problem by having covered the instructional material in the preceding chapters. This enables us, in this chapter, to minimize the background material as we go through the cases. We provide you with page numbers to make it easier to find the appropriate reference. If you need clarification on how to perform a skill or why a particular drug is indicated, just refer to the appropriate section of the book.

The Core Cases

To be consistent with the American Heart Association's ACLS course, we will emphasize the core cases. Each case follows a standard format:

Overview: An overview of the case and a list of the algorithms that are used
Psychomotor Skills: A list of the skills that are covered
Background Patient Information: Background information on the hypothetical patient who is at the center of the case
Assessment and Management Priorities: The pertinent assessment findings and appropriate management of the patient. In real life, assessment and management are often done concurrently. It is difficult to represent this fact by words printed on paper. The following icons will be used to organize the flow of the case.

   assessment icon

   management icon

Key Points: The major considerations for this kind of case.
In this scenario, you MUST: These are considered the critical actions and skills necessary to maximize the patient's chance for survival.
Unacceptable Actions: Actions that represent common mistakes made in managing these situations. Any of these reduce the patient's probability of survival and are considered to be unacceptable.

An important note: Patient care is *not* linear. Assessment and management, especially in emergency situations, occur simultaneously. Multiple individuals perform skills and interventions concurrently. The ACLS cases, by design, attempt to describe a non-linear process in a linear fashion.

This textbook is intended to be used interactively. Use a note card or ruler to cover the management steps as you read each case. At each step, think of what you would do based on the assessment information.

Respiratory Arrest with a Pulse

Overview
This case is used to emphasize progressive and sequential airway management, ventilatory support, and IV access for the patient in respiratory arrest. The order of airway management techniques in the patient in respiratory arrest is identical to that for the patient in cardiac arrest. Using the patient

in respiratory arrest as an example offers you an opportunity to focus on airway management and IV priorities and skills.

This case uses the following algorithm to establish these priorities:

- Universal Algorithm: see Chapter 10, Figure 10-1

Psychomotor Skills

- Noninvasive airway techniques
  - pocket face mask
  - bag-valve mask
  - oropharyngeal airway
  - barrier methods
  - oxygen delivery systems
- Invasive airway techniques
  - endotracheal intubation
- Intravenous access

Background Patient Information

A 70-year-old-female presents with a long history of heavy smoking and a past medical history of COPD. She has experienced 3 hours of severe dyspnea, which has been refractory to her prescription medications. Immediately upon your arrival and questioning of the patient, she stops breathing. You are by yourself (and feel extremely lonely right now).

Assessment and Management

Time		Assessment and Management	See Pages
01:12	A	ABCD Survey: The patient is unconscious and unresponsive.	15, 286-87
01:12	M	Get help! Activate your code team or call 911. Open the patient's airway using the head-tilt, chin-lift method. If available, use an oral or nasal airway to maintain the airway. If not available, maintain an open airway with the head-tilt, chin-lift.	16-19
01:12	A	Breathing: You look, listen, and feel. The patient is not breathing.	19-21
01:13	M	You must ventilate the patient immediately. With any luck, you will have some adjunctive equipment to use. The best course of action is to use a bag-valve-mask, mouth-to-mask, or a barrier device. Ventilate the patient twice.	74-80
01:13	A	Circulation: The patient has a carotid pulse. Therefore, you realize, defibrillation or compressions are not appropriate.	21
01:15	M	Continue to ventilate the patient with high-percent oxygen. Definitively manage the patient's airway. Quickly prepare the intubation equipment and intubate the patient.	43-58

Time		Assessment and Management	See Pages
01:16	A	You reassess the airway once you have intubated. You make sure to confirm tube placement.	56
01:19	M	Establish an IV lifeline. This is a routine part of advanced life support and should be performed as soon as possible. Often, other people can start an IV while you are intubating.	98-99
01:21	A	You obtain complete vital signs and a history, perform a physical exam, attach the monitor, and obtain a 12 lead ECG.	
01:34	M	Consider suspected causes and use the appropriate algorithm. Transfer the patient to a critical care unit and provide ventilator support.	

Key Points

- The assessment of and attention to the airway are a major priority in any unconscious patient.
- Use the Universal Algorithm.
- Use the primary ABCD survey to establish the basic priorities of management in the arrested and nonarrested patient.
- Use noninvasive airway techniques for the initial management of the airway. These include manual positioning, oropharyngeal airways, and suctioning.
- Basic techniques are used to initially ventilate the nonbreathing patient. These include barrier devices, bag-valve mask, pocket face mask.
- Venturi masks, nonrebreathing masks, and nasal cannulas are used to provide supplemental oxygen to the breathing patient.
- Invasive airway management is used for the definitive management of the airway.
- Peripheral IV of normal saline or lactated Ringer's is preferred in emergency situations.
- Continued assessment is required in every scenario.
- IV, cardiac monitor, vital signs, history, physical, 12 lead ECG, and labs are part of the routine assessment and management of cardiac emergencies.

In this Scenario, You MUST

1. Perform the steps of the primary ABCD survey.
2. Use the Universal Algorithm.
3. Open the airway and initiate ventilation.
4. Reassess the adequacy of ventilations and trouble shoot problems.
5. Intubate the patient.
6. Assess the placement of the endotracheal tube and the adequacy of ventilation.

7. Establish IV access.

8. Perform or refer the patient for a complete workup.

9. Make arrangements for mechanical ventilation.

Unacceptable Actions

- Failure to adequately assess the patient
- Initiating an intervention before appropriate assessment
- Performing external chest compressions
- Interruption in ventilation except for intubation or reassessment
- Failure to deliver high concentration oxygen
- Using an inappropriate oxygen delivery device (e.g., a nasal cannula, simple face mask)
- Failure to identify a malpositioned endotracheal tube
- Taking more than 30 seconds to intubate the trachea

Witnessed Ventricular Fibrillation, Adult Cardiac Arrest

Overview

One of the major goals of the ACLS course is to treat ventricular fibrillation. It is important that you start to think about ventricular fibrillation as a survivable rhythm and treat it aggressively. The most important intervention for the patient in ventricular fibrillation is defibrillation. The possibility of survival drops with every second that passes. This case emphasizes the use of the automated external defibrillator.

This case uses the following algorithms:

- Universal Algorithm: see Chapter 10, Figure 10-1
- AED Algorithm: see Chapter 6, Figure 6-4

Psychomotor Skills

- Cardiopulmonary resuscitation
- Automated defibrillation
- Noninvasive airway techniques

Background Patient Information

A 58-year-old male patient suddenly clutches his chest and falls to the floor in the waiting room of his family physician's office. There are two of you, and an AED is located down the hall.

Assessment and Management

Time		Assessment and Management	See Pages
10:48	A	ABCD Survey: One rescuer performs the survey and finds that the patient is unconscious and unresponsive. He is not breathing and has no pulse.	15, 286-87
10:48	M	Have one rescuer begin initial management of the ABCs while the other retrieves the defibrillator.	18-21

Time		Assessment and Management	See Pages
10:49	M	Immediately upon arrival of the AED, place the pads on the patient and stop CPR. The AED is turned on and (if necessary) the rhythm analyzed.	21-23, 149-52
10:49	A	The AED signals that a shock is indicated.	
10:50	M	Press the shock button and deliver up to three shocks if the patient remains in a shockable rhythm.	
10:51	A	Following the initial three shocks, the patient has a pulse but is not breathing. The blood pressure is 98/60.	
10:52	M	DO NOT continue CPR, but ventilate the patient once every 5 seconds.	

Key Points

- Use the Universal and AED Algorithms.
- Use the ABCD assessment for every cardiac arrest scenario.
- The use of the AED is a psychomotor skill that requires regular practice with the equipment that you will be using. You must be familiar with the operation, method of attachment of the pads, safety, shock delivery, and troubleshooting of the defibrillator.
- You must know how to turn on the power, attach the AED, analyze the ECG, and safely deliver the shock.
- If the patient regains a pulse, immediately measure the blood pressure.
- Pulseless ventricular tachycardia is treated like ventricular fibrillation.

In this Scenario, You MUST

1. Perform the initial ABCD assessment.
2. Use the Universal and AED Algorithms.
3. Initiate proper CPR if a defibrillator is not immediately available.
4. Deliver the first defibrillation within 90 seconds of arrival of the AED.
5. Maintain the airway and ventilate the patient.
6. Check the pulse. If the patient has a pulse, check blood pressure.
7. Support ventilations after the return of a pulse.

Unacceptable Actions

- Unsafe operation of the AED
- Failure to clear during AED attempts

Adult Ventricular Fibrillation/Pulseless Ventricular Tachycardia

Overview

The management of ventricular fibrillation and pulseless ventricular tachycardia are major focuses of ACLS. Many patients who have VF or pulseless VT have little or no myocardial damage and can survive and live long, productive lives after their cardiac event.

This case uses the following algorithms:

- Universal Algorithm: see Chapter 10, Figure 10-1
- Ventricular Fibrillation/Pulseless Ventricular Tachycardia (VF/VT) Algorithm: see Chapter 10, Figure 10-2
- AED Algorithm: see Chapter 6, Figure 6-4

Psychomotor Skills

- CPR during cardiac arrest
- Assessment and reassessment of the cardiac arrest patient
- Recognition of VF or pulseless VT
- Repeated defibrillation with a standard manual defibrillator
- Attachment and use of monitoring ECG leads
- Leading a cardiac arrest team
- Use of the endotracheal tube to deliver medications
- Use of alternative airway skills if endotracheal intubation is unsuccessful
- Gaining IV access and delivering medications to the patient in cardiac arrest
- Use of epinephrine, lidocaine, bretylium, magnesium sulfate, procainamide, and sodium bicarbonate in cardiac arrest

Background Patient Information

A 45-year-old male is applying for a job as an electrician at the local hospital. He collapses in the human resources waiting room. The HR office is just down the hall from the cardiac exercise lab. You respond alone, with your AED in one hand and pocket mask in the other.

Assessment and Management

Time		Assessment and Management	See Pages
15:37	A	ABCD Survey: The patient is unconscious, unresponsive, apneic, and pulseless.	15-16, 18-21, 286-87
15:37	M	Assure that the code team is activated. Since you have an AED immediately available, attach the pads. If the AED indicates a shockable rhythm, deliver 3 shocks in rapid sequence. (Most AEDs are set to deliver the initial three shocks at 200 J, 200-300 J, and 360 J.)	21-23, 149-52
15:39	A	The patient is still pulseless and apneic.	
15:39	M	Begin ventilation and external cardiac chest compressions.	21, 79-80

Time		Assessment and Management	See Pages

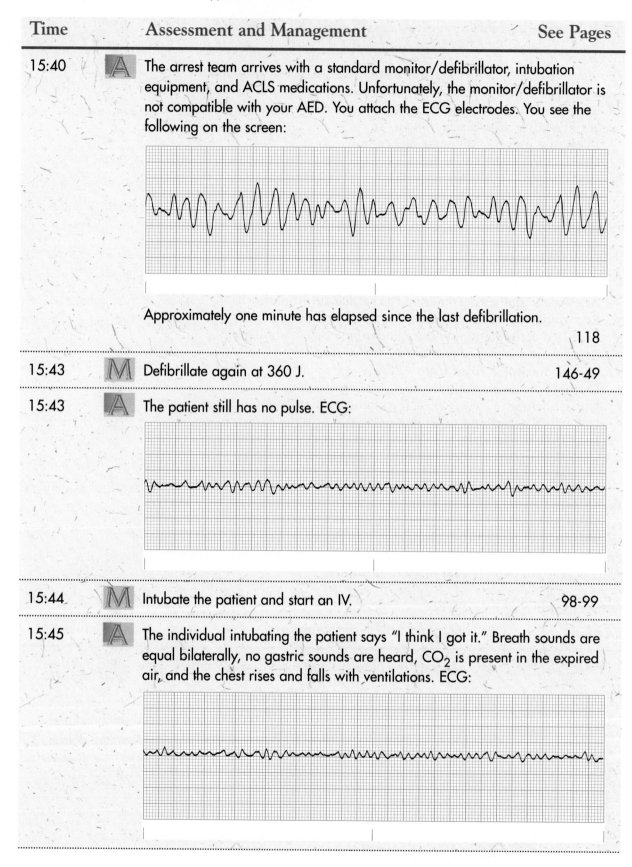

15:40   A   The arrest team arrives with a standard monitor/defibrillator, intubation equipment, and ACLS medications. Unfortunately, the monitor/defibrillator is not compatible with your AED. You attach the ECG electrodes. You see the following on the screen:

Approximately one minute has elapsed since the last defibrillation.

118

15:43   M   Defibrillate again at 360 J.   146-49

15:43   A   The patient still has no pulse. ECG:

15:44   M   Intubate the patient and start an IV.   98-99

15:45   A   The individual intubating the patient says "I think I got it." Breath sounds are equal bilaterally, no gastric sounds are heard, CO_2 is present in the expired air, and the chest rises and falls with ventilations. ECG:

Time		Assessment and Management	See Pages

15:46   M   Secure the tube. Administer 2.0–2.5 mg epinephrine endotracheally. Wait 30–60 seconds and defibrillate again at 360 J.   171-74

15:47   A   The patient has no pulse. ECG:

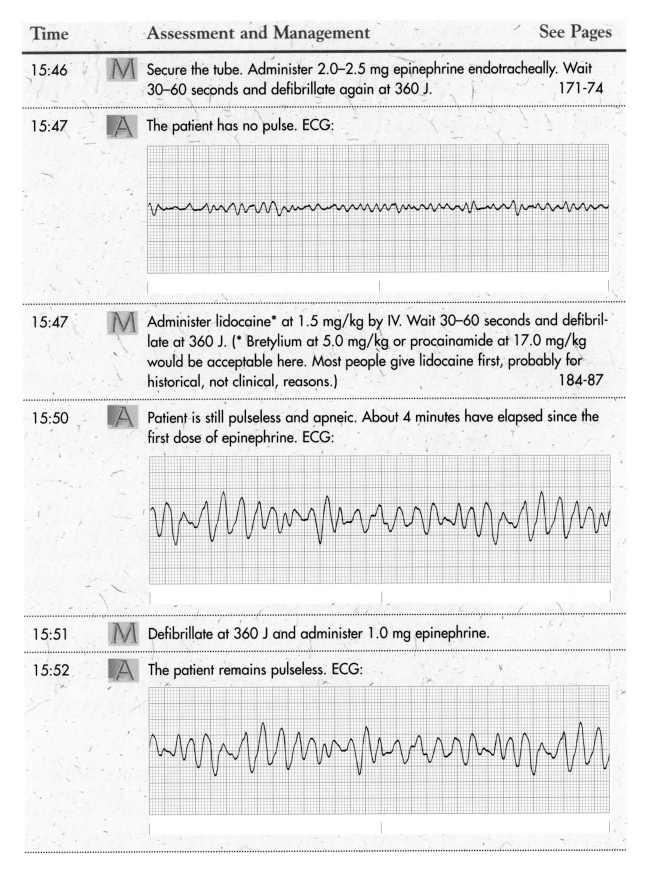

15:47   M   Administer lidocaine* at 1.5 mg/kg by IV. Wait 30–60 seconds and defibrillate at 360 J. (* Bretylium at 5.0 mg/kg or procainamide at 17.0 mg/kg would be acceptable here. Most people give lidocaine first, probably for historical, not clinical, reasons.)   184-87

15:50   A   Patient is still pulseless and apneic. About 4 minutes have elapsed since the first dose of epinephrine. ECG:

15:51   M   Defibrillate at 360 J and administer 1.0 mg epinephrine.

15:52   A   The patient remains pulseless. ECG:

Time	Assessment and Management	See Pages
15:55	**M** Administer a repeat dose of epinephrine at 1.0 mg and an initial dose of bretylium* at 5.0 mg/kg by IV. Wait 30–60 seconds and defibrillate. (* A repeat dose of lidocaine at 1.5 mg/kg or an initial dose of procainamide at 17.0 mg/kg would be acceptable here, but most people give bretylium.)	189-91
15:56	**A** The patient has a pulse! His blood pressure is 90/50. ECG:	
15:57	**M** Start a bretylium drip, and get him to the CCU as soon as possible!	

Key Points

- Use the Universal, VF/VT, and AED Algorithms.
- Follow the ABCD survey sequence.
- Immediately intubate the patient who is refractory to the first three defibrillatory shocks.
- An IV of normal saline or lactated Ringer's should be started for the patient in cardiac arrest. Drugs in cardiac arrest should be followed by a 20 cc fluid flush.
- Defibrillate 30–60 seconds after each drug administration.
- Perform CPR between each shock.

In this Scenario, You MUST

1. Initially perform the ABCs and frequently reassess the patient's condition.
2. Follow the Universal, VF/VT, and AED Algorithms.
3. Assure uninterrupted chest compressions and ventilations.
4. Attach the ECG monitor.
5. Recognize ventricular fibrillation.
6. Direct the code team.
7. Deliver defibrillation at the proper energy setting and in the proper sequence.
8. Deliver shocks 30–60 seconds after drug administration.
9. Demonstrate the proper transfer of care from BLS to ALS.
10. Intubate and obtain IV access at the proper time in the arrest management.
11. Administer the proper sequence and dose of pharmacological agents.

Unacceptable Actions

- Failure to perform CPR when indicated
- Failure to effectively ventilate the apneic patient
- Failure to intubate the patient at the appropriate time
- Any unsafe or ineffective operation of the defibrillator
- Failure to clear during AED attempts
- Failure to shock after each drug
- Medication errors
- Failure to assess pulse after rhythm conversion

Pulseless Electrical Activity

Overview

Pulseless electrical activity (PEA) is not a specific dysrhythmia. PEA is used to describe the situation when a cardiac rhythm does not produce mechanical evidence of contraction. There are a number of causes of this condition, including electromechanical dissociation (EMD), pseudo-EMD, idioventricular rhythms, ventricular escape rhythms, bradyasystolic rhythms, and post defibrillation idioventricular rhythms. The prognosis for survival from PEA is very poor. The best chance for resuscitation is to find and treat the cause of the PEA. The patient history and your physical exam provide clues to the underlying problems.

This case uses the following algorithm:

- Universal Algorithm: see Chapter 10, Figure 10-1
- Pulseless Electrical Activity (PEA) Algorithm: see Chapter 10, Figure 10-3

Psychomotor Skills

- Physical examination for hypovolemia, pericardial tamponade, and tension pneumothorax
- Fluid resuscitation
- Pericardiocentesis
- Needle chest decompression

Background Patient Information

You are treating a 28-year-old female who was shot in the right anterior chest with a small-caliber handgun. There is an entrance wound at the level of the fourth intercostal space just lateral to the mid clavicular line. You cannot find an exit wound.

Assessment and Management

Time		Assessment and Management	See Pages
00:14	A	ABCD Survey: The patient is pulseless and apneic. There is about 100 cc of external blood loss.	18-21, 286-87
00:14	M	Manually control the airway and immediately begin ventilation and external chest compressions.	35-37, 74-81

Time	Assessment and Management	See Pages
00:15	Ⓐ You "quick look" at the patient's cardiac rhythm. You see:	111-12
00:16	Ⓜ Attach monitoring electrodes for continuous ECG monitoring. Intubate immediately, obtain IV access, and administer 1.0 mg of epinephrine.	286-88
00:16	Ⓐ You hear heart tones, absent breath sounds on the right side, the neck veins are flat, trachea is deviated to the left, and the ventilatory compliance is poor.	
00:17	Ⓜ Place a 14 gauge IV catheter in the 2nd intercostal space, midclavicular line.	292
00:18	Ⓐ You are relieved to hear a rush of air and the patient regains a pulse. The blood pressure is 80/50.	
00:18	Ⓜ Continue ventilating with 100 percent oxygen and consider fluid resuscitation to improve the blood pressure.	

Key Points

- Use the Universal and PEA Algorithms.
- Follow the ABCD survey sequence.
- Search for one of the reversible causes of PEA (hypovolemia, hypoxia, cardiac tamponade, tension pneumothorax, hypothermia, massive pulmonary embolism, drug overdose, hyperkalemia, acidosis, massive myocardial infarction).
- Epinephrine is used to increase myocardial and cerebral blood flow during the resuscitation of patients in PEA.
- Atropine is used to treat absolute or relative bradycardia in patients who are in PEA.

In this Scenario, You MUST

1. Perform the primary ABCD survey.
2. Use the Universal and PEA Algorithms.
3. Initiate CPR.

4. Properly operate and attach the monitor.

5. Recognize pulseless electrical activity.

6. Direct the team members to intubate and start an IV.

7. Be able to list the common conditions which cause PEA, the signs/symptoms and emergency treatment for each.

Unacceptable Actions

- Failure to assess the patient
- Failure to consider the various causes of PEA
- Treating PEA only with epinephrine
- Failure to properly ventilate the patient or failure to intubate quickly
- Failure to volume resuscitate the patient
- Defibrillating the patient
- Failure to perform proper CPR

Asystole

Overview

Asystole is an ominous cardiac rhythm. Although it may represent the end point of resuscitative efforts, it may also result from a variety of reversible causes. One of the main considerations in the treatment of asystole is to search for reversible causes. When asystole results or persists after a prolonged resuscitation effort, you should consider terminating the code.

This case uses the following algorithms:

- Universal Algorithm: see Chapter 10, Figure 10-1
- Asystole Algorithm: see Chapter 10, Figure 10-4

Psychomotor Skills

- Recognition of the role of ventilation on acid-base balance in cardiac arrest
- Assessment of causes of asystole
- Identifying the appropriate point to terminate the resuscitation

Background Patient Information

A 37-year-old male has taken an overdose of his antidepressant medication.

Assessment and Management

Time	Assessment and Management	See Pages
20:54	**A** ABCD Survey: The patient is unresponsive, pulseless and apneic. Quick look reveals the following:	15-16, 18-21, 122, 286-87

Time		Assessment and Management	See Pages
20:54	M	Confirm the rhythm in two leads. Initiate ventilation with 100% oxygen and perform external chest compressions. Intubate and obtain IV access.	294-95
20:58	A	You consider the differential diagnosis of asystole (hypoxia, hyperkalemia, hypokalemia, preexisting acidosis, drug overdose, hypothermia).	295
20:59	M	Immediately attach the transcutaneous pacer (TCP) and administer 1.0 mg epinephrine.	157-62, 171-74
21:02	A	There is no response. The patient remains pulseless and apneic.	
21:04	M	Administer atropine at 1.0 mg.	192-96
21:08	A	There is still no response.	
21:10	M	Repeat epinephrine at 1.0 mg every 3–5 minutes and atropine at 1.5 mg to a total cumulative dose of 0.04 mg/kg. Consider alternative epinephrine doses. Consider termination of resuscitation if no response.	171-74

Key Points

- Use the Universal and Asystole Algorithms.
- Follow the ABCD survey sequence.
- Proper ventilation is the best way to maintain acid-base balance in cardiac arrest.
- Search for treatable causes of asystole.
- Asystole is usually considered an endpoint of resuscitation. If no treatable cause is identified, consider termination of the resuscitation.
- The reversible causes of asystole are: hypoxia, hyperkalemia, hypokalemia, acidosis, drug overdose, hypothermia, and an extension of progressive bradycardia.
- Transcutaneous pacing should be instituted as soon as possible in the resuscitation.
- Epinephrine, atropine, and sodium bicarbonate are used in the management of asystole.

In this Scenario, You MUST

1. Perform all of the steps of the primary ABCD survey.
2. Use the Universal and Asystole Algorithms.
3. Initiate CPR.
4. Recognize and confirm asystole.
5. Recognize the role of ventilation in acid-base balance.
6. Properly monitor the IV access site.
7. List and describe the treatment for the causes of asystole.

8. List the proper dose of epinephrine, atropine, and sodium bicarbonate.

9. Perform TCP early and concurrently with medications.

10. Perform a pulse check with every rhythm change.

11. Describe the considerations in terminating the resuscitation.

Unacceptable Actions

- Diagnosing asystole in only one lead
- Use of TCP too late or without the concurrent use of medications.

Acute Myocardial Infarction

Overview

Most of the ACLS course focuses on reversing cardiac arrest. The remaining algorithms are designed to *prevent* cardiac arrest. Recent therapeutic options have lead to a significant reduction in the morbidity and mortality from acute myocardial infarction.

This case uses the following algorithms:

- Universal Algorithm: see Chapter 10, Figure 10-1
- Acute Myocardial Infarction Algorithm: see Chapter 8, Figure 8-7

Psychomotor Skills

- Rhythm diagnosis
- 12 lead ECG

Background Patient Information

This scenario begins as a 56-year-old car salesman begins to have chest discomfort while closing a deal that would make him Bob Smith's Salesman of the Year. He is thinking of the all-expense-paid trip to Hawaii when he starts to look dusky and sweaty, and the caring customers insist that he sit down and rest. When he feels no relief after 2 minutes, some concerned coworkers insist that they "call first, call fast." They dial 911.

Assessment and Management

Time	Assessment and Management	See Pages
At the outset of the case, you take the role of a responding paramedic.		
10:22	**A** ABC Survey: The patient is conscious, alert, and oriented. He is complaining of severe, "squeezing" chest pain, radiating into his left arm. He says it started about 10 minutes ago. He is pale and diaphoretic. He is having some shortness of breath. He has no pertinent medical history.	
10:23	**M** Oxygen–IV–monitor–vital signs: Since the patient is having shortness of breath, apply oxygen by nonrebreather at 12 lpm, place him on the cardiac monitor, obtain baseline vital signs, and start an IV of NS at a KVO rate.	286-88

Time		Assessment and Management	See Pages
10:26	A	The vitals are: Pulse: 80 strong and regular, Respirations: 16 and unlabored, BP: 154/88, SaO$_2$ 98%. You see the following on the monitor:	111-12

Time		Assessment and Management	See Pages
10:28	M	Administer1 tablet or spray of 0.3–0.4 mg nitroglycerin and contact medical control for consultation. Medical control requests that you repeat the nitroglycerin and requests a 12 lead ECG. Load the patient into the ambulance and begin transport.	205-6, 242-43
10:30	A	The pain is not relieved. Vitals are unchanged. The 12 lead ECG indicates a probable acute inferior wall myocardial infarction. (See Figure 11-1.) The patient is in severe discomfort.	233-36
10:32	A	Transmit the ECG to the hospital by cellular phone and recontact medical control. Medical control requests that you screen the patient for thrombolytic therapy and administer narcotics for pain control.	
10:34	A	You question the patient from a predefined checklist about his medical history. He has no contraindications to thrombolytic therapy.	244-46
10:36	M	Administer 2.0 mg of morphine sulfate for pain control, contact the receiving hospital, and inform them that the patient qualifies for thrombolysis. Have him chew an aspirin.	203-4, 243-44

At this point in the case, you take the role of the physician in the emergency department

Time		Assessment and Management	See Pages
10:41	A	On arrival in the emergency department, the patient is still conscious, alert, and oriented. He still has some chest discomfort, but "the medicine they gave me sure did help." The blood pressure is 150/90, SaO$_2$ is 99%. The focused history shows a previously healthy male with acute onset of severe chest pain, no history or physical-exam findings excluding this patient as a candidate for thrombolysis.	
10:44	M	Start a nitroglycerin drip at 10–20 µg/min, administer beta blockers, and repeat morphine at 1.0–3.0 mg to keep him comfortable. The thrombolytics have arrived from the pharmacy (you requested them based on the paramedic's report and the transmitted ECG).	242-48

Time	Assessment and Management	See Pages
10:46	A Repeat 12 lead confirms an acute, transmural inferior wall MI.	
10:55	M Begin thrombolytics and heparin	244-47
11:24	M Transfer the patient to the CCU.	

Key Points

- Use the Universal and Acute Myocardial Infarction Algorithms.
- Follow the ABC survey steps.
- The most effective strategy for decreasing the morbidity and mortality from AMI is early recognition and early care.
- Learn your local protocols for managing a suspected AMI patient.
- The prehospital interventions for the suspected AMI patient are:
  - oxygen–IV–continuous cardiac monitor–vital signs
  - nitroglycerin
  - pain relief with narcotics
  - 12 lead ECG
  - informing the receiving facility
  - rapid transport to an appropriate facility
  - screening of patients to receive thrombolytics.
- In the emergency department, a team approach should be used to decrease the "door-to-drug" time of thrombolytics to appropriate patients.
- Emergency departments must determine in advance who will make the decision about who is eligible to receive thrombolytics.
- The emergency department interventions for the suspected AMI patient are:
  - IV–continuous cardiac monitor–vital signs–oxygen saturation
  - 12 lead ECG
  - targeted history and physical exam
  - decision as to the eligibility and appropriateness of thrombolytic therapy
  - chest x-ray, blood studies, consultations as needed
- You should be able to list the actions, indications, dosage, and precautions for:
  - oxygen
  - nitroglycerin
  - morphine
  - thrombolytic agents
  - aspirin
  - heparin
  - lidocaine
  - beta blockers
  - magnesium sulfate
  - coronary angioplasty (PTCA)

FIGURE 11-1 12-lead ECG indicating acute inferior wall myocardial infarction.

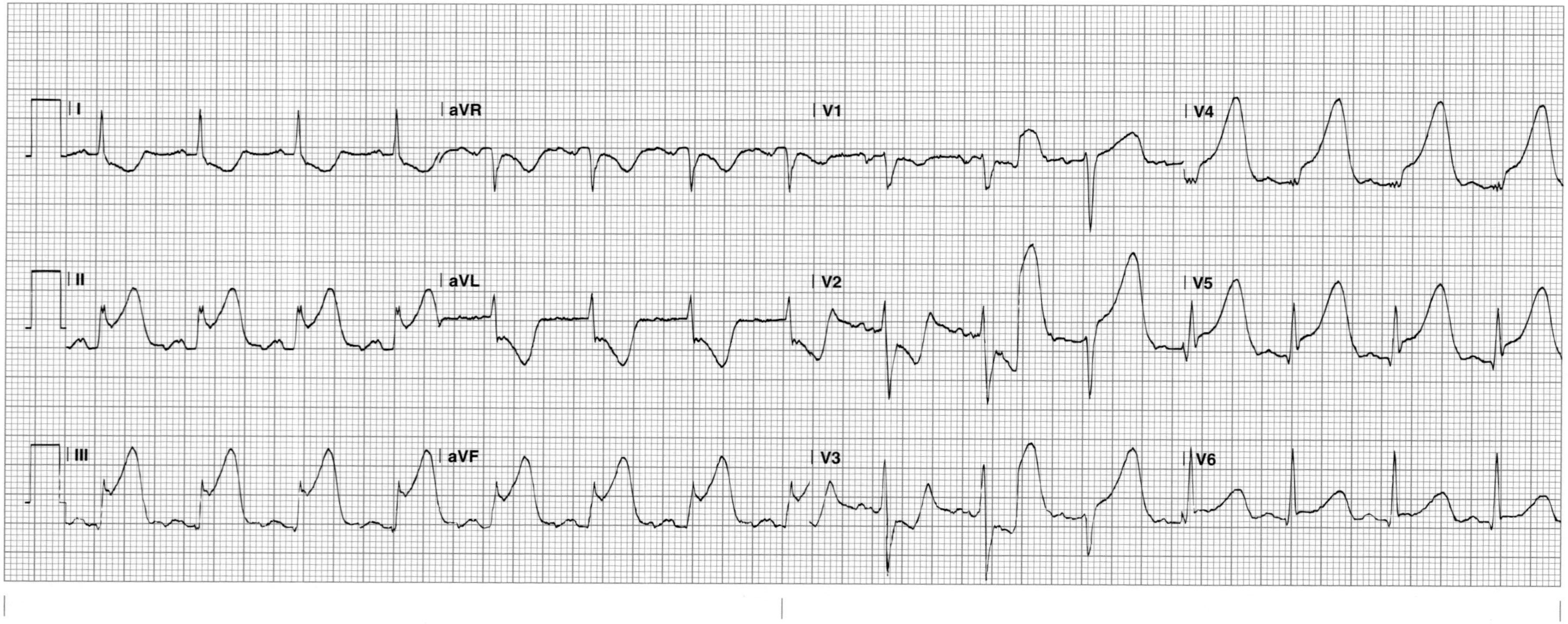

- You should be able to treat the following dysrhythmias in the setting of the AMI patient:
  - normal sinus rhythm, sinus bradycardia, sinus tachycardia
  - AV nodal blocks: first degree, second degree (Mobitz I and II), and third degree block
  - multiple PACs, atrial tachycardia, atrial tachycardia with block, atrial flutter with various degrees of block, PVCs, and ventricular ectopy
  - ventricular fibrillation and ventricular tachycardia

In this Scenario, You MUST

1. Perform a rapid, focused history and physical exam including vitals and 12 lead ECG.
2. Use the Universal and Acute Myocardial Infarction Algorithms.
3. List the major indications, including ECG criteria, and exclusion criteria for thrombolytic therapy.
4. List the major actions, indications, and contraindications for the medications used to treat a suspected acute myocardial infarction.
5. Identify and treat dysrhythmias in the setting of a myocardial infarction.

Unacceptable Actions

- Failure to consider and properly evaluate a patient with acute chest pain consistent with an AMI
- Failure to obtain a 12 lead ECG in a timely fashion
- Failure to administer oxygen and other indicated medications
- Failure to control pain
- Failure to recognize exclusion criteria for thrombolytics
- Administering contraindicated medications

Bradycardia

Overview

Bradycardic rhythms are common pre- and postarrest presentations. Properly managing bradycardias can prevent cardiac arrest and reduce the possibility that a patient will re-arrest. The most important management interventions in bradycardias are atropine and transcutaneous pacing.

This case uses the following algorithms:

- Universal Algorithm: see Chapter 10, Figure 10-1
- Bradycardia Algorithm: see Chapter 10, Figure 10-5

Psychomotor Skills

- Operation of the transcutaneous pacer
- Administering a dopamine and epinephrine drip
- Interpretation of bradycardias

Background Patient Information:

You are seeing a 62-year-old female who is complaining of severe weakness and dizziness. She gets "really lightheaded" if she sits up. She has some minor chest discomfort and moderate shortness of breath.

Time		Assessment and Management	See Pages
11:33	A	ABC Survey: The patient is conscious, but disoriented. Pulse 49; blood pressure 72/48; respirations 26 and labored.	
11:35	M	Administer high flow oxygen, start an IV, attach a cardiac monitor, pulse oximeter, and automatic blood pressure monitor.	286-87
11:37	A	SaO$_2$ 84%, BP 70/50, cardiac monitor shows	114-15

Time		Assessment and Management	See Pages
11:40	M	Administer atropine at 0.5 to 1.0 mg, apply the pacer pads and prepare the transcutaneous pacer.	299-302
11:42	A	The patient's heart rate is 52, BP is 72/50.	
11:45	M	Set the heart rate on the TCP to 80 bpm and gradually increase the output until you have electrical capture.	159-60
11:48	A	At 60 mA, you note that the patient's heart rate is 80, blood pressure is 86/64 and her level of consciousness is improving. She is complaining about the pain from the pacer.	
11:53	M	Administer small amounts of narcotics or benzodiazepines for analgesia/sedation.	

Key Points

- Use the Universal and Bradycardia Algorithms. The bradycardia algorithm is used to treat relative and absolute bradycardias.
- Follow the ABC survey steps.
- Bradycardia should be treated only if it is symptomatic. Symptomatic bradycardia causes any of the following: chest pain, dyspnea, weakness/dizziness, syncope, decreased level of consciousness, hypotension, ventricular ectopy.
- Atropine is used in the initial management of symptomatic bradycardia.
- The transcutaneous pacer is set up while you are awaiting the actions of atropine.
- Dopamine or epinephrine infusions are used if the patient is unresponsive to atropine and the transcutaneous pacer is unavailable or fails to produce mechanical capture.

- Isoproterenol is rarely used.
- Do not use lidocaine to treat a ventricular escape rhythm.

In this Scenario, You MUST

1. Recognize symptomatic bradycardia from your assessment and physical exam findings.
2. Use the Universal and Bradycardia Algorithms.
3. Obtain IV access and place the patient on oxygen and a cardiac monitor.
4. Administer the appropriate dose of atropine.
5. Apply the transcutaneous pacer while awaiting the actions of the atropine.
6. Know the dose for a dopamine infusion.
7. Identify second degree type II and third degree AV blocks.
8. Recognize the need for transcutaneous pacing.
9. Order a 12 lead ECG.
10. Consider the use of thrombolytics if the patient has signs and symptoms suggestive of AMI.

Unacceptable Actions

- Failure to organize transcutaneous pacing while waiting for atropine to work
- Failure to recognize the importance of transvenous pacing for second degree type II block
- Inappropriately using isoproterenol, dopamine, or epinephrine
- Using lidocaine to treat ventricular escape rhythms
- Treating an asymptomatic bradycardia

Unstable Tachycardia

Overview

The management of any unstable tachycardia, regardless of its type, is by synchronized cardioversion. The only pitfall is treating sinus tachycardia with an underlying problem like a reentry dysrhythmia. The patient history will help you avoid this mistake. The differentiation of types and origination of reentry tachycardias are only needed if the patient is stable. Do not allow yourself to become distracted by ECG interpretation of tachycardias in unstable patients. The treatment is the same: cardioversion.

This case uses the following algorithms:

- Universal Algorithm: see Chapter 10, Figure 10-1
- Tachycardia Algorithm: see Chapter 10, Figure 10-6
- Electrical (Synchronized) Cardioversion Algorithm: see Chapter 6, Figure 6-5

Psychomotor Skills

- Identification of unstable tachycardia
- Synchronized cardioversion
- Switching from synchronized to unsynchronized cardioversion.

Background Patient Information

A 38-year-old female suddenly became "faint" and had a syncopal episode while at work. She is dizzy and lightheaded and is complaining of a "funny feeling" in her chest.

Assessment and Management

Time	Assessment and Management	See Pages
14:02	**A** ABC Survey: Skin is pale, weak pulse at 180, minor shortness of breath, BP is 72/40.	
14:05	**M** Administer high flow oxygen, start an IV, attach a continuous ECG monitor, pulse oximeter, and automatic blood pressure monitor.	286-87
14:05	**A** SaO_2 is 92%; BP is 74/44; monitor shows:	122-23

14:07	**M** Prepare suction equipment and intubation equipment.	
14:09	**A** The patient is very lightheaded and has a syncopal episode every time she tries to sit up.	302-9
14:10	**M** Administer a sedative agent.	
14:13	**A** Patient is sleepy but easily awakened.	
14:14	**M** Perform synchronized cardioversion at 100 joules.	153-55
14:16	**A** The heart rate is 118, blood pressure is 86/64.	

14:18	**M** Administer a bolus of lidocaine at 1.0–1.5 mg/kg or bretylium at 5.0 mg/kg and then start a lidocaine infusion at 2.0 mg/min or a bretylium infusion at 1.0–2.0 mg/min.	184-87, 189-91

Key Points

- Use the Universal, Tachycardia, and Electrical (Synchronized) Cardio-version Algorithms.
- Follow the ABC survey steps.
- Tachycardic patients who present with chest pain, dyspnea, decreased level of consciousness, hypotension, shock, pulmonary congestion, or CHF are unstable and need to be cardioverted immediately.
- Approximately 80% of wide complex tachycardias are ventricular.
- Be sure to become familiar with the operation of the defibrillator that you will be using; specifically, learn where the synchronize button is located.

In this Scenario, You MUST

1. Perform the initial assessment including ABCs, attach the cardiac monitor, and take baseline vital signs.
2. Use the Universal, Tachycardia, and Electrical (Synchronized) Cardioversion Algorithms.
3. Identify patients who are unstable and tachycardic.
4. Reassess the patient (pulse, respiration, blood pressure) and administer anti-dysrhythmic agents after cardioversion.
5. Administer oxygen, start an IV, and place the patient on continuous cardiac monitoring.
6. Change from synchronized cardioversion to unsynchronized cardioversion if the patient goes into ventricular fibrillation or if delays in cardioversion occur because of difficulty with synchronization.

Unacceptable Actions

- Failure to resynchronize the defibrillator after cardioversion
- Failure to differentiate between stable and unstable tachycardia
- Failure to attempt to determine the cause of the tachycardia after treatment
- Failure to provide antidysrhythmic therapy after cardioversion

Stable Tachycardia

Overview

At first, the stable tachycardia algorithm looks very intimidating. When you dissect it to its most basic parts, it is very logical. We will use two patient scenarios to illustrate the clinical decision making for the patient with stable tachycardia.

These cases use the following algorithms:

- Universal Algorithm: see Chapter 10, Figure 10-1
- Tachycardia Algorithm: see Chapter 10, Figure 10-6

Psychomotor Skills

- Rhythm diagnosis
- Vagal maneuvers
- Synchronized cardioversion

Background Patient Information: Stable Tachycardia #1

A 52-year-old female is complaining about a sudden onset of heart palpitations. She is conscious, alert, and oriented and in no distress. She denies chest discomfort or dyspnea.

Assessment and Management

Time	Assessment and Management	See Pages
14:14	**A** ABC Survey: The patient has had similar episodes in the past and is taking verapamil at home. Her blood pressure is 128/82, heart rate is 180, respirations are 14 and unlabored.	
14:16	**M** Place the patient on low flow oxygen, start an IV, place the patient on a cardiac monitor, pulse oximeter, and automatic blood pressure monitor.	286-87
14:18	**A** The blood pressure is 130/80; SaO_2 98%. The monitor shows:	

The patient has no carotid bruits.   119-22

Time	Assessment and Management	See Pages
14:19	**M** Attempt vagal maneuvers.	302-9
14:21	**A** ECG:	

The blood pressure is 132/80.

Time	Assessment and Management	See Pages
14:24	**M** Administer adenosine at 6.0 mg rapid IV bolus.	196-97

Time		Assessment and Management	See Pages

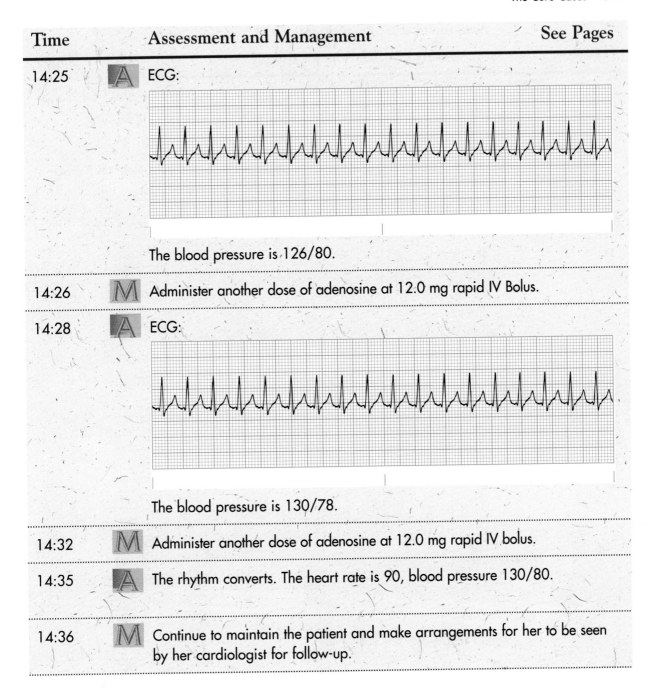

14:25 A ECG:

The blood pressure is 126/80.

14:26 M Administer another dose of adenosine at 12.0 mg rapid IV Bolus.

14:28 A ECG:

The blood pressure is 130/78.

14:32 M Administer another dose of adenosine at 12.0 mg rapid IV bolus.

14:35 A The rhythm converts. The heart rate is 90, blood pressure 130/80.

14:36 M Continue to maintain the patient and make arrangements for her to be seen by her cardiologist for follow-up.

Background Patient Information: Stable Tachycardia patient #2
A 52-year-old female is complaining about a sudden onset of heart palpitations. She is conscious, alert, and oriented and in no distress. She denies chest discomfort or dyspnea. (Same patient information as for Patient #1. Variations in treatment result from the history, not the presentation.)

Assessment and Management

Time	Assessment and Management	See Pages
22:58	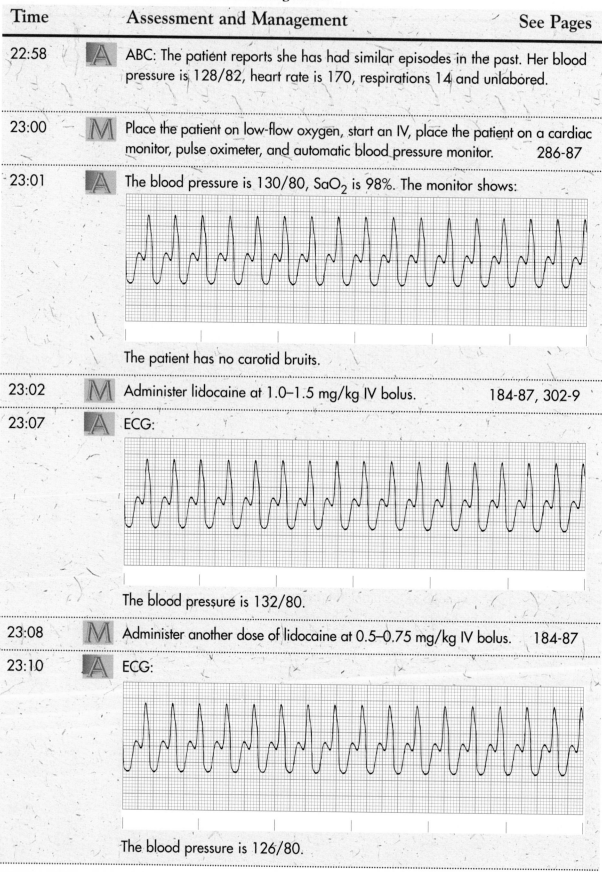 ABC: The patient reports she has had similar episodes in the past. Her blood pressure is 128/82, heart rate is 170, respirations 14 and unlabored.	
23:00	Ⓜ Place the patient on low-flow oxygen, start an IV, place the patient on a cardiac monitor, pulse oximeter, and automatic blood pressure monitor.	286-87
23:01	Ⓐ The blood pressure is 130/80, SaO₂ is 98%. The monitor shows: The patient has no carotid bruits.	
23:02	Ⓜ Administer lidocaine at 1.0–1.5 mg/kg IV bolus.	184-87, 302-9
23:07	Ⓐ ECG: The blood pressure is 132/80.	
23:08	Ⓜ Administer another dose of lidocaine at 0.5–0.75 mg/kg IV bolus.	184-87
23:10	Ⓐ ECG: The blood pressure is 126/80.	

Time		Assessment and Management	See Pages
23:11	M	Administer adenosine at 6.0 mg rapid IV bolus.	196-97
23:12	A	ECG:	

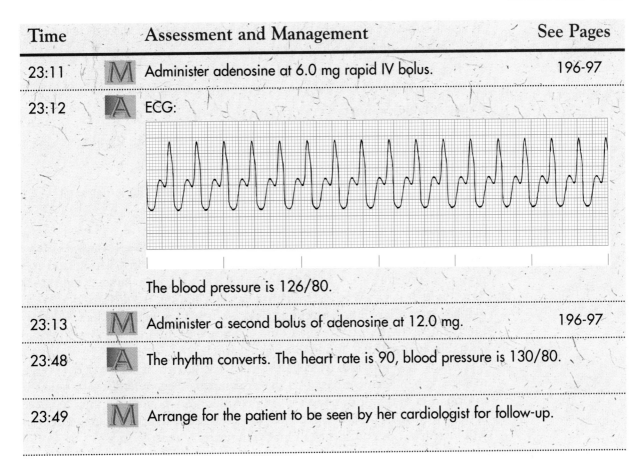

The blood pressure is 126/80.

23:13	M	Administer a second bolus of adenosine at 12.0 mg.	196-97
23:48	A	The rhythm converts. The heart rate is 90, blood pressure is 130/80.	
23:49	M	Arrange for the patient to be seen by her cardiologist for follow-up.	

Key Points

- Use the Universal and Tachycardia Algorithms.
- Follow the ABC survey steps.
- The first step in the algorithm is to rule out instability. Stable tachycardia may be sinus tachycardia, PSVT, atrial fibrillation, atrial flutter, wide-complex tachycardia of uncertain origin, or ventricular tachycardia.
- Know the indications, actions, dosing, and complications of the following drugs that are used to treat tachycardia: adenosine, verapamil, diltiazem, lidocaine, procainamide, bretylium, and beta blockers.
- If a wide complex tachycardia is of uncertain type, administer lidocaine first. If there is no response, use a trial of adenosine to rule out supraventricular tachycardia with aberrant conduction. If there is no response to the adenosine, begin a procainamide infusion. If the procainamide is not successful in converting the rhythm, administer bretylium. A maintenance infusion should be initiated if lidocaine, procainamide, or bretylium was successful in converting the rhythm.

In this Scenario, You MUST

1. Perform initial assessment, including ABCs, monitor, and vital signs.
2. Use the Universal and Tachycardia Algorithms.
3. Determine the category of the tachycardia.
4. Assess the cardiovascular stability of the tachycardic patient.

5. Perform pharmacology and electrical cardioversion to manage tachycardia.
6. Correctly perform synchronized cardioversion.
7. Reassess the patient after synchronized cardioversion.

Unacceptable Actions

- Failure to perform an initial survey and determine the stability of the patient
- Incorrect rhythm interpretation
- Failure to listen for a carotid bruit prior to carotid sinus massage

SUMMARY

This chapter has introduced the concept of case-based instruction and has presented the core case studies from the AHA ACLS course: Respiratory Arrest with a Pulse; Witnessed Ventricular Fibrillation, Adult Cardiac Arrest; Adult Ventricular Fibrillation/Pulseless Ventricular Tachycardia; Pulseless Electrical Activity; Asystole; Adult Myocardial Infarction; Bradycardia; Unstable Tachycardia; and Stable Tachycardia.

Each case provides a scenario with a sequence of interwoven assessments and management based on the assessments. Page references to relevant information in the prior chapters are provided. Key points and unacceptable actions for each case are listed. This kind of practical, applicable instruction will increase your confidence in managing cardiac emergencies.

REVIEW QUESTIONS

1. What is the first step that should be taken any time you recognize an unconscious patient and you are alone?
   a. Get help.
   b. Open the airway.
   c. Assess the breathing.
   d. Assess the pulse.

2. What is the initial method of opening the airway for any non-trauma patient?
   a. oropharyngeal airway
   b. endotracheal intubation
   c. chin lift without head tilt
   d. head tilt, chin lift

3. You must be able to deliver the first defibrillation within _____ seconds of the arrival of an AED.
   a. 30
   b. 60
   c. 90
   d. 120

4. If you have an AED immediately available, what should you do once you determine that an unresponsive patient is pulseless?
   a. Get help.
   b. Begin 1 minute of CPR and then defibrillate.
   c. Assure that the airway is open and the patient is being ventilated.
   d. Attach the AED pads and defibrillate.

5. What is the first step after inflating the cuff of the endotracheal tube?
   a. Confirm tube placement by pulse oximetry.
   b. Confirm tube placement by inspection and auscultation.
   c. Secure the tube.
   d. Insert a bite block.

6. How long should you wait to defibrillate after administering a medication to a patient in ventricular fibrillation.
   a. immediately
   b. 15–30 seconds
   c. 30–60 seconds
   d. 60–90 seconds

7. Which of the following is **not** an appropriate antidysrhythmic in the first line pharmacological treatment of ventricular fibrillation?
   a. procainamide
   b. bretylium
   c. lidocaine
   d. adenosine

8. Which of the following is used in cardiac arrest of any origin or presenting rhythm?
   a. epinephrine
   b. lidocaine
   c. atropine
   d. sodium bicarbonate

9. What is the likely cause of PEA in a patient with chest trauma, distended neck veins, and muffled heart tones?
   a. tension pneumothorax
   b. hypovolemia
   c. hypoxia
   d. cardiac tamponade

10. What should you do if a patient in asystole fails to respond to transcutaneous pacing and atropine?
    a. Administer sodium bicarbonate.
    b. Consider the termination of resuscitation.
    c. Use high dose epinephrine.
    d. Administer a 300 cc fluid bolus.

11. What should guide the **initial** amount of oxygen delivered to a patient with signs and symptoms of an acute myocardial infarction?
    a. blood gasses
    b. pulse oximetry
    c. the level of respiratory distress
    d. All patients should receive high flow oxygen.

12. What is the most effective strategy for decreasing the morbidity and mortality from AMI?
    a. early recognition and care
    b. thrombolytics
    c. PTCA
    d. nitroglycerin

13. At what heart rate should you set the pacer to treat symptomatic bradycardia?
    a. 60
    b. 70
    c. 80
    d. 90

14. What is the treatment for unstable wide complex tachycardia?
    a. lidocaine
    b. adenosine
    c. verapamil
    d. cardioversion

15. Which of the following is the pharmacological treatment of stable narrow complex tachycardia refractory to adenosine?
    a. lidocaine
    b. verapamil
    c. procainamide
    d. bretylium

Chapter**Twelve**

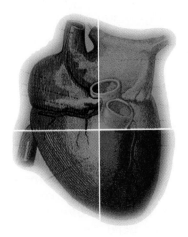

Special Resuscitation Situations

Not every cardiac arrest is precipitated by a problem with the heart. When a person suffers cardiac arrest from a non-cardiac cause, such as trauma or hypothermia, resuscitation must be attempted, just as for any patient in arrest from a cardiac cause. In addition, however, special consideration must be given to the condition that caused the arrest. This is a patient who probably has a healthy heart and has an excellent chance of successful resuscitation if the underlying cause is identified and treated.

Topics that will be covered in this chapter are:

- Traumatic Cardiac Arrests
- Cardiac Arrest and Pregnancy
- Lightning Strikes
- Hypothermia and Near Drowning
- Toxicologic Cardiac Emergencies and Arrest

CASE STUDY

It is a cold day in late January, and you are outside your house taking down your Christmas decorations and lights. As you are coiling up a string of lights, you hear the faint pitch of a siren approaching your neighborhood. The siren gets louder and louder until you realize that the ambulance is turning onto your street. You quickly glance around to the neighbors' houses—trying to see if anything looks awry—when you see your neighbors two houses down waving frantically at the approaching ambulance. They are new to the neighborhood, and you briskly walk across the front yards to ask Mrs. Tieche if you can help.

Through her tears she tells you her nephew David has fallen through the ice in the pond behind the neighbors' house. The paramedics grab their gear and walk past you as Mrs. Tieche leads them behind the house. Since you have completed a course in advanced life support, you offer the paramedics your help. As soon as you get to the backyard, you see the limp, blue, cold body of a young man lying supine on the frozen ground. Mr. Tieche is performing CPR.

How would you proceed to assess and care for this patient? In this chapter, you will learn about special patient considerations that may necessitate a change in your routine management for cardiovascular emergencies. Later, we will return to the case study and apply the procedure learned.

Introduction

This book emphasizes the cardiac arrest that is precipitated by a failure or disturbance in the myocardium itself. This emphasis is deliberate, because the majority of cardiac arrests do occur in an older population who have some form of cardiac disease.

However, it is important to realize that *not all cardiac arrests are caused primarily by heart disease*. The subset of patients who suffer cardiac arrest from other etiologies is small. However, it is extremely important to recognize these patients and understand the physiology behind their arrests—and then understand why they require special assessment and management considerations—in order to appropriately and effectively manage the emergency. It is important to remember that many of the patients in this category may still have a healthy heart. And successful resuscitation is likely if they are provided the appropriate treatment aimed at the cause of their arrest.

This chapter is designed to introduce you to these special resuscitation considerations, and provide you with a functional knowledge of how to handle these special emergencies requiring resuscitation.

Traumatic Cardiac Arrests

Assessing and treating a patient in cardiac arrest from a traumatic incident can be most frustrating to the care provider. Unlike the majority of patients with cardiac arrest from a cardiac problem, traumatic arrests can occur from a host of diverse etiologies. Too often care providers look at the patient in terms of *how* he came to be in arrest (e.g., car crash, fall, gunshot), rather than by what *organ systems* have been involved in that traumatic incident. This narrow approach may cause one to overlook certain injuries, or to provide a "knee-jerk" itinerary of interventions that may (or may not) be 100% appropriate for the patient.

The best approach is to first find out how the person was traumatized (the mechanism of injury), and then relate that to the organ system(s) that may be involved in the trauma. This approach will allow you to focus your attention appropriately on the real causative agent(s) of the arrest. Remember these two points regarding traumatic arrests: (1) *The traumatic incident is what caused the organ system failure*, and (2) *the organ system failure is what caused the cardiac arrest*.

Understand, also, that a variety of mechanisms of injury that *seem* to be different are essentially the same and produce similar injuries. Take, for example, an unrestrained driver who crashes his car and sustains severe chest wall injuries. He may go into arrest from a pulmonary injury that causes profound hypoxia, or from pericardial tamponade, or even from acute hemorrhaging into the thorax from a torn aorta. But yet the same chest injuries could be anticipated in a different patient who sustains his injuries when a car falls off a jack-stand and lands on his chest. The point is simply this: Use the mechanism of injury *only* as a clue to give you insight to the organs that are probably involved in the trauma, then focus your assessment and management energy on correcting those deficits.

Table 12-1 lists potential causes of arrest following trauma.

Approach to the Traumatic Cardiac Arrest Patient

The causes of traumatic cardiac arrest are numerous. The trauma patient with multiple organ hemorrhage has such profound damage that even the best medicine today is rarely capable of correcting the problems and preventing death. Both blunt and penetrating etiologies of traumatic cardiac arrest carry an extremely poor prognosis. These patients rarely survive. But since it is virtually impossible to fully assess the extent of damage in the out-of-hospital and emergency department phases, the patient should be extended full cardiopulmonary resuscitation focused on replacing or supporting lost vital functions and correcting underlying abnormalities in oxygenation and circulation.

TABLE 12-1 POTENTIAL CAUSES OF TRAUMATIC CARDIAC ARREST

- Acute internal hemorrhage from an abdominal or thoracic injury

- Profound hypoxia from a disturbance of airway patency, or pulmonary efficacy (airway obstruction, laryngeal fracture, pneumothorax, open chest wall injury)

- Severe CNS damage from cervical spinal cord injury or head injury

- Direct trauma to vital organs (lungs, heart, great blood vessels)

- Inadequate cardiac output from excessive mechanical pressure on the heart (tension pneumothorax, pericardial tamponade)

- Acute external hemorrhage (arterial and large venous) from soft tissue injury

TABLE 12-2 TRAUMATIC ARRESTS IN WHICH RESUSCITATION IS UNLIKELY

- Hemicorporectomy or decapitation

- Full body burns

- Severe blunt trauma with absence of all of the following:
  - pupillary response (and)
  - vital signs (and)
  - shockable cardiac rhythms

- Deeply penetrating cranial injury(ies)

- Penetrating cranial and/or truncal wound(s) with prolonged (>15 min) transport time to a health care facility

The limitation to providing full resuscitation to the traumatized cardiac arrest patient is when the cardiac arrest exists in conjunction with a severed head or trunk, full body burns, severe blunt trauma with no pupillary response, no vital signs and no shockable cardiac rhythm, deeply penetrating wound to the cranium, or penetrating cranial or trunk wounds with anticipated transport time of 15 minutes or more (Table 12-2). In these patients, the extent of damage is so grave that attempts at resuscitation are often futile. Since the exact criteria for withholding or initiating resuscitation vary across the nation, it is up to you to become familiar with and adhere to the policy and protocols established in your area.

Treatment of the Traumatic Cardiac Arrest Patient

Specifically, initial out-of-hospital management of the trauma cardiac arrest should include the following:

- Spinal immobilization until radiography rules out spinal injury
- Airway management with close attention to supporting inadequate breathing with positive pressure ventilation, oxygen, and endotracheal intubation
- Control of external hemorrhage
- Application and interpretation of the ECG monitor, shocking ventricular fibrillation, if present, according to the V-fib algorithm
- Intravenous access with an isotonic crystalloid (lactated Ringer's or normal saline) and fluid boluses of 20 ml/kg if hypovolemia is known or suspected.
- Assessment for, and treatment of, injuries leading to the arrest
- Fluid replacement
- Decompression of tension pneumothorax
- Correction of oxygenation and ventilation deficits
- Administration of medications and nonpharmacologic interventions as appropriate for the presenting cardiac ECG tracing

If the trauma patient goes into or is in arrest while in the emergency department, the following may be considered by the emergency department physician:

- Surgical airway procedures if the airway cannot be maintained with an endotracheal tube
- Thoracic decompression
- Administration of blood products
- Relief of cardiac tamponade by pericardiocentesis
- Emergency thoracotomy as appropriate, to allow
  - direct cardiac massage
  - relief of cardiac tamponade
  - direct cardiac volume loading
  - aortic cross clamping
  - control of intrathoracic hemorrhage
- Central venous access, arterial sampling
- Administration of medications and nonpharmacologic interventions as appropriate for the presenting cardiac ECG tracing

In conclusion, decisions about appropriate management of the traumatic cardiac arrest must be made in light of the underlying organ failure. In some instances, simple correction of an occluded airway, relief of a tension pneumothorax, or control of external hemorrhage may be all that is necessary to achieve a successful resuscitation. It is of utmost importance for the care provider to assess the mechanism of injury to determine probable body organs involved, and then perform the assessment and treatment necessary to support and/or replace lost functions. However, the care provider must also recognize those situations in which resuscitation of the traumatic arrest patient is futile and would result in a needless expenditure of resources.

Cardiac Arrest and Pregnancy

Assessment and treatment of a pregnant woman is different than for the nonpregnant patient because of changes in cardiovascular and respiratory systems that take place during pregnancy. These changes (as discussed below) result in an altered presentation of the common signs and symptoms of certain medical emergencies. When you understand the basic changes in physiology, you can provide more appropriate and efficient assessment and care.

Briefly, the most prominent changes in the female's body during pregnancy are increases in blood volume, resting heart rate and cardiac output, resting respiratory rate and oxygen consumption, decreased blood pressure, loosening of hip joints, displacement of abdominal organs, and increased pressure on the inferior vena cava (Table 12-3).

These changes result in an increase in susceptibility to cardiovascular and respiratory emergencies, while at the same time they reduce the patient's ability to compensate for the insult.

Finally, it is also extremely important to realize that you have two patients: the mother and her unborn child. Treatment you administer to the mother must, therefore, serve the twin goals of reversing the mother's

TABLE 12-3 PHYSICAL CHANGES IN A PREGNANT WOMAN
• Increase in blood volume by approximately 50%
• Increase in resting heart rate and cardiac output
• Decrease in blood pressure (more pronounced near term)
• Increase in resting respiratory rate
• Overall increase in oxygen consumption
• Loosening of hip joints (leads to increased trauma from falls)
• Displacement of abdominal organs from the gravid uterus
• Increased pressure on the inferior vena cava by the uterus

emergency as well as ensuring uninterrupted and sufficient oxygenation and circulation to the fetus. While there are numerous factors that can lead to fetal complications, the number one cause of fetal death is maternal death.

Treatment of the Pregnant Cardiac Arrest Patient

Cardiac arrest in a pregnant female, while relatively rare, is possible from medical and traumatic causes. And when it does occur, the resuscitative interventions and medication normally used during an arrest should be administered. This includes electrical therapy, closed chest compressions, and ventilatory management with intubation.

It is also important to take measures that will help reduce the pressure of the gravid uterus on the inferior vena cava to avoid a decrease in venous return to the heart as the weight of the fetus collapses the inferior vena cava between the uterus and the sacrum. The resulting drop in preload will reduce arterial pressure. This "supine hypotensive syndrome" can result in hypotension by itself, or it can worsen any hypotension that may already be present from the initial traumatic or medical insult. To minimize this effect, place the patient on her left side at a 15–20-degree angle. This will help displace the uterus off the vena cava and improve venous return. Manual displacement is another option, but it is physically tiring and is not any more effective.

If the pregnant patient is in cardiac arrest and her fetus is viable, it may become necessary to perform an emergency cesarean section to save the baby. This should be an option only after the following measures have been proven unsuccessful in restoring effective spontaneous circulation in the mother:

- Properly performed artificial circulation (CPR)
- Displacement of the gravid uterus to the left
- Fluid therapy for vascular volume
- Medication therapy appropriate to the presenting cardiac rhythm

The decision to perform an emergency cesarean section is one that should not be taken lightly. Numerous additional factors need to be taken into consideration—for example, the factors that precipitated the maternal arrest, availability of personnel capable of performing the procedure, the gestational age of the fetus, and the amount of time since the onset of the maternal arrest. Optimally, the procedure should be performed within 5 minutes of the arrest; however successful infant survival has been documented after 20 minutes of maternal arrest. In the out-of-hospital phase of arrest management, the possibility that the baby may survive even if the mother cannot be saved underscores the importance of proper oxygenation, ventilations, compressions, IV therapy, and medication administration.

Specifically, initial management of the pregnant cardiac arrest patient should include the following:

- Performance of CPR with the patient rolled to her left at 20 degrees. This may be best accomplished by placing the patient on a backboard and supporting it with pillows or blankets.
- Airway management with intubation, ventilation, and maximal oxygenation
- Pharmacological support and fluid therapy as appropriate for the patient's cardiac rhythm and physiological condition
- Consider the feasibility of emergency cesarean section

In summary, treatment of the pregnant female who suffers cardiac arrest includes appropriate treatment for the mother while ensuring the best opportunity for survival of the fetus should the mother fail to have a return of spontaneous circulation. To this end, proper treatment of the cardiac arrest is essential. The care provider should administer the normal modalities for the arrest, as well as specific interventions discussed above for the pregnant female. Remember, also, that the mother is still the best incubator for the fetus, and all efforts should be extended to reverse the cardiac arrest and return normal circulation.

Lightning Strikes

Lightning strikes are the number one cause of deaths from natural environmental phenomena. Hundreds of persons die from lightning strikes every year, while many others sustain injuries, and numerous survivors of lightning strikes have residual effects.

The mortality rate from lightning strikes is about 30%. It is actually an interesting question why more people do *not* die, considering that a lightning strike delivers over 100 million volts. One reason for the relatively high survival rate is thought to be the "flash-over" effect. The theory is that the energy of a lightning strike is delivered in such a brief instant that most of it "flashes over" the outside of the body. Since a relatively small amount of electricity actually enters the body, there is a relatively good chance for survival.

Despite the "flash-over" theory, some individuals apparently receive a flow of energy through their body that is high enough to disrupt normal cardiac and respiratory activity, or it may be that certain individuals are more susceptible than others to the effects of a lightning strike. In either case, the primary cause of death from a lightning strike is asystole or ventricular fibrillation, usually secondary to prolonged apnea.

With a lightning strike, the electrical current flow acts like a massive direct current defibrillation which depolarizes the heart, producing asystole. In numerous instances, following this depolarization, the heart is able to repolarize appropriately and restore normal electrical activity. Unfortunately, however, there is also depression of the brain stem secondary to the lightning strike that causes prolonged periods of apnea. As a result, the patient may develop spontaneous electrical activity of the heart producing blood flow, but then, since the apnea may persist, degrade into ventricular fibrillation or asystole secondary to hypoxia.

Treatment of the Patient in Cardiac Arrest from a Lightning Strike

The management goals for a patient in cardiac arrest following a lightning strike are similar to those for a patient who has experienced a cardiac arrest under more "normal" circumstances. The purpose of your treatment should be to provide aggressive ventilation or oxygenation and perfusion to the heart and brain until cardiac activity is restored and ventilatory efforts again become spontaneous.

Specifically, initial management of the patient in cardiac arrest from a lightning strike should include the following:

- Precautionary spinal immobilization
- Cardiac monitoring, and administration of defibrillation if necessary
- Securing the airway with endotrachael intubation
- Oxygenation and positive pressure ventilation
- IV therapy for medication administration; limit fluid bolusing unless necessary
- Appropriate stabilization of related injuries secondary to the strike (e.g., fractures, burns)

In a situation where numerous people are injured in the same lightning strike, it behooves the out-of-hospital care provider to alter his assessment format to allow those who "look dead" to be treated first. This way, you will be sure to provide ventilation, oxygenation, and artificial circulation to those individuals until a perfusing rhythm and spontaneous respirations return. In the instance where you have a patient displaying only apnea after the strike, the provision of ventilation and oxygenation will help prevent secondary hypoxic cardiac arrest.

Hypothermia and Near Drowning

Hypothermia and Near Drowning in Association with Arrest

Both hypothermia and near drowning are often associated with cardiopulmonary arrest. Special considerations for the management of patients suffering hypothermia and/or near drowning are discussed in the following sections.

Hypothermia

Hypothermia in association with respiratory and cardiac arrest deserves special discussion, because the body tends to decrease all metabolic and related activity as the core temperature decreases, and this in turn allows the body to survive longer periods of arrest. It has been documented that under certain circumstances of hypothermia, patients have full neurological recovery despite prolonged arrest.

Physiologic changes that accompany hypothermia include:

- Decreased metabolic rate
- Decreased cardiac activity
- Decreased respiratory activity
- Decreased mental function (confusion)
- Hypotension
- Flaccid muscles
- Eventual unconsciousness and cardiac arrest

Near Drowning

Even though near drowning is a distinctly different medical emergency from hypothermia, it is mentioned in this section because almost all near drowning victims have some degree of hypothermia. For this reason, the treatment of the two is very similar. As with hypothermia, the physical appearance of the near-drowning victim may be deceiving, presenting much like death. Oftentimes, the exact length of time underwater is not known, so attempts at resuscitation should be started immediately unless grossly obvious signs of death are present (such as rigor mortis, dependent lividity, or putrefaction).

In near drowning, in addition to hypothermia other physiological factors increase the likelihood of successful resuscitation with neurological recovery. The "mammalian diving reflex" occurs in any person who dives into cold water (<68 degrees F). This reflex causes:

- Inhibition of breathing
- Slowing of heart rate
- Vasoconstriction of peripheral vessels
- Constant blood flow maintained to heart/brain
- About a 50% drop in metabolic activity

Hypothermia and Near Drowning Commonalities

In both the hypothermic patient and near-drowning patient, resuscitative measures should be instituted as soon as it is safe to do so, with less attention paid to the length of time in arrest than in other arrest situations. How long can the period of arrest be, and still have neurologic recovery? There is no concrete answer to that question since there are so many variables that play a role in eventual recovery. The length of time submerged or exposed to the cold environment, the exact temperature of the environment, the age of the patient, the general health condition of the victim, presence of associated trauma, and length of time till rewarming is initiated—all factor into the potential for a successful resuscitation.

Basic-Life-Support Treatment

Both the drowning patient and the hypothermic patient may still be in an environment that may be dangerous to the provider of initial emergency care. In a hazardous situation like this, rescue must be carried out by trained and experienced experts. It is your responsibility to keep not only yourself and your team safe, but also to keep eager bystanders safe should they want to "jump-in" and help with the rescue. The goal here is to minimize the risk of danger to yourself, your coworkers, and the bystanders, as well as to avoid additional harm to the patient.

The first goal of management is to assess and support lost vital functions. Assess vital signs in any hypothermic patient for about 30–45 seconds. This is to assure that you will not miss an extremely bradypneic or bradycardic rhythm. Airway maintenance and rescue breathing or ventilations with a BVM should be initiated as early *as safely possible* when the spontaneous respirations are lost or diminished. Concurrently, full spinal immobilization should be maintained, since many times there is trauma associated with the emergency. This is especially true with diving emergencies, since the patient may have struck his head while diving into shallow or unknown water. In these instances, immobilization needs to be carried out while the patient is still in the water. Even if trauma isn't confirmed, immobilization is recommended until x-rays rule out any spinal injury.

Chest compressions for the hypothermic or near-drowning patient should be carried out according to normal CPR standards. Another intervention appropriate during the initial management is to remove any wet garments, and to protect the patient from heat loss by shielding the patient from the environment and/or wrapping the patient in dry material.

When hypothermia is present, as confirmed by a temperature recording, rewarming interventions may be indicated. The degree of hypothermia may predispose the patient to the "after-drop" phenomenon. (After-drop is the sudden return of cold, acidic blood to the heart from the cold extremities after the extremities have been rewarmed and the peripheral vessels begin to dilate.) However, after-drop can be mitigated by rewarming the patient according to the hypothermia algorithm (Figure 12-1). Remember, however, that a cold heart is also very susceptible to the irritability caused by rough handling of the patient. During treatment, be cautious and handle the patient gently to avoid precipitating ventricular fibrillation.

Advanced-Life-Support Treatment

Treatment goals and interventions for the near-drowning patient in cardiac arrest are the same as for any other cardiac arrest patient: Early intubation, defibrillation, IV access, and drug therapy are appropriate. Often, it may be impossible to determine the exact length of submersion. Therefore, the patient should be provided with full advanced cardiac life support on scene and en route to the hospital, where the emergency department physician can decide whether or not to maintain resuscitative efforts. If the resuscitation is successful, the patient should be transported to a health care facility regardless of patient stability.

Treatment for the hypothermic patient in cardiac arrest is slightly different than for patients in arrest from other causes. As mentioned earlier, many physical manipulations and interventions (e.g., moving the patient, intubating, pacing) have been shown to precipitate ventricular fibrillation in a hypothermic patient who is not yet in full cardiac arrest. While these interventions must never be withheld when needed, it is important to keep this in mind when dealing with hypothermic patients.

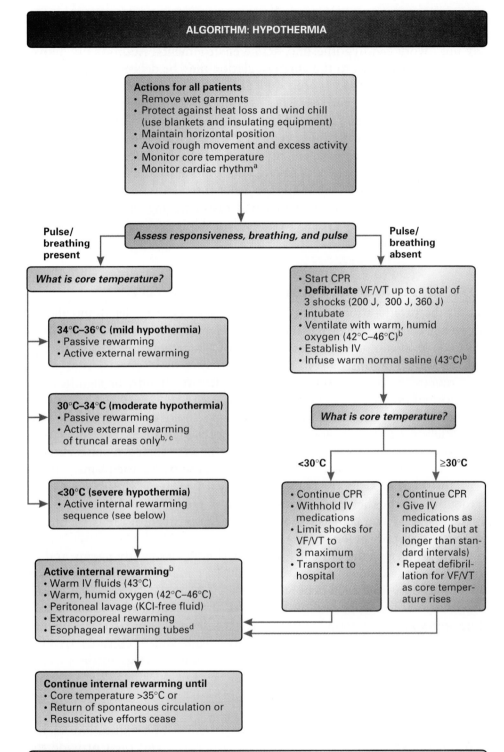

FIGURE 12-1
Algorithm for treatment of hypothermia. Adapted with permission. Journal of the American Medical Association, October 28, 1992, Volume 268, No. 16, *Guidelines for Cardiopulmonary Resuscitation and Emergency Cardiac Care*, p.2245. ©1992 American Medical Association.

ALGORITHM: HYPOTHERMIA

Actions for all patients
• Remove wet garments
• Protect against heat loss and wind chill (use blankets and insulating equipment)
• Maintain horizontal position
• Avoid rough movement and excess activity
• Monitor core temperature
• Monitor cardiac rhythm[a]

Assess responsiveness, breathing, and pulse

Pulse/breathing present

What is core temperature?

34°C–36°C (mild hypothermia)
• Passive rewarming
• Active external rewarming

30°C–34°C (moderate hypothermia)
• Passive rewarming
• Active external rewarming of truncal areas only[b, c]

<30°C (severe hypothermia)
• Active internal rewarming sequence (see below)

Active internal rewarming[b]
• Warm IV fluids (43°C)
• Warm, humid oxygen (42°C–46°C)
• Peritoneal lavage (KCl-free fluid)
• Extracorporeal rewarming
• Esophageal rewarming tubes[d]

Continue internal rewarming until
• Core temperature >35°C or
• Return of spontaneous circulation or
• Resuscitative efforts cease

Pulse/breathing absent

• Start CPR
• **Defibrillate** VF/VT up to a total of 3 shocks (200 J, 300 J, 360 J)
• Intubate
• Ventilate with warm, humid oxygen (42°C–46°C)[b]
• Establish IV
• Infuse warm normal saline (43°C)[b]

What is core temperature?

<30°C
• Continue CPR
• Withhold IV medications
• Limit shocks for VF/VT to 3 maximum
• Transport to hospital

≥30°C
• Continue CPR
• Give IV medications as indicated (but at longer than standard intervals)
• Repeat defibrillation for VF/VT as core temperature rises

a. This may require needle electrodes through the skin

b. Many experts think these interventions should be done only in-hospital, though practice varies.

c. Methods include electric or charcoal warming devices, hot water bottles, heating pads, radiant heat sources, and warming beds.

d. Esophageal rewarming tubes are widely used internationally and should become available in the United States.

The severely hypothermic heart may not be as responsive to cardiac drug and electrical therapy as the normothermic heart. Also, medications may not "work" in hypothermic, acidic environments. Additionally, movement of IV push drugs to the core circulation may be delayed by peripheral vasoconstriction, sludged blood, and diminished perfusion pressures with CPR. The concern is that the drugs will accumulate to toxic levels in the extremities and then be "dumped" on the heart as rewarming begins. Thus the primary treatment for the severely hypothermic patient (core temp <30 degrees C) is aimed at internal rewarming until the core temperature is brought up to a range where the body will respond to more aggressive therapy. Once this has been achieved, the other interventions and therapies as indicated in Figure 12-1 may be carried out. Utilizing this approach will afford the hypothermic cardiac arrest patient the greatest chances for a successful resuscitation.

Toxicologic Cardiac Emergencies and Arrest

Due to the proliferation of drug use in our society, both legal and illegal, emergency cardiac care providers need to become aware that certain drugs at a toxic level can interfere not only with CNS activity but can be cardiotoxic as well. For this reason, patients suffering toxic effects from drugs often require specific treatments that may deviate slightly, or significantly, from normal practices.

For example, tricyclic antidepressants (TCAs) are extremely cardiotoxic at high levels. Because it interferes with neurochemical transmitters, a TCA overdose can have profound effects on the heart, ranging from tachydysrhythmias to axis deviations to ventricular irritability. Yet the primary treatment for TCA toxicity is not geared toward treating the dysrhythmia. Rather the specific therapy here is to alkalinize the blood with sodium bicarbonate. This, as you can see, is a major deviation from normal advanced-cardiac-life-support practice.

The problem is the difficulty, or impossibility, of identifying any and all drugs with cardiac side effects. Realistically, it is impossible and unnecessary to try to discuss how each drug will affect the body. Such extensive knowledge is beyond the scope and purpose of this text. (Table 12-4 does identify some of the more common cardiotoxic overdoses and their basic treatment).

As an alternative however, the authors want you to consider treating the toxicologic emergency from a "process" point of view. In the process method, approach all toxicologic patients the same way, have certain management goals, and access information centers that will have the information you need to treat the specific overdose.

In the process method, approach the patient with the question "What vital functions have been lost that need support?" and then provide the appropriate care for these functions as your initial stabilization. Despite the specific type of cardiac emergency, all patients should receive initial stabilization of the ABCs until specific treatments for the toxin have been identified.

Poison Control Centers (PCCs) have been established across the United States and Canada to assist in the treatment of toxicologic emergencies. Officials at the Center can assist you in setting priorities and formulating an

TABLE 12-4 POTENTIALLY CARDIOTOXIC OVERDOSES AND TREATMENT CONSIDERATIONS

Toxin	Specific Antidote	Adjunctive Therapy
benzodiazepine	flumazenil	airway maintenance
beta-blocker	—	saline, epinephrine, glucagon
Ca++ channel blocker	calcium	saline, epinephrine, glucagon
carbon monoxide	oxygen	hyperbaric chamber
cocaine	—	benzodiazepine, labetalol
tricyclic antidepressant	—	bicarbonate, saline
digitalis	fab fragment antibodies	airway care, supportive care
ethanol	—	supportive care
isoniazid (INH)	pyridoxine	diazepam
narcotic	naloxone	airway maintenance
organophosphate	atropine	protopam sulfate, supportive care

effective treatment plan. PCC officials can also provide information about any available antidote that may be appropriate for the patient.

Calls to the PCC are typically toll-free, and most are staffed by professionals 24 hours a day to assist health care providers as well as the public. Staffed by experienced professionals, each center is also connected to a network of nationwide consultants who can answer questions about almost any poison. In addition, information on the poison center's computer is updated every 90 days to provide the latest information on treatment options and antidotes.

Be prepared to tell the poison center officials the patient's approximate age and weight. Summarize the patient's condition, including level of responsiveness, level of activity, skin color, vomiting, cardiac activity, and other pertinent physical findings. Any directions from a poison control center should be administered in consultation with the responsible physician overseeing the patient's care.

SUMMARY

For the majority of cardiac arrests and other cardiac emergencies, treatment is essentially the same. Considerations must be given however, to those situations where the normal and accepted practices of advanced life support need to be modified to accommodate the patient's specific situation. In this

CASE STUDY FOLLOW-UP

Assessment

As you follow the paramedics to the rear of your neighbor's home, Mrs. Tieche tells you her nephew was walking on the ice to "test" it—making sure it was safe for the kids to play on. She added that when he didn't return into the house, she looked outside and saw the hole in the ice where he had apparently fallen through. "Somehow," she added, "my husband must have pulled him out while I was around front waiting for the ambulance." Estimating, she adds that her nephew must have been under the water for about 15 or 20 minutes.

Even though the patient looks clinically dead, you and the paramedics begin your assessment. Paramedic Lago assesses for a pulse and respirations for a full 30 seconds while Paramedic Davis readies the "quick-look" paddles of the cardiac monitor. To assist in confirming pulselessness, you assess for heart tones as well. As you touch the patient's skin, you note it to be very cold to the touch, with some minor abrasions to the forehead from falling through the ice.

Treatment

With no signs of life present, and the cardiac monitor displaying an idioventricular rhythm, Paramedic Lago initiates compressions while her partner goes for the immobilization equipment. After hyperventilating the patient with a BVM, you intubate the patient and resume ventilations with warmed and humidified oxygen, all the time maintaining cervical spine control. Immobilization is completed rapidly, and a tympanic-membrane temperature reveals a temperature of 32 degrees Celsius. CPR is maintained.

Since the back-up crew has not yet arrived, you decide to assist the paramedics in the back of the ambulance. Once there, you complete the removal of wet clothing. Since the patient is cold and has poor peripheral veins, the decision is made to initiate an external jugular vein IV. This, you reason, should help speed the drugs to the core circulation, since the jugular vein is physically closer to the core than an arm vein.

The monitor reveals fine ventricular fibrillation, so electrical therapy is applied—without success, as the patient remains in ventricular fibrillation. One mg of epinephrine is administered, and the patient is now en route to the receiving hospital. The onboard oxygen being delivered to the patient is humidified and warmed to assist in internal warming as heating packs are prepared and placed at the groin, axillary, and neck regions. Since the transport time is short, about 10 minutes, there is time to administer only one additional dose of epinephrine along with one dose of lidocaine. Defibrillation is again unsuccessful. Additional medication and electrical therapy are withheld until the core temperature rises.

Upon arrival at the emergency department, the ED staff assess the core temperature to be 33 degrees C. They maintain your rewarming techniques and start to administer warmed IV fluids, as well as initiating additional rewarming techniques. After a short period of time, the core temperature has increased, and defibrillation converts the patient into a bradycardic rhythm with a pulse and systolic pressure.

With continued rewarming, the patient's heart rate and systolic blood pressure continues to rise without the assistance of further pharmacological therapy. Care providers are being careful not to aggressively handle the patient. By the time you leave to return home, the patient is physiologically more stable with a core temperature of 36 degrees C. However, the patient has yet to show any sings of neurological recovery.

chapter, we have looked at traumatic cardiac arrests, cardiac arrest and pregnancy, cardiac emergencies associated with lightning strikes, CVA and TIAs, cardiac arrest in the hypothermic or near-drowning patient, and cardiac emergencies associated with toxic drug effects. Emergency cardiac care providers should note carefully the differences in these emergencies with respect to triage, emphasis of treatment, and techniques.

REVIEW QUESTIONS

1. Which of the following traumatic injuries could lead to cardiac arrest?
   a. massive arterial hemorrhage
   b. spinal cord injury
   c. cardiac tamponade
   d. a and c
   e. a, b, and c

2. What treatment must be provided to any cardiac arrest victim from trauma?
   a. spinal immobilization
   b. nasotracheal intubation
   c. IV therapy of D_5W
   d. oxygen at 10 liters per minute

3. What is the proper fluid bolus amount for the trauma victim in need of fluid replacement?
   a. 10 ml/kg
   b. 20 ml/kg
   c. 30 ml/kg
   d. 40 ml/kg

4. Which patient should **not** receive cardiopulmonary resuscitation with advanced life support?
   a. 25-year-old trauma arrest in a PEA rhythm of 60/minute
   b. 63-year-old trauma arrest with full body burns
   c. 51-year-old trauma arrest with hypovolemia
   d. 33-year-old trauma arrest with a tension pneumothorax

5. Which one of these physiological changes in the pregnant female may mask early signs of shock?
   a. gravid uterus
   b. increased pulmonary function
   c. increased metabolic activity and oxygen consumption
   d. increased resting heart rate and cardiac output
   e. c and d

6. The number one cause of fetal death is
   a. trauma to the uterus.
   b. tearing of the placenta.
   c. maternal hypertension.
   d. maternal death.

7. What causes supine hypotensive syndrome in the pregnant female?
   a. pressure on the pulmonary veins
   b. pressure on the descending aorta
   c. pressure on the inferior vena cava
   d. pressure on the iliac arteries and veins

8. The administration of medications used in cardiac arrest should be altered in what way when treating a pregnant female?
   a. Administer half the dose normally used.
   b. Administer the normal dose, but lengthen the repeat times.
   c. Do not administer anything through a central line.
   d. None. Utilize the medications as appropriate for any other arrest.

9. A patient has been struck by lightning while playing golf. What would be the immediate concern regarding treatment?
   a. intubation
   b. positive pressure ventilation
   c. compressions
   d. IV initiation

10. Your lightning victim has been found in ventricular fibrillation. You should
    a. defibrillate at 360 joules.
    b. defibrillate at 300 joules.
    c. defibrillate at 200 joules.
    d. defibrillate at 100 joules.

11. What is the most likely mechanism causing death in the victim struck by lightning?
    a. apnea resulting from depression of the brain stem
    b. persistent ventricular fibrillation that is refractory to drugs
    c. associated trauma from being thrown
    d. extensive burns from the lightning

12. Would it be appropriate to provide spinal immobilization to the cardiac arrest victim who was struck by lightning while providing initial management?
    a. yes   b. no

13. Which of the following changes is **not** seen in the victim of hypothermia?
    a. slowing heart rate
    b. increasing respiratory rate
    c. redirection of blood flow to heart and brain
    d. drop in metabolic activity

14. What is the **primary** concern when dealing with victims of hypothermia or near-drowning?
    a. personal safety during the rescue
    b. early initiation of mouth-to-mouth ventilations
    c. rapid defibrillation
    d. oxygenation

15. Which of the following is true regarding medication administration in the severely hypothermic cardiac arrest patient (core temp < 30 degrees C)?
    a. You should delay administration of drugs until the core temperature rises.
    b. Drugs may not be effective on the hypothermic heart.
    c. Drugs lose their effectiveness when they are chilled by the blood.
    d. Drug dosages should be doubled since they are less effective.

16. All toxicologic cardiac arrests should receive
    a. endotrachael intubation.
    b. defibrillation.
    c. specific antidotes for the drug they ingested.
    d. nasogastric tube for gastric evacuation.

17. Poison Control Centers (PCCs) provide
    a. up-to-date treatment plans.
    b. tracking of emerging toxicologic trends.
    c. follow-up to patient treatment.
    d. specific antidotes when necessary.
    e. all of the above

Chapter**Thirteen**

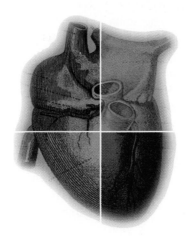

Special Treatment Considerations

After a cardiac emergency, the patient will be stabilized by health care providers in the out-of-hospital setting and in the emergency department. Ultimately, the patient will still require definitive care—care that focuses on correcting the underlying problem and restoring the patient, as nearly as possible, to good health. This level of care can best be provided in the coronary care and other units the patient will inhabit until he is well enough to go home from the hospital. Although they are beyond the normal scope of advanced cardiac life support training, some of these considerations of definitive care—and other considerations that are not an inherent part of advanced cardiac life support—are briefly introduced in this chapter.

The topics to be covered are:

- Cerebral Resuscitation
- Advanced Monitoring Interventions for Cardiac Arrest Patients
- Adjuncts for Artificial Circulation

CASE STUDY

Freshly armed with additional knowledge and skills you acquired in a recent advanced cardiac life support class, you arrange to do some "ride-along" time with a local EMS service, an experience that will allow you to apply your new knowledge as well as serve toward completion of your required continuing education hours.

That day, your ride-along happens to be with two seasoned paramedics, Joe and Rich. The day drags by slowly. After completing 11 hours of your 12-hour shift, you have yet to get even one trip. Finally, about 15 minutes before it's time for you to leave, a call comes in for a "man-down."

When you arrive on scene about 4 minutes later, you see a collapsed man, on his back, with the first responders performing two-person CPR. You think you understood what you learned in your ACLS class, but your heart is pounding anyway as you follow Joe and Rich toward the patient.

How would you proceed to assess and care for this patient? This chapter will describe the assessment and necessary treatment of a patient with a cardiac emergency which may require special treatment considerations. Later, we will return to the case and apply the procedures learned.

Introduction

We begin this chapter by reiterating that the goal of advanced cardiac life support is to temporarily correct (or supplement) altered physiological processes until definitive care can be provided. It is important for you to realize that care rendered in the out-of-hospital and emergency department setting are temporizing measures. Rarely would a patient be cured (let alone discharged) from an emergency department visit after suffering a cardiac arrest. It is not that this level of care is impossible in the ED, but rather that it is reserved for care providers who have the special training and the day-to-day experience and resources to manage patients during that extremely delicate post arrest period.

The obvious example is the typical progression of a cardiac arrest victim through the health care system. First, out-of-hospital resuscitation provides early CPR, defibrillation, drug therapy, and airway maintenance while the patient is transported to the emergency department. Secondly, the emergency department staff focuses on patient stabilization with subsequent transport to a coronary care unit. It is in the coronary care unit and step-down units that definitive care takes place.

The following discussion is intended to provide you with an introduction to some of the special treatment considerations that, for the most part, are a part of definitive cardiac care. A full explanation of these concerns is well beyond the scope of this text. The authors recommend that health care providers who need additional information regarding these topics seek the support of the specialty areas of the hospital where these procedures and technologies are more commonplace, and refer to texts devoted specifically to them. (Enlist the help of cardiologists and internal medicine physicians for references.) The authors hope that this approach will encourage you to expand your knowledge of these special areas while keeping the essential purposes of advanced cardiac life support in focus.

Cerebral Resuscitation

Since the brain is the foundation on which the body must rely, once the heart has been resuscitated it is imperative to restore cerebral blood flow to near normal levels and to correct any concerns of hypoxemia and acidosis. It is a certainty that if the brain is not being properly oxygenated or perfused, it is just a matter of time until cardiac arrest will recur.

After cardiac arrest occurs and cerebral blood flow (CBF) ceases, humans will lose consciousness in about 15 seconds. As the residual levels of glucose and adenosine triphosphate (ATP) are exhausted, the respirations become agonal and the pupils become fixed and dilated. This deterioration of cerebral functioning occurs rapidly, with irreversible damage occurring in roughly 6 minutes. (However, be aware that more recent research has indicated some cerebral neurons may be more resistant to ischemia than previously believed.) It is during this period of clinical death that advanced cardiac life support attempts to restore cerebral perfusion by compensating for and/or correcting the effects of cardiac arrest.

The restoration of cerebral perfusion after cardiac arrest is not problem-free. For a period of some hours, in fact, additional brain damage may occur. This "postresuscitation syndrome," as it is called by the American Heart Association, is marked by a cerebral blood flow that is still inadequate despite the return of spontaneous cardiac output. While the exact cause of the postresuscitation syndrome is yet unknown, some hypotheses point to the possibility of reflex vasoconstriction due to abnormal calcium movement, platelet clumping (aggregation), red blood cell deformity, and/or capillary bed edema.

Regardless of the cause of the syndrome, the key for health care providers is to remember that the normal ability of the brain to maintain its perfusion seems to be diminished or lost during a period of time that may last up to 24 hours after a cardiac arrest has been corrected. They must be attuned to certain physiologic considerations and procedures aimed toward ensuring adequate CBF and maximal cerebral outcome for the patient (Figure 13-1).

Cerebral Perfusion Pressures

Under normal circumstances, the brain has the ability to autoregulate its own blood flow. This means that, when there are fluctuations in the systolic pressure, the brain will adjust its vascular tone to maintain a constant CBF. However, as a result of the tissue damage and accumulation of acids and metabolites common to cardiac arrest, this ability of autoregulation is temporarily diminished. During the postresuscitation period, CBF is more dependent upon systolic blood pressure. For the care provider, this means that the systolic pressure must be returned to levels that are similar to, or slightly higher than, those observed prior to the cardiac arrest. This should be accomplished by using vasopressors and fluid therapy as appropriate.

Oxygenation

Optimal oxygenation will provide the cells with sufficient oxygen to support their metabolic activity. As a guide, maintaining the PaO_2 above 100 mmHg

FIGURE 13-1 Postresuscitation care: cerebral resuscitation considerations.

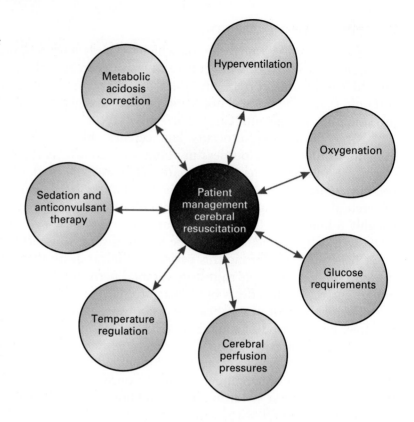

should allow for proper oxygenation. Since there may be pulmonary damage as a result of the arrest that may interfere with oxygen diffusion, positive end-expiratory pressure (PEEP) may be utilized to assure oxygenation across the alveolar wall. During the oxygenation, be sure to administer the lowest concentration of oxygen possible with carefully titrated PEEP, as lung damage can occur with long-term use of high concentration oxygen. The goal is to maintain a PaO_2 of 100 mmHg, using the minimal necessary amounts of oxygen and PEEP.

Hyperventilation

Hyperventilation has been shown to have two main benefits to the post cardiac arrest patient. First, hyperventilation should help eliminate excessive accumulations of CO_2 (especially after sodium bicarbonate administration) via the lungs, helping to reverse tissue acidosis that is common during arrest. Secondly, some research has indicated that, by lowering the $PaCO_2$ through controlled hyperventilation, there is a reflexive constriction of cerebral vessels. The enhanced vasoconstriction, in turn, lowers intracranial pressure (ICP) by decreasing the amount of blood flow through the brain.

While the concept of vasoconstriction may seem contradictory to improving cerebral perfusion, in those individuals with high ICP, the vasoconstriction can actually enhance cerebral perfusion pressure by lowering ICP. (Review the information on intracranial pressure as a factor in cerebral perfusion pressure in Chapter 9 on stroke.) This effect is only temporary, however. The body's normal acid-base adjustment systems start to compensate for the drop in $PaCO_2$ and the effects diminish after about 4 hours.

Metabolic Acidosis Correction

The longer a person is in cardiac arrest, the worse the acidosis becomes. While hyperventilation will help eliminate the carbon dioxide created during the body's buffering of metabolic acidosis, the buffering mechanism can easily become overwhelmed by massive cellular acidosis. In the post arrest patient, the continued acidosis depresses myocardial activity and contributes to eventual death. To help correct this, proper ventilation should be continued with endotracheal intubation and an adequate minute ventilation. The administration of sodium bicarbonate should be guided by blood gas analysis and occur secondary to establishment of proper ventilation.

Temperature Regulation

An often-overlooked aspect of patient management, temperature control can be a benefit to post arrest management or become a detriment if left unattended. Research has shown how an increase in core temperature causes an increase in metabolic rate and oxygen demand. As the cerebral metabolic rate increases, it requires an additional flow of oxygenated blood to meet metabolic demands. This increase may be enough to aggravate the already poor balance between supply and demand in a post arrest brain.

Conversely, hypothermia is a widely accepted way to depress cerebral metabolic activity and, consequently, blood-flow requirements. However, in the post arrest scenario, hypothermia also contributes to increased blood viscosity and a drop in cardiac output—both of which are a detriment to cerebral perfusion after cardiac arrest. Researchers cannot agree as to the therapeutic benefits of inducing hypothermia for a post arrest patient. For now, the best guide is to protect the patient from environmental extremes and maintain normothermia.

Glucose Requirements

Glucose levels can have a significant impact on successful cardiac arrest management. Normal levels of blood glucose should be assured by routine monitoring of the blood glucose level (BGL). Excessively high levels and excessively low levels of glucose have both been shown to be detrimental to patient outcomes. Therefore, normal levels should be maintained to allow adequate stores of energy for the body during the repair process following the arrest.

Sedation and Anticonvulsant Therapy

An important consideration while managing a patient who has been successfully resuscitated from cardiac arrest is preventing activities that may increase the cerebral metabolic rate. For example, although comatose, a portion of the brain may still respond with heightened metabolic activity in response to external stimuli (for example a sternal rub or suctioning). This causes a localized need for increased perfusion in the face of a diminished supply. The imbalance can then result in a localized deficit and additional damage. It should be a rule, then, to minimize external stimuli to the comatose post arrest patient. Administering sedatives or relaxants may help achieve this end.

Seizure activity, an ever-present danger to the post arrest patient, needs special consideration. A single seizure has the potential of increasing cerebral metabolic activity 300% to 400%. The sudden requirement for increased blood supply and oxygenation will cause a detrimental shift in the balance of supply and demand and worsen neurologic outcomes. While researchers disagree as to the benefit of prophylactic anticonvulsant therapy, all agree that any seizures that occur should be quickly and aggressively terminated. To achieve this, normal anticonvulsant drugs (e.g., diazepam, dilantin, barbiturates) may be employed.

Brain Resuscitation after Cardiopulmonary Arrest

In light of the advancing knowledge about the etiologies that underlie the postresuscitation syndrome, more and more therapeutic modalities are being hypothesized and tested in controlled studies to determine their value. As yet, however, there are no drugs that can be recommended for routine treatment of post arrest brain damage.

Advanced Monitoring Interventions for Cardiac Arrest Patients

The following section is an introduction to invasive monitoring techniques. These techniques are typically not required during the early stages of advanced cardiac life support, and information about them is considered to be supplemental to the ACLS course. Should you be assigned to a work area where these more advanced techniques are practiced, you should locate and study an appropriate text on invasive monitoring techniques.

Arterial Cannulation

Arterial cannulation is a process of placing an indwelling catheter into an appropriate artery. Typically, site preferences include the radial artery, femoral artery, axillary artery, or possibly the dorsal pedal artery. It is important to note that there must be evidence of adequate collateral circulation at the chosen site in case the artery should occlude.

Arterial cannulation allows continual and accurate monitoring of arterial pressure. It also allows for sampling of arterial blood without repeated arterial sticks and, to a lesser extent, determination of cardiac output with indocyanine green dye.

Cannulation of the Pulmonary Artery

Cannulation of the pulmonary artery is accomplished by inserting a catheter with a balloon tip into the central circulation until it passes through the right side of the heart and eventually is placed in the pulmonary artery. This placement allows for determination of pulmonary wedge pressures and cardiac output and for sampling of pulmonary arterial blood (which is actually mixed venous blood).

With the data obtained, the care provider can make determinations about left and right ventricular functions, determine mitral valve function, differentiate cardiogenic from noncardiogenic pulmonary edema, and detect the presence of a ruptured intraventricular septum. Additionally, the effectiveness of interventions can be determined, since serial measurements can be performed.

Arterial Puncture

Arterial puncture is the insertion of a needle into an artery to secure an arterial blood specimen. Lab tests are done on the sample to determine such things as arterial gas levels, carbon monoxide levels, or lactate. As noted earlier, if repeated sampling is necessary, placement of an indwelling arterial catheter may be preferred to avoid the discomfort and complications of repeated sticks.

Adjuncts for Artificial Circulation

CPR is now generally considered to be a temporizing measure whose chief benefit is to provide some degree of cardiac output and oxygenation to vital organs until more definitive care (e.g., defibrillation, drugs, intubation) can be provided to the cardiac arrest victim. In essence, CPR delays biological death (irreversible cell death) in the face of clinical death (cessation of heartbeat and respirations). With this goal in mind, proposed new interventions and techniques that make compressions more effective should result in increased blood flow and oxygenation to vital organs and ultimately lead to improvements in cardiac arrest survival.

Alternative Techniques to Compressions

Since no newly proposed technique has been shown to consistently improve cardiac arrest survival rates, none has been recommended to replace the standard CPR technique. However, some of these alternative techniques may improve the hemodynamics of compressions.

Interposed abdominal compressions have been shown to improve blood flow, although not consistently in all studies. In this technique, the abdomen is compressed during the relaxation phase of chest compressions. The theory is that this improves blood flow by increasing the aortic diastolic pressure and, as a result, coronary perfusion. This technique requires three people—one to provide ventilations, one to perform chest compressions, and one to perform abdominal compressions—and should be conducted after endotracheal intubation is completed. The risks of abdominal injuries, poor ventilation (due to increases in intra-abdominal pressure with compressions), and aspiration must be further considered before interposed abdominal compressions are recommended as a standard.

Simultaneous ventilation-compression CPR is another new technique that attempts to increase cardiac output. This technique uses the entire thorax as a pump by inflating the lungs (which put pressure on the lateral aspects of the heart), while depressing the sternum (which provides anteroposterior pressure). In hypothesis, this would improve artificial blood flow by providing more complete circumferential pressure to the heart. While promising in theory, studies have not shown improved survivability for cardiac arrest, and therefore this technique has not been recommended as routine.

High-frequency (or rapid manual) CPR is yet another alternative chest-compression technique. In this technique, the standard external compression rates are dramatically increased. The theory is that if the heart rate is increased (artificially with the compressions) then cardiac output should improve. (This presumes that the stroke volume, or amount of blood ejected with each compression, stays the same or even improves slightly.) Some laboratory studies, but not all, have shown this to be the case. So while high-frequency CPR shows some potential benefits, additional studies of outcomes for patients in cardiac arrest need to be conducted to determine its efficacy.

Mechanical Devices for CPR

A number of mechanical devices have been devised that provide compressions and/or ventilations to the cardiac arrest patient. They are designed to standardize CPR technique, reduce rescuer fatigue, ensure adequacy of compressions, and free up rescuers to attend to other aspects of advanced life support. To date, these devices are intended only for the adult in cardiac arrest.

The cardiac press device has a hinged arm that swings over the patient's thorax and is positioned so the press is over the sternum and adjusted to the proper depth. This permits the device, which is manually operated, to deliver consistent compressions.

The automatic resuscitator is a gas-powered device that is programmed to deliver ventilations and compressions. While larger and heavier than other mechanical devices, it allows rescuers to attend to other aspects of patient care during arrest management. This is beneficial in those instances when care providers are few.

Vest CPR is an experimental method that compresses the thorax pneumatically with a perithoracic vest. In essence, this device operates under the same hemodynamic principles as simultaneous ventilation-compression CPR. While some preliminary studies have indicated that the vest-CPR device does improve hemodynamic status, there has not yet been enough research on humans to confidently recommend it.

Finally, active compression-decompression CPR is an adjunct that attaches to the thorax via a large suction cup and provides active compression and decompression (or upstroke). Further outcome assessments are being conducted, but initial studies are promising.

Invasive CPR

Direct cardiac massage (which was performed routinely prior to the introduction of closed-chest compressions), has been shown to provide better blood flow and perfusion pressures than closed-chest compressions. The applicability to routine cardiac arrests, the majority of which occur outside the hospital, is limited. However, certain patients who are already in the hospital prior to arrest may benefit from this technique.

Cardiopulmonary bypass, used normally in cardiac surgery, has also been shown to be beneficial in cardiac arrest care. However, like direct cardiac massage, its applicability is mainly in-hospital and requires a coordinated resuscitation team with the appropriate training and technology. As such, it is not a consideration for routine cardiac arrest management.

CPR Assessment

Other than outcome studies (how many patients died vs. how many were successfully resuscitated), there are actually few ways to reliably assess the effectiveness of CPR.

Most commonly, pulses are felt to assess the effectiveness of compressions. Femoral pulses felt during compressions are very misleading since you may actually be feeling venous backflow rather than arterial flow. For this reason, femoral pulses should be assessed during spontaneous pulse checks only. And since femoral pulses tend to be fainter than carotid pulses, the carotid is still the preferred site to check for a spontaneous pulse as well as to check effectiveness of compressions. Doppler ultrasound may detect spontaneous blood flow that cannot be discerned by palpation of pulse points and may also be useful during the arrest management, especially in patients in pulseless electrical activity.

While a carotid pulse may indicate forward blood flow, research continues to find methods that can more accurately determine the effectiveness of CPR. Respiratory gas measurement via capnometry shows some promise as a reliable test of CPR adequacy. Since expired CO_2 is dependent upon pulmonary perfusion, end tidal CO_2 monitoring has been shown to accurately estimate adequacy of CPR and cardiac output. Experimental models have shown a positive correlation between successful resuscitation from cardiac arrest and higher expired CO_2 levels. Capnometry readings improve prior to successful resuscitation and may be used to indicate the return of spontaneous circulation. Despite these promising findings, research is still being conducted to assess its usefulness in clinical practice.

CASE STUDY FOLLOW-UP

Having just finished your ACLS course, you are doing a "ride-along" with an experienced team when a call comes in for a "man down." Arriving on scene, you discover two first responders doing CPR on a supine male.

Assessment

As soon as the ambulance is positioned, you, Joe, and Rich grab the necessary equipment and walk toward the patient. Arriving at the patient's side, you quickly confirm pulselessness while Joe prepares to obtain a "quick look" with the monitor. Rich kneels down beside you and says bystanders report the patient was complaining of chest pain when he suddenly became unresponsive.

Treatment

After doing a "quick-look," Joe says out loud that the patient is in a bradydysrhythmic rhythm. You add, "It must be PEA since there is no palpable pulse." Rich concurs and initiates CPR again while Joe starts hyperventilating the patient with an oropharyngeal airway and BVM. He asks you to prepare a 8.0 mm ET tube with the #3 MacIntosh laryngoscope blade and handle.

After about 6 minutes on scene, you are prepared for transport. The patient has been placed on a backboard and has been successfully intubated by Joe. Rich has administered the first epinephrine and atropine down the endotracheal tube. Before pulling away from the scene, Joe

(continued)

motions for you to take the BVM and ventilate the patient. He adds that he needs to set up the cardiac press with Rich before he starts driving to the hospital.

You recall that one problem with postresuscitation is the management of cerebral edema. To help minimize this, you elect to maintain hyperventilation of the patient, which in turn will allow elimination of excess carbon dioxide promote cerebral vasoconstriction. You watch the end tidal CO_2 monitor as it displays the amount of carbon dioxide expired with each ventilation. By this time, Rich has initiated and IV and the ambulance is moving with resuscitation continuing en route. You are fascinated to watch the cardiac press administering compressions because you've never seen one in use before.

When you arrive at the hospital, unfortunately, despite all the advanced cardiac life support interventions, the patient is still in arrest. Since the cardiac press is mobile, it is transferred with the patient into the emergency department. It continues to administer compressions as the ED staff takes over treatment of the patient. Joe and Rich then converse with the ED physician, giving him a brief overview of the events.

Afterward, Joe and Rich commend you on your performance. Although the arrest was not a "save," you are pleased you had an opportunity to exercise your ACLS skills.

SUMMARY

This chapter has been an introduction to some considerations of definitive cardiac care and several techniques and technologies now being studied that may enhance the chances of restoring the cardiac patient to good health.

Of paramount concern is cerebral resuscitation, taking various measures to compensate for postresuscitation syndrome, the brain's diminished ability to regulate its own cerebral perfusion during a period of 24 hours or so after correction of a cardiac arrest. These measures include oxygenation and hyperventilation, correction of metabolic acidosis, temperature and glucose regulation, and anti-convulsant therapy as needed.

Additional special considerations include advanced invasive monitoring interventions such as arterial cannulation and adjuncts, techniques, and technologies to improve and measure the effectiveness of CPR compressions.

REVIEW QUESTIONS

1. In relation to cardiac arrest, what does "postresuscitation syndrome" refer to?
   a. the period of time preceding cardiac arrest when the patient is experiencing chest pain
   b. the period of time following the return of spontaneous circulation when the patient exhibits seizures
   c. the period of time following the return of spontaneous circulation when the patient is still hypotensive
   d. the period of time following cardiac arrest when the brain is hypoperfused despite spontaneous circulation

2. What factors can help alleviate the postresuscitation syndrome?
   a. glucose regulation
   b. hyperventilation
   c. temperature regulation
   d. a and b
   e. a, b, and c

3. Seizures are an ever-present danger during the postresuscitation period. They are best managed by
   a. prophylactic administration of an anticonvulsant prior to the onset of a seizure.
   b. administration of valium or barbiturates to terminate the seizures should they occur.
   c. allowing seizures to occur since the medication to stop them is more likely to worsen the postresuscitation syndrome than the seizure itself.
   d. a and b

4. Which advanced monitoring intervention allows for continual monitoring of arterial pressures or sampling of arterial blood?
   a. arterial cannulation
   b. arterial puncture
   c. saphenous line placement
   d. pulmonary artery cannulation

5. By what general principle(s) do the alternative adjuncts for artificial circulation offer an improvement in the performance of CPR for the cardiac arrest patient?
   a. they help reduce rescuer fatigue
   b. they improve the hemodynamics of compressions
   c. they are less likely to administer inappropriate compressions
   d. all the above

6. What is the **currently** approved way to assess the effectiveness of the compressions during CPR?
   a. assessment of the carotid pulse
   b. assessment of the femoral pulse
   c. monitoring end tidal CO_2 readings
   d. monitoring pulse oximetry

7. Drug therapies are currently available that can reverse post-arrest brain damage.
   a. true
   b. false

Appendix

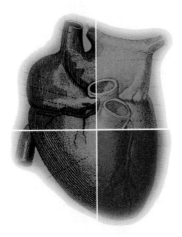

Recommendations of the American College of Cardiology and the American Heart Association on Practice Guidelines for the Management of Patients with Acute Myocardial Infarction

Ryan TJ, Anderson JL, Antman EM, Braniff BA, Brooks NH, Califf, RM, Hillis LD, Hiratzka LF, Rapaport E, Riegel BJ, Russell RO, Smith EE III, Weaver WD.

ACC/AHA guidelines for the management of patients with acute myocardial infarction: a report of the American College of Cardiology/American Heart Association Task Force on Practice Guidelines (Committee on Management of Acute Myocardial Infarction). *J Am Coll Cardiol.* 1996: 28: 1328-1428.

Recommendations

The following is a listing of the recommendations made by the ACC/AHA Task Force on Practice Guidelines in the ACC/AHA Task Force Report "ACC/AHA Guidelines for the Management of Patients with Acute Myocardial Infarction." More detailed information regarding the evidence and the rationale for these recommendations can be found in the full text of the guidelines themselves, which appears in the November 1996 issue of the *Journal of the American College of Cardiology*.

Explanation of Classes

As in previous guidelines, the American College of Cardiology and the American Heart Association have used the following classification system in which indications for a diagnostic procedure, a particular therapy, or intervention are designated as:

Class I: Conditions for which there is evidence for and/or general agreement that a given procedure or treatment is beneficial, useful, and effective.

Class II: Conditions for which there is conflicting evidence and/or a divergence of opinion about the usefulness/efficacy of a procedure or treatment.

Class IIa: Weight of evidence/opinion is in favor of usefulness/efficacy.

Class IIb: Usefulness/efficacy is less well established by evidence/opinion.

Class III: Conditions for which there is evidence and/or general agreement that a procedure/treatment is not useful/effective and in some cases may be harmful.

Prehospital Issues

Class I

1. Availability of 911 access.

2. Availability of an emergency medical services (EMS) system staffed by persons trained to treat cardiac arrest with defibrillation if indicated and to triage patients with ischemic-type chest discomfort.

Class IIa

1. Availability of a first-responder defibrillation program in a tiered response system.

2. Healthcare providers educate patients/families about signs and symptoms of acute MI, accessing EMS, and medications.

Class IIb

1. Twelve-lead telemetry.

2. Prehospital thrombolysis in special circumstances (e.g., transport time greater than 90 minutes).

Initial Recognition and Management in the Emergency Department

Class I

1. Emergency department acute MI protocol that yields a targeted clinical examination and a 12-lead ECG within 10 minutes and a door-to-needle time that is less than 30 minutes.

Routine Measures

1. Supplemental oxygen, intravenous access, and continuous electrocardiographic monitoring should be established in all patients with acute ischemic-type chest discomfort.

2. An ECG should be obtained and interpreted within 10 minutes of arrival in the ED in all patients with suspected acute ischemic-type chest discomfort.

Oxygen

Class I

1. Overt pulmonary congestion.

2. Arterial oxygen desaturation (SaO_2 less than 90%).

Class IIa

1. Routine administration to all patients with uncomplicated MI during the first 2 to 3 hours.

Class IIb

1. Routine administration of supplemental oxygen to patients with uncomplicated MI beyond 3 to 6 hours.

Intravenous Nitroglycerin

Class I

1. For the first 24 to 48 hours in patients with acute MI and CHF, large anterior infarction, persistent ischemia, or hypertension.

2. Continued use (beyond 48 hours) in patients with recurrent angina or persistent pulmonary congestion.

Class IIa

None.

Class IIb

1. For the first 24 to 48 hours in all patients with acute MI who do not have hypotension, bradycardia, or tachycardia.

2. Continued use (beyond 48 hours)[a] in patients with a large or complicated infarction.

Class III

1. Patients with systolic blood pressure less than 90 mm Hg or severe bradycardia (less than 50 bpm).

Aspirin

Class I

1. A dose of 160 to 325 mg should be given on day 1 of acute MI and continued indefinitely on a daily basis thereafter.

Class IIb

1. Other antiplatelet agents such as dipyridamole or ticlopidine may be substituted if true aspirin allergy is present.

---

[a] Oral or topical preparation may be substituted.

Atropine

Class I

1. Sinus bradycardia with evidence of low cardiac output and peripheral hypoperfusion or frequent premature ventricular complexes at onset of symptoms of acute MI.

2. Acute inferior infarction with type I second- or third-degree atrioventricular (AV) block associated with symptoms of hypotension, ischemic discomfort, or ventricular arrhythmias.

3. Sustained bradycardia and hypotension after administration of nitroglycerin.

4. For nausea and vomiting associated with administration of morphine.

5. Ventricular asystole.

Class IIa

1. Symptomatic patients with inferior infarction and type I second- or third-degree heart block at the level of the AV node (i.e., with narrow QRS complex or with known existing BBB [bundle branch block]).

Class IIb

1. Administration concomitant with (before or after) administration of morphine in the presence of sinus bradycardia.

2. Asymptomatic patients with inferior infarction and type I second-degree heart block or third-degree heart block at the level of the AV node.

3. Second- or third-degree AV block of uncertain mechanism when pacing is not available.

Class III

1. Sinus bradycardia greater than 40 bpm without signs or symptoms of hypoperfusion or frequent premature ventricular contractions.

2. Type II AV block and third-degree AV block and third-degree AV block with new wide QRS complex presumed due to acute MI.

Thrombolysis

Class I

1. ST elevation (greater than 0.1 mV, two or more contiguous leads),[b] time to therapy 12 hours or less,[c] age less than 75 years.

2. Bundle branch block (obscuring ST-segment analysis) and history suggesting acute MI.

Class IIa

1. ST elevation,[b] age 75 years or older.

Class IIb

1. ST elevation,[b] time to therapy greater than 12 to 24 hours.[c]

2. Blood pressure on presentation greater than 180 mm Hg systolic and/or greater than 110 mm Hg diastolic associated with high-risk MI.

Class III

1. ST elevation,[b] time to therapy greater than 24 hours,[c] ischemic pain resolved.

2. ST-segment depression only.

Primary PTCA

Class I

1. As an alternative to thrombolytic therapy only if performed in a *timely fashion by individuals skilled in the procedure*[d] *and supported by experienced personnel in high volume centers.*[e]

Class IIa

1. As a reperfusion strategy in patients who are candidates for reperfusion but who have a *risk of bleeding* contraindication to thrombolytic therapy.

2. Patients in cardiogenic shock.

Class IIb

1. As a reperfusion strategy in patients who fail to qualify for thrombolytic therapy for reasons other than a risk of bleeding contraindication.

Early Coronary Angiography in the ST-Segment Elevation or Bundle Branch Block Cohort Not Undergoing Primary PTCA

Class I

None.

Class IIa

1. Patients with cardiogenic shock or persistent hemodynamic instability.

Class IIb

1. Patients with evolving large or anterior infarcts treated with thrombolytic agents in whom it is believed that the artery is not patent and adjuvant PTCA is planned.

Class III

1. Routine use of angiography and subsequent PTCA within 24 hours of administration of thrombolytic agents.

Emergency or Urgent Coronary Artery Bypass Graft Surgery

Class I

1. Failed angioplasty with persistent pain or hemodynamic instability in patients with coronary anatomy suitable for surgery.

2. Acute MI with persistent or recurrent ischemia refractory to medical therapy in patients

---

[b] Repeat ECGs recommended during medical observation in clinical settings when initial ECG is nondiagnostic of ST elevation.

[c] Time of symptom onset is defined as beginning of continuous persistent discomfort that brought the patient to the hospital.

[d] Individuals who perform more than 75 PTCA procedures per year.

[e] Centers that perform more than 200 PTCA procedures per year.

with coronary anatomy suitable for surgery who are not candidates for catheter intervention.

3. At the time of surgical repair of postinfarction VSD [ventricular septal defect] or mitral valve insufficiency.

Class IIa

1. Cardiogenic shock with coronary anatomy suitable for surgery.

Class IIb

1. Failed PTCA and small area of myocardium at risk; hemodynamically stable.

Class III

1. When the expected surgical mortality rate equals or exceeds the mortality rate associated with appropriate medical therapy.

Early Coronary Angiography and/or Interventional Therapy in Non-ST-Segment Elevation Cohort

Class I

1. Patients with recurrent (stuttering) episodes of spontaneous or induced ischemia or evidence of shock, pulmonary congestion, or LV dysfunction.

Class IIa

1. Patients with persistent ischemic-type discomfort despite medical therapy and an abnormal ECG or two or more risk factors for coronary artery disease.

2. Patients with chest discomfort, hemodynamic instability, and an abnormal ECG.

Class IIb

1. Patients with chest discomfort and an unchanged ECG.

2. Patients with ischemic-type chest discomfort and a normal ECG and more than two risk factors for coronary artery disease.

Hospital Management

Early, General Measures

Class I

1. Selection of electrocardiographic monitoring based on infarct location and rhythm.

2. Bed rest with bedside commode privileges for initial 12 hours in hemodynamically stable patients free of ischemic-type chest discomfort.

3. Avoidance of Valsalva.

4. Careful attention to maximum pain relief.

Class IIb

1. Routine use of anxiolytics.

Class III

1. Prolonged bed rest (more than 12 to 24 hours) in stable patients without complications.

Identification and Treatment of the Patient at High Risk

Management of Recurrent Chest Discomfort

Class I

1. Aspirin for pericarditis.

2. ß-Adrenoceptor blockers intravenously, then orally for ischemic-type chest discomfort.

3. (Re)administration of thrombolytic therapy (alteplase) for patients with recurrent ST elevation.

4. Coronary arteriography for ischemic-type chest discomfort recurring after hours to days of initial therapy and associated with objective evidence of ischemia in patients who are candidates for revascularization.

Class IIa

1. Nitroglycerin intravenously for 24 hours, then topically or orally for ischemic-type chest discomfort.

Class IIb

1. Corticosteroids for pericarditis.

2. Indomethacin for pericarditis.

Hemodynamic Monitoring

Balloon Flotation Right-Heart Catheter Monitoring

Class I

1. Severe or progressive CHF or pulmonary edema.

2. Cardiogenic shock or progressive hypotension.

3. Suspected mechanical complications of acute infarction, i.e., VSD, papillary muscle rupture, or pericardial tamponade.

Class IIa

1. Hypotension that does not respond promptly to fluid administration in a patient without pulmonary congestion.

Class III

1. Patients with acute infarction without evidence of cardiac or pulmonary complications.

Intra-arterial Pressure Monitoring

Class I

1. Patients with severe hypotension (systolic arterial pressure less than 80 mm Hg) and/or cardiogenic shock.

2. Patients receiving vasopressor agents.

Class IIa

1. Patients receiving intravenous sodium nitroprusside or other potent vasodilators.

Class IIb

1. Hemodynamically stable patients receiving intravenous nitroglycerin for myocardial ischemia.

2. Patients receiving intravenous inotropic agents.

Class III

1. Patients with acute infarction who are hemodynamically stable.

Intra-aortic Balloon Counterpulsation

Class I

1. Cardiogenic shock not quickly reversed with pharmacological therapy as a stabilizing measure for angiography and prompt revascularization.

2. Acute mitral regurgitation or VSD complicating MI as a stabilizing therapy for angiography and repair/revascularization.

3. Recurrent intractable ventricular arrhythmias with hemodynamic instability.

4. Refractory post-MI angina as a bridge to angiography and revascularization.

Class IIa

1. Signs of hemodynamic instability, poor LV function, or persistent ischemia in patients with large areas of myocardium at risk.

Class IIb

1. In patients with successful PTCA after failed thrombolysis or those with three-vessel coronary disease to prevent reocclusion.

2. In patients known to have large areas of myocardium at risk with or without active ischemia.

Rhythm Disturbances

Atrial Fibrillation

Class I

1. Electrical cardioversion for patients with severe hemodynamic compromise or intractable ischemia.

2. Rapid digitalization to slow a rapid ventricular response and improve LV function.

3. Intravenous ß-adrenoceptor blockers to slow a rapid ventricular response in patients without clinical LV dysfunction, bronchospastic disease, or AV block.

4. Heparin should be given.

Class IIa

Either diltiazem or verapamil intravenously to slow a rapid ventricular response if ß-adrenoreceptor blocking agents are contraindicated or ineffective.

Ventricular Tachycardia/Ventricular Fibrillation

Class I

1. Ventricular fibrillation (VF) should be treated with an unsynchronized electric shock with an initial energy of 200 J; if unsuccessful, a second shock of 200 to 300 J should be given, and, if necessary, a third shock of 360 J.

2. Sustained (more than 30 seconds or causing hemodynamic collapse) polymorphic ventricular tachycardia (VT) should be treated with an unsynchronized electric shock using an initial energy of 200 J; if unsuccessful, a second shock of 200 to 300 J should be given, and, if necessary, a third shock of 360 J.

3. Episodes of sustained monomorphic VT associated with angina, pulmonary edema, or hypotension (blood pressure less than 90 mm Hg) should be treated with a synchronized electric shock of 100 J initial energy. Increasing energies may be used if not initially successful.

4. Sustained monomorphic VT not associated with angina, pulmonary edema, or hypotension (blood pressure less than 90 mm Hg) should be treated with one of the following regimens:

a. Lidocaine; bolus 1.0 to 1.5 mg/kg. Supplemental boluses of 0.5 to 0.75 mg/kg every 5 to 10 minutes to a maximum of 3 mg/kg total loading dose may be given as needed. Loading is followed by infusion of 2 to 4 mg/min (30 to 50 µg/kg per minute).

b. Procainamide; 20 to 30 mg/min loading infusion, up to 12 to 17 mg/kg. This may be followed by an infusion of 1 to 4 mg/min.

c. Amiodarone; 150 mg infused over 10 minutes followed by a constant infusion of 1.0 mg/min for 6 hours and then a maintenance infusion of 0.5 mg/min.

d. Synchronized electrical cardioversion starting at 50 J (brief anesthesia is necessary).

Class IIa

1. Infusions of antiarrhythmic drugs may be used after an episode of VT/VF but should be discontinued after 6 to 24 hours and the need for further arrhythmia management assessed.

2. Electrolyte and acid-base disturbances should be corrected to prevent recurrent episodes of VF when an initial episode of VF has been treated.

Class IIb

1. Drug-refractory polymorphic VT should be managed by aggressive attempts to reduce myocardial ischemia, including therapies such as ß-adrenoceptor blockade, intra-aortic balloon pumping, and emergency PTCA/CABG surgery. Amiodarone, 150 mg infused over 10 minutes followed by a constant infusion of 1.0 mg/min for up to 6 hours and then a maintenance infusion of 0.5 mg/min may also be helpful.

Class III

1. Treatment of isolated ventricular premature beats, couplets, runs of accelerated idioventricular rhythm, and nonsustained VT.

2. Prophylactic administration of antiarrhythmic therapy when using thrombolytic agents.

Bradyarrhythmias and Heart Block

Atropine

Class I

1. Symptomatic sinus bradycardia (generally, heart rate less than 50 bpm associated with hypotension, ischemia, or escape ventricular arrhythmia).

2. Ventricular asystole.

3. Symptomatic AV block occurring at the AV nodal level (second-degree type I or third degree with a narrow-complex escape rhythm).

Class IIa

None.

Class III

1. Atrioventricular block occurring at an infra-nodal level (usually associated with anterior MI with a wide-complex escape rhythm).

2. Asymptomatic sinus bradycardia.

Temporary Pacing

Placement of Transcutaneous Patches[f] and Active (Demand) Transcutaneous Pacing[g]

Class I

1. Sinus bradycardia (rate less than 50 bpm) with symptoms of hypotension (systolic blood pressure less than 80 mm Hg) unresponsive to drug therapy.[g]

2. Mobitz type II second-degree AV block.[g]

3. Third-degree heart block.[g]

4. Bilateral BBB (alternating BBB, or RBBB and alternating left anterior fascicular block [LAFB], left posterior fascicular block [LPFB]) (irrespective of time of onset).[f]

5. Newly acquired or age-indeterminate LBBB, LBBB and LAFBa, RBBB, and LPFBa.[f]

6. RBBB or LBBB and first-degree AV block.[f]

Class IIa

1. Stable bradycardia (systolic blood pressure greater than 90 mm Hg, no hemodynamic compromise, or compromise responsive to initial drug therapy).[f]

2. Newly acquired or age-indeterminate RBBB.[f]

Class IIb

1. Newly acquired or age-indeterminate first-degree AV block.[f]

Class III

1. Uncomplicated acute MI without evidence of conduction system disease.

[f] Transcutaneous patches applied; system may be attached and activated within a brief time if needed. Transcutaneous pacing may be very helpful as an urgent expedient. Because it is associated with significant pain, high-risk patients likely to require pacing should receive a temporary pacemaker.

[g] Apply patches and attach system; system is in either active or standby mode to allow immediate use on demand as required. In facilities in which transvenous pacing or expertise are not available to place an intravenous system, consideration should be given to transporting the patient to one equipped and competent in placing transvenous systems.

Temporary Transvenous Pacing[h]

Class I

1. Asystole.

2. Symptomatic bradycardia (includes sinus bradycardia with hypotension and type I second-degree AV block with hypotension not responsive to atropine).

3. Bilateral BBB (alternating BBB or RBBB with alternating LAFB/LPFB) (any age).

4. New or indeterminate-age bifascicular block (RBBB with LAFB or LPFB, or LBBB) with first-degree AV block.

5. Mobitz type II second-degree AV block.

Class IIa

1. RBBB and LAFB or LPFB (new or indeterminate).

2. RBBB with first-degree AV block.

3. LBBB, new or indeterminate.

4. Incessant VT, for atrial or ventricular over-drive pacing.

5. Recurrent sinus pauses (greater than 3 seconds) not responsive to atropine.

Class IIb

1. Bifascicular block of indeterminate age.

2. New or age-indeterminate isolated RBBB.

Class III

1. First-degree heart block.

2. Type I second-degree AV block with normal hemodynamics.

3. Accelerated idioventricular rhythm.

4. Bundle branch block or fascicular block known to exist before acute MI.

Permanent Pacing After Acute Myocardial Infarction

Class I

1. Persistent second-degree AV block in the His Purkinje system with bilateral BBB or complete heart block after acute MI.

2. Transient advanced (second- or third-degree) AV block and associated BBB.[i]

3. Symptomatic AV block at any level.

Class IIb

1. Persistent advanced (second- or third-degree) block at the AV node level.

[h] It should be noted that in choosing an intravenous pacemaker system, patients with substantially depressed ventricular performance, including right ventricular infarction, may respond better to atrial/AV sequential pacing than ventricular pacing.

[i] An electrophysiology study should be considered to assess the site and extent of heart block in uncertain cases.

Class III

1. Transient AV conduction disturbances in the absence of intraventricular conduction defects.

2. Transient AV block in the presence of isolated LAFB.

3. Acquired LAFB in the absence of AV block.

4. Persistent first-degree AV block in the presence of BBB that is old or age indeterminate.

Other Surgical Interventions

Emergency or Urgent Cardiac Repair of Mechanical Defects

Class I

1. Papillary muscle rupture with severe acute mitral insufficiency.

2. Postinfarction VSD or free wall rupture and pulmonary edema or cardiogenic shock (emergency or urgent).

3. Postinfarction ventricular aneurysm associated with intractable ventricular tachyarrhythmias and/or pump failure (urgent).

Class III

1. Acute infarctectomy in hemodynamically stable patients.

Rationale and Approach to Pharmacotherapy

Antithrombotics/Anticoagulants

Heparin

Class I

1. Patients undergoing percutaneous or surgical revascularization.

Class IIa

1. Intravenously in patients undergoing reperfusion therapy with alteplase.

2. Subcutaneously (7500 U twice daily) (intravenous heparin is an acceptable alternative) in all patients not treated with thrombolytic therapy who do not have a contraindication to heparin. In patients who are at high risk for systemic emboli (large or anterior MI, atrial fibrillation [AF], previous embolus, or known LV thrombus), intravenous heparin is preferred.

3. Intravenously in patients treated with nonselective thrombolytic agents (streptokinase, anistreplase, urokinase) who are at high risk for systemic emboli (large or anterior MI, AF, previous embolus, or known LV thrombus).

Class IIb

1. Patients treated with nonselective thrombolytic agents, not at high risk, subcutaneous heparin, 7500 U to 12,500 U twice a day until completely ambulatory.

Class III

1. Routine intravenous heparin within 6 hours to patients receiving a nonselective fibrinolytic agent (streptokinase, anistreplase, urokinase) who are not at high risk for systemic embolism.

β-Adrenoceptor Blocking Agents

Early Therapy

Class I

1. Patients without a contraindication to β-adrenoceptor blocker therapy who can be treated within 12 hours of onset of infarction, irrespective of administration of concomitant thrombolytic therapy.

2. Patients with continuing or recurrent ischemic pain.

3. Patients with tachyarrhythmias, such as AF with a rapid ventricular response.

Class IIb

1. Non-Q-wave MI.

Class III

1. Patients with moderate or severe LV failure or other contraindications to β-adrenoceptor blocker therapy.

Agiotensin Converting Enzyme Inhibitors

Class I

1. Patients within the first 24 hours of a suspected acute MI with ST-segment elevation in two or more anterior precordial leads or with clinical heart failure in the absence of significant hypotension or known contraindications to use of ACE inhibitors.

2. Patients with MI and LV ejection fraction less than 40% or patients with clinical heart failure on the basis of systolic pump dysfunction during and after convalescence from acute MI.

Class IIa

1. All other patients within the first 24 hours of a suspected or established acute MI, provided significant hypotension or other clear-cut contraindications are absent.

2. Asymptomatic patients with mildly impaired LV function (ejection fraction 40% to 50%) and a history of old MI.

Class IIb

1. Patients who have recently recovered from MI but have normal or mildly abnormal global LV function.

Calcium Channel Blockers

Class I

None.

Class IIa

1. Verapamil or diltiazem may be given to patients in whom β-adrenoceptor blockers are ineffective or contraindicated (i.e., bronchospastic disease) for relief of ongoing ischemia or control of a rapid ventricular response with AF after acute MI in the absence of CHF, LV dysfunction, or AV block.

Class IIb

1. In non-ST-elevation infarction, diltiazem may be given to patients without LV dysfunction, pulmonary congestion, or CHF. It may be added to standard therapy after the first 24 hours and continued for 1 year.

Class III

1. Nifedipine (short acting) is generally contraindicated in routine treatment of acute MI because of its negative inotropic effects and the reflex sympathetic activation, tachycardia, and hypotension associated with its use.

2. Diltiazem and verapamil are contraindicated in patients with acute MI and associated LV dysfunction or CHF.

Magnesium

Class I

None.

Class IIa

1. Correction of documented magnesium (and/or potassium) deficits, especially in patients receiving diuretics before onset of infarction.

2. Episodes of torsades de pointes-type VT associated with a prolonged QT interval should be treated with 1 to 2 g magnesium administered as a bolus over 5 minutes.

Class IIb

1. Magnesium bolus and infusion in high-risk patients such as the elderly and/or those for whom reperfusion therapy is not suitable.

Preparation for Discharge from the Hospital

Noninvasive Evaluation of Low-Risk Patients

Stress ECG

Class I

a. Before discharge for prognostic assessment or functional capacity (submaximal at 4 to 6 days or symptom limited at 10 to 14 days).

b. Early after discharge for prognostic assessment and functional capacity (14 to 21 days)

c. Late after discharge (3 to 6 weeks) for functional capacity and prognosis if early stress was submaximal.

2. Exercise, vasodilator stress nuclear scintigraphy, or exercise stress echocardiography when baseline abnormalities of the ECG compromise interpretation.[j]

Class IIa

1. Dipyridamole or adenosine stress perfusion nuclear scintigraphy or dobutamine echocardiography before discharge for prognostic assessment in patients judged to be unable to exercise.

2. Exercise two-dimensional echocardiography or nuclear scintigraphy (before or early after discharge for prognostic assessment).

Class III

1. Stress testing within 2 to 3 days of acute MI.

2. Either exercise or pharmacological stress testing at any time to evaluate patients with unstable postinfarction angina pectoris.

3. At any time to evaluate patients with acute MI who have uncompensated CHF, cardiac arrhythmia, or noncardiac conditions that severely limit their ability to exercise.

4. Before discharge to evaluate patients who have already been selected for cardiac catheterization. In this situation an exercise test may be useful after catheterization to evaluate function or identify ischemia in distribution of a coronary lesion of borderline severity.

Assessment of Ventricular Arrhythmia—Routine Testing

Class I

None.

Class IIa

None.

Class IIb

1. Ambulatory (Holter) monitoring, signal-averaged ECG, heart rate variability, baroreflex sensitivity monitoring, alone or in combination with these or other tests, including functional tests (ejection fraction, treadmill testing) for risk assessment after MI, especially in patients at higher perceived risk, when findings might influence management issues, or for clinical research purposes.

Invasive Evaluation

Coronary Angiography and Possible PTCA

Class I

1. Patients with spontaneous episodes of myocardial ischemia or episodes of myocardial ischemia provoked by minimal exertion during recovery from infarction.

2. Before definitive therapy of a mechanical complication of infarction such as acute mitral regurgitation, VSD, pseudonaneurysm, or LV aneurysm.

3. Patients with persistent hemodynamic instability.

---

[j] Marked abnormalities in the resting ECG such as LBBB, LV hypertrophy with strain, ventricular pre-excitation, or a ventricular paced rhythm render a displacement of ST segments virtually uninterpretable. For patients taking digoxin or who have less than 1 mm ST depression on their resting tracing who undergo standard stress electrocardiographic testing, it must be realized that further ST depression with exercise may have minimal diagnostic significance.

Class IIa

1. When MI is suspected to have occurred by a mechanism other than thrombotic occlusion at an atherosclerotic plaque. This would include coronary embolism, certain metabolic or hematological diseases, or coronary artery spasm.

2. Survivors of acute MI with depressed LV systolic function (LV ejection fraction less than or equal to 40%), CHF, prior revascularization, or malignant ventricular arrhythmias.

3. Survivors of acute MI who had clinical heart failure during the acute episode but subsequently demonstrated well-preserved LV function.

Class IIb

1. Coronary angiography performed in all patients after infarction to find persistently occluded infarct-related arteries in an attempt to revascularize the artery or to identify patients with three-vessel disease.

2. All patients after a non-Q wave MI.

3. Recurrent VT or VF or both, despite antiarrhythmic therapy in patients without evidence of ongoing myocardial ischemia.

Class III

1. Routine use of coronary angiography and subsequent PTCA of the infarct-related artery within days after receiving thrombolytic therapy.

2. Survivors of MI who are thought not to be candidates for coronary revascularization.

Routine Coronary Angiography and PTCA After Successful Thrombolytic Therapy

Class I

None.

Class IIa

None.

Class III

1. Routine PTCA of the stenotic infarct-related artery immediately after thrombolytic therapy.

2. Percutaneous transluminal coronary angioplasty of the stenotic infarct-related artery within 48 hours of receiving a thrombolytic agent in asymptomatic patients without evidence of ischemia.

Secondary Prevention

Management of Lipids

Class I

1. The AHA Step II diet, which is low in saturated fat and cholesterol (less than 7% of total calories as saturated fat and less than 200 mg/d cholesterol), should be instituted in all patients after recovery from acute MI.

2. Patients with LDL cholesterol levels greater than 125 mg/dL despite the AHA Step II diet should be placed on drug therapy with the goal of reducing LDL to less than 100 mg/dL.

3. Patients with normal plasma cholesterol levels who have a high-density lipoprotein HDL cholesterol level less than 35 mg/dL should receive non-pharmacological therapy (e.g., exercise) designed to raise it.

Class IIa

1. Drug therapy may be added to diet in patients with LDL cholesterol levels less than 130 mg/dL but greater than 100 mg/dL after an appropriate trial of the AHA Step II diet alone.[k]

2. Patients with normal total cholesterol levels but HDL cholesterol less than 35 mg/dL despite diet and other nonpharmacological therapy may be started on drugs such as niacin to raise HDL levels.

Class IIb

1. Drug therapy using either niacin or gemfibrozil may be added to diet regardless of LDL and HDL levels when triglyceride levels are greater than 400 mg/dL.

Long-Term β-Adrenoceptor Blocker Therapy in Survivors of Myocardial Infarction

Class I

1. All but low-risk patients without a clear contraindication to β-adrenoceptor blocker therapy. Treatment should begin within a few days of the event (if not initiated acutely) and continue indefinitely.

Class IIa

1. Low-risk patients without a clear contraindication to β-adrenoceptor blocker therapy.

Class III

1. Patients with a contraindication to β-adrenoceptor blocker therapy.

Anticoagulants

Long-Term Anticoagulation After Acute Myocardial Infarction

Class I

1. For secondary prevention of MI in post-MI patients unable to take daily aspirin.[l]

---

[k] HmG CoA reductase drugs provide the greatest lowering of LDL cholesterol. Niacin is less effective in lowering LDL, although it is more effective in raising HDL levels. Resins are rarely sufficiently effective to be used alone, but they may be used to supplement lowering LDL with either niacin or HmG CoA reductase drugs.

[l] See "Initial Recognition and Management in the Emergency Department," "Aspirin," in "ACC/AHA Guidelines for the Management of Patients with Acute Myocardial Infarction: Executive Summary" in the *Journal of the American College of Cardiology*, 1996: 28: 1328-1428.

2. Post-MI patients in persistent AF.

3. Patients with LV thrombus.

Class IIa

1. Post-MI patients with extensive wall motion abnormalities.

2. Patients with paroxysmal AF.

Class IIb

1. Post-MI patients with severe LV systolic dysfunction with or without CHF.

Estrogen Replacement Therapy (ERT) and Myocardial Infarction

Class IIa

1. All postmenopausal patients who have an MI should be carefully counseled about the potential beneficial effects of ERT and offered the option of ERT if they desire it.

Answers and Rationales

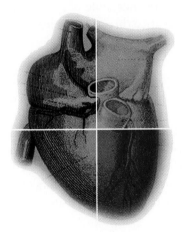

Review Questions
Answers and Rationales

Chapter 1—Key Concepts of Advanced Cardiac Life Support

1. **(a)** In cardiac arrest management, it is necessary to treat the patient as a whole and not just treat the rhythm. The rhythm may be a result of a pre-cardiac-arrest condition, such as a tension pneumothorax resulting in pulse-less electrical activity, that is reversible. Just treating the PEA rhythm without needle decompression to relieve the pneumothorax will result in a futile resuscitation attempt. However, decompression of the chest may provide immediate results with a favorable outcome. Electrical therapy, in cases such as ventricular fibrillation and ventricular tachycardia, takes precedence as an initial treatment over medications and endotracheal intubation.

2. **(c)** The amount of time that elapses between cardiac arrest and defibrillation is the most critical factor related to patient survival. The energy level and amount of transthoracic resistance do influence successful defibrillation; however, time delay is the most significant variable in successful defibrillation.

3. **(c)** Early prevention is not a link in the chain of survival. Early defibrillation is the missing link.

4. **(d)** The patient must be deemed competent and capable of making a rational decision in order to refuse medical care. Terminal illness or approval from family members, physicians, or hospital administrators does not determine the patient's right or ability to refuse care. If the patient is deemed incompetent or incapable of making a rational decision, the physician relies on advance directives or legal surrogates, if any, in the decision-making process.

5. **(b)** If a question exists regarding a do-not-resuscitate order, it is necessary to begin full resuscitation to the standard of care that would be provided if no order existed. That is, you treat the patient as if there had never been an order. That means initiating advanced life support until the order may be clarified. If the resuscitation is not initiated and the order turns out to be invalid, critical time has elapsed and unsuccessful resuscitation may be directly attributed to your delay in action. Also, emergency care providers must be aware of whether the laws of their state whether advance directives can be applied in emergency situations.

Chapter 2—Systematic Approach to Emergency Cardiac Care: The Primary and Secondary Surveys

1. **(c)** Establishing unresponsiveness by shaking and shouting (or talking and touching for a trauma patient) is the first step once you are at the patient's side. However, you must ensure your own safety first before approaching the patient or scene.

2. **(a)** As a health care provider trained in basic and advanced cardiac life support, it is assumed that you have much more training and experience in dealing with medical emergencies. Thus, you need to be decisive and take the most appropriate action based on the presenting situation. It is most appropriate in this situation to establish unresponsiveness, open the airway, and attempt to ventilate, even though you have a high index of suspicion that the patient is choking. If the patient is choking, it is more important for you, as a health care provider, to attempt to relieve the obstruction than to leave the patient and call for help. You would not begin the foreign body airway obstruction maneuvers until you have confirmed an airway obstruction. Chest compressions will not be performed until the airway is cleared and pulselessness is established.

3. **(b)** Any time you suspect possible cervical spinal trauma, it is necessary to open the airway using a jaw-thrust maneuver while the head and neck are maintained in a neutral in-line position. The head-tilt, chin-lift maneuver will cause hyperextension and manipulation of the cervical spine, possibly aggravating an injury. Keeping the head in a neutral position without performing a jaw thrust will not create an open airway.

4. **(a)** The procedures conducted in the primary survey are basic skills, including defibrillation. Initiation of an intravenous line, endotracheal intubation, and administration of medication are all considered components of the secondary survey.

5. **(c)** The time to defibrillation is the most critical factor influencing the success rate of defibrillation. Delays in defibrillation are paralleled by an

increasingly hypoxic and acidotic myocardium which directly decreases the success of defibrillation. Even though airway management, endotracheal intubation, and medication administration are critical in resuscitation, initial defibrillation takes precedence.

6. **(a)** When conducting the secondary survey, you should first perform endotracheal intubation and assess adequacy of ventilation, then initiate an intravenous line and administer medication, then consider the differential diagnosis.

7. **(c)** Bretylium is not an acceptable drug to be administered down the endotracheal tube. Drugs used in resuscitation that can be administered down the endotrachael tube are lidocaine (Xylocaine), epinephrine, atropine, and naloxone (Narcan). These can be remembered by remembering the mnemonic LEAN.

8. **(b)** Normal saline is the preferred intravenous solution in the cardiac arrest patient. It is an isotonic volume expander. Any dextrose-containing solutions should be avoided because of potential postarrest neurological sequelae.

9. **(c)** When administering medications by the endotracheal route, it is necessary to give 2 to 2.5 times the standard dose to assure sufficient and timely absorption, distribution, and action.

10. **(b)** The differential diagnosis should be conducted as part of the secondary survey following the initiation of drug therapy. However, there may be times when consideration of a differential diagnosis may occur much earlier to dictate the appropriate patient management. For example, a trauma patient needs more aggressive fluid therapy, which may be initiated earlier in the secondary survey based on the mechanism of injury.

Chapter 3—Airway Management, Ventilation, and Oxygen Therapy

1. **(b)** Sonorous sounds usually indicate a partial airway occlusion at the level of the pharynx. The tongue is commonly the cause of obstruction. Wheezing indicates an increase in airway resistance in the bronchioles. Laryngeal obstruction, from edema or other material, produces stridor or a crowing-type sound. A gurgling sound is heard when secretions, blood, or vomitus is present in the airway.

2. **(c)** Even with an oropharyngeal or nasopharyngeal airway in place, a manual airway maneuver must be maintained. Tracheobronchial suctioning cannot be performed through an oropharyngeal airway. If the airway stimulates a gag reflex upon insertion, because of its hard-plastic construction, it will continue to stimulate the gag reflex when it is in place.

3. **(d)** Stimulation of the sympathetic nervous system may result from endotracheal intubation, but it is a complication, not an advantage, of this procedure. Stimulation of the sympathetic nervous system may increase myocardial oxygen demand due to an increase in myocardial workload resulting from tachycardia and an increased contractile force. This may precipitate dysrhythmias and increased intracranial hypertension. Lidocaine, epinephrine, atropine, and naloxone may be given down the endotracheal tube, therefore, it may serve as a drug route. Asynchronous ventilation to

chest compression may occur with the endotracheal tube in place. The major advantage of the endotracheal tube is that it protects the airway by isolating it from aspiration of foreign material.

4. **(a)** The curved blade is designed to fit in the vallecula. With an upward and forward lifting motion on the laryngoscope handle, the epiglottis is indirectly lifted, exposing the glottic opening. The straight blade is placed under the epiglottis and is used to directly lift it up to expose the glottic opening.

5. **(c)** In an emergency situation, a 7.5 mm i.d. endotracheal tube would be appropriate for both a male and female. Women usually require a 7.0–to–8.0 mm i.d. tube, whereas males usually take an 8.0–to–8.5 mm i.d. tube.

6. **(a)** When inserting an endotracheal tube, the best indicator to use to determine the proper tube depth is to continue until the proximal end of the cuff has passed 1 to 2.5 cm beyond the level of the cords. The centimeter marker is only used as a guide to monitor tube depth once proper placement has occurred, since the depth will vary with each patient. The tip of the tube should sit midway between the level of the carina and larynx.

7. **(b)** With the first ventilation following tube placement, the chest should be inspected for rise and fall while auscultating over the epigastrium for sounds. Auscultation is done in this sequence to prevent unnecessary air from inflating the stomach while bilateral breath sounds are being assessed with each ventilation. If the tube is in the esophagus while breath sounds are checked, the practitioner may provide several ventilations before then auscultating the epigastrium and realizing that the tube is misplaced. By auscultating over the epigastrium first, you lessen the amount of air insufflation in the stomach and reduce the incidence of possible gastric distention, regurgitation, and aspiration. Condensation in the tube or centimeter marker is not an acceptable method to determine tube placement.

8. **(c)** Patients with blunt trauma to the face have a high incidence of cervical and other spinal injury. Therefore, the head and neck of a patient with facial trauma must be maintained in a neutral in-line position while airway management is being performed, including endotracheal intubation. Hyperventilation is indicated in patients with suspected increases in intracranial pressure from head injury. Typical cuff volume is 10 ml of air and has no bearing on facial trauma or spinal injury. With the distal end of the cuff at the level of the cords, the tip of the tube will not be positioned midway between the carina and larynx. This will lead to easy dislodgement and misplacement, possibly in the esophagus, upon movement of the patient.

9. **(a)** If the esophageal obturator airway (EOA) is inserted in a patient greater than 7 feet tall, the cuff of the tube will not be seated below the level of the carina. When the cuff is inflated with 30–35 ml of air, it will possibly cause compression of the soft posterior tracheal wall and result in tracheal obstruction. The device should only be used in patients greater than 16 years of age and those with no gag reflex who are completely unresponsive. Narcotic drug overdose is not a contraindication as long as the patient has no gag reflex and is completely unresponsive.

10. **(c)** The cricothyroid membrane is located inferior to the thyroid cartilage (Adam's apple) and superior to the cricoid cartilage, the large bulky circumferential ring that is the most inferior part of the larynx.

11. **(b)** When providing positive pressure ventilation, regardless of the technique or type of device being used, 10 to 15 ml/kg of tidal volume must be delivered with each breath.

12. **(c)** Because the flow-restricted oxygen-powered ventilation device provides high rates and volumes of airflow, barotrauma and subsequent pneumothorax may result. The device uses oxygen as its source of power; therefore, 100% oxygen is delivered with each ventilation. Because of the high rate and volume of delivered air, the device is intended for adult patients only.

13. **(a)** The suction should be set at between –80 and –120 mmHg when performing tracheobronchial suctioning to reduce the risk of trauma to the mucosa and other tissue. When performing oropharyngeal suctioning, the pressure should be set at greater than –120 mmHg. The patient should be hyperventilated prior to and after any suction procedure. Suction is only applied while withdrawing the catheter; it is never applied while inserting the catheter down the tube. Suction should not be applied for greater than 15 seconds.

14. **(d)** Hypoxemia is the most serious complication associated with tracheobronchial suctioning. When suction is applied, the functional residual volume is removed from the lungs. Along with an interruption in ventilation, both of these lead to serious hypoxemia. Therefore, it is imperative that the patient be hyperventilated prior to and after all suction procedures.

15. **(b)** If the liter flow is set at less than 6 lpm, the patient will begin to rebreathe his exhaled gas, resulting in a reduction in FiO_2 and potential increases in carbon dioxide. At 8-to-10 lpm, the FiO_2 is about 60%. The simple face mask has no reservoir; the nonrebreather mask does. Oxygen masks are not typically well tolerated by pediatric patients.

Chapter 4—Gaining Intravenous Access

1. **(a)** Catheter over the needle is by far the most common IV catheter used for peripheral vein cannulation. Through-the-needle catheters and hollow needles are less commonly used. An intraosseous catheter would be inserted into the medulla of a bone, not a vein.

2. **(c)** Normal saline is preferred to keep the vein open in cardiac arrest. Fluids for resuscitation in cardiac arrest should not contain dextrose. Sterile water should never be used as an IV fluid because it is severely hypotonic.

3. **(b)** Delivery of medication to the central circulation is *less* rapid from a peripheral than from a central site. However, peripheral cannulation is an easier skill to master, the peripheral veins are easier to find, and peripheral cannulation can usually be accomplished during CPR, whereas central cannulation would require interruption of CPR.

4. **(d)** The antecubital fossa (or the external jugular vein) is preferred because, in cardiac arrest, peripheral venous circulation is compromised, and it is important to introduce medications as close to the central

circulation as possible. The hand vein and saphenous vein of the leg are peripheral veins, but farther from the central circulation. The subclavian vein is central, not peripheral.

5. Two strategies for improving delivery of medications to the central circulation in cardiac arrest are: (a) raise the extremity, and (b) follow each medication with a saline flush of 20–50 ml.

6. Limit IV attempts for a patient who may be a candidate for thrombolysis because thrombolytics act to dissolve clots and will therefore increase the risk of or aggravate bleeding or hematomas.

Chapter 5—Dysrhythmia Recognition

1. **(d)** Myocardial tissue is the only muscle tissue that possesses the property of automaticity. Automaticity is the ability of the muscle tissue to contract on its own, without nervous control. All muscle cells in the body depolarize, repolarize, and contract.

2 **(c)** The three specialized types of myocardial cells are pacemaker, conduction, and working cells.

3. **(b)** Pacemaker cells depolarize at regular intervals, causing a depolarization of adjacent muscle tissue. All myocardial tissue contracts when a wave of depolarization reaches it. Repolarization occurs as the ions that flow out of the cell are pumped back in. The delay in conduction between the atria and the ventricles is caused by the AV node.

4. **(a)** The main pacemaker of the healthy heart is the SA node, which depolarizes at a rate of 60–100 times a minute.

5. **(c)** The AV node depolarizes spontaneously at a rate of 40–60 times a minute and functions as a back-up mechanism if the SA node fails to fire.

6. **(c)** Myocardial working cells are responsible for the mechanical contraction of the heart. The pacemaker cells depolarize at regular intervals and cause the regular contraction of the working cells. The conduction cells serve as a conductive pathway to carry the impulse to depolarize from the pacemakers to the working cells.

7. **(c)** The QRS complex is caused by the depolarization of ventricular cells, which results in ventricular contraction. Atrial depolarization and contraction are represented by the P wave. Ventricular repolarization is seen as the T wave. The delay between atrial and ventricular contraction would be represented by the distance between the P wave and the QRS complex.

8. **(a)** A variance of greater than .04 second between R waves is the definition of irregularity. Automaticity is the ability to contract without nervous control. Ectopy is when beats originate at sites other than the pacemakers of the heart. A dysrhythmia is any disturbance in the normal rhythm of the heart.

9. **(b)** A bundle branch block widens the QRS complex because conduction is delayed on one side of the heart. Hypernatremia causes peaked T waves;

hypothermia causes J waves; and acute myocardial infarctions cause ST segment changes.

10. **(c)** All narrow QRS complexes have followed the normal conduction pathways *below* the level of the AV node and, therefore, must have originated above the ventricles—at the AV node or higher. Impulses generated above the ventricles *may* have wide QRS complexes if they have aberrant conduction. The narrow QRS complex *may* have originated in the SA node and traveled the internodal pathways to the AV node, but it may also have originated at the AV node and not traveled the internodal pathways.

11. **(c)** The maximum normal P-R interval is .20 seconds.

12. **(a)** The only "red flag" for sinus tachycardia is a rate above 100 beats per minute.

13. **(b)** The only "red flag" for sinus dysrhythmia is irregularity.

14. **(d)** Atrial fibrillation is the only dysrhythmia that is *irregularly* irregular. Second degree, Type I heart block and sinus rhythm with PVCs are *regularly* irregular due to beats being dropped from a regular underlying rhythm. Third degree heart block is often regular.

15. **(f)** b and d—Atrial fibrillation is irregular and has no discernible P waves. The baseline is wavy with fibrillatory (f) waves.

16. **(a)** Atrial fibrillation is not a reentry dysrhythmia. Supraventricular tachycardia, atrial flutter, and ventricular tachycardia are all reentry dysrhythmias.

17. **(d)** Atrial flutter has no P waves but has a sawtooth, or picket fence, baseline caused by flutter (F) waves.

18. **(f)** a and d—Supraventricular tachycardia is a very fast rhythm with no discernible P waves.

19. **(f)** a, c, and d—Ventricular tachycardia is a very fast rhythm with a wide QRS complex and no discernible P waves.

20. **(e)** The only "red flag" in first degree AV block is a P-R interval greater than .20 seconds.

21. **(f)** d and e—Third degree heart block is identified by lack of a consistent relationship between P waves and the QRS complexes (hence an inconsistent P-R interval).

22. **(c)** Since all PVCs originate within the ventricles, they always have wide QRS complexes. Supraventricular ectopic beats (PACs and PJCs) usually have narrow QRS complexes but can have wide QRS complexes if there is aberrant conduction.

23. **(c)** Most PVCs have a compensatory pause because the SA node does not sense the PVC and continues to fire, unaffected. Most PACs reset the SA node and, therefore, have a noncompensatory pause.

24. **(a)** The term that means PVCs every third beat is *trigeminy*. *Bigeminy* is PVCs every other beat. *Multifocal* PVCs are those that are morphologically different from each other. *Salvos* are more than one PVC in a row.

25. Answer: ventricular tachycardia.

Rationale:

Rate	180	
Regularity	Regular	
QRS Complex Do all of the QRS complexes look alike? What is the width of the QRS complex?	 Yes Wide	
P Waves Is there a P wave before every QRS complex? Is there a QRS after every P wave?	No P waves NA NA	
P-R Interval What is the P-R interval? Is the P-R interval constant?	 NA NA	

26. Answer: atrial fibrillation

Rationale:

Rate	90	
Regularity	Irregular	
QRS Complex Do all of the QRS complexes look alike? What is the width of the QRS complex?	 Yes Narrow	
P Waves Is there a P wave before every QRS complex? Is there a QRS after every P wave?	No P waves NA NA	
P-R Interval What is the P-R interval? Is the P-R interval constant?	 NA NA	

27. Answer: normal sinus rhythm

Rationale:

Rate	80
Regularity	Regular
QRS Complex	
Do all of the QRS complexes look alike?	Yes
What is the width of the QRS complex?	Narrow
P Waves	
Is there a P wave before every QRS complex?	Yes
Is there a QRS after every P wave?	Yes
P-R Interval	
What is the P-R interval?	0.16
Is the P-R interval constant?	Yes

28. Answer: ventricular fibrillation

Rationale:

Rate	0	⚑
Regularity	NA	
QRS Complex	No QRS complexes	⚑
Do all of the QRS complexes look alike?	NA	
What is the width of the QRS complex?	NA	
P Waves	No P waves	⚑
Is there a P wave before every QRS complex?	NA	
Is there a QRS after every P wave?	NA	
P-R Interval		
What is the P-R interval?	NA	
Is the P-R interval constant?	NA	

29. Answer: supraventricular tachycardia

Rationale:

Rate	180	⚑
Regularity	Regular	
QRS Complex		
Do all of the QRS complexes look alike?	Yes	
What is the width of the QRS complex?	Narrow	
P Waves	No P waves	⚑
Is there a P wave before every QRS complex?	NA	
Is there a QRS after every P wave?	NA	
P-R Interval		
What is the P-R interval?	NA	
Is the P-R interval constant?	NA	

30. Answer: normal sinus rhythm with PVCs

Rationale:

Rate	70	
Regularity	Irregular	⚑
QRS Complex		
Do all of the QRS complexes look alike?	No	⚑
What is the width of the QRS complex?	The QRS complexes from the underlying rhythm are narrow. The premature beats are wide.	⚑
P Waves		⚑
Is there a P wave before every QRS complex?	No	
Is there a QRS after every P wave?	Yes	
P-R Interval		
What is the P-R interval?	Not consistent	⚑
Is the P-R interval constant?	No	⚑

Chapter 6—Electrical Therapy

1. **(c)** Defibrillation (otherwise known as asynchronous cardioversion) is the treatment of choice for a heart in ventricular fibrillation. It is not used in bradycardic rates these patients mainly need drug therapy to control the rate. Defibrillation is not warranted in asystole confirmed in multiple leads. Atrial fibrillation is not life threatening in and of itself, so it is also controlled by drug therapy, and occasionally by synchronized cardioversion.

2. **(c)** Regarding successful cardioversion, the general rule is the earlier it is provided the greater the chance for successful conversion. After that, it is important to take steps necessary to reduce transthoracic resistance. In this instance, timing the countershock with end expiration will reduce the distance from the paddles to the heart, thereby allowing more energy to reach the myocardium. Since the delivery of electrical therapy is time-dependent in the unstable patient, it is often indicated prior to any drugs or other interventions.

3. **(a)** Asynchronous cardioversion is known more commonly as defibrillation. Synchronous cardioversion is the preferred treatment of tachydysrhythmias and starts with lower energy levels of 50–100 joules. Remember also that all forms of cardioversion need to use conductive medium. Lastly, the energy levels must be tailored for pediatrics when defibrillation is necessary.

4. **(d)** Defibrillation of asystolic hearts is actually damaging, because it can cause a profound increase in vagal tone. This may result in the elimination of any spontaneous initiation of an impulse.

5. **(c)** Defibrillation is carried out in a step-wise sequence of increasing energy levels. The initial stack of three shocks is administered at 200, 200–300, then 360 joules.

6. **(a)** Automated external defibrillators (AEDs) are indicated for cardiac arrest patients in ventricular fibrillation, regardless of the underlying cause of cardiac arrest. Since defibrillation is time-dependent, it should be applied as early as possible.

7. **(a)** The AED is preprogrammed to administer a stack of three shocks after the analysis mode has determined that VF is still present each time. This differs from the manual defibrillator, which the operator should use to administer only one countershock each time after the initial stack of three. The energy levels are the same for the two types of defibrillators, and studies have shown that the AED is just as effective as the manual defibrillator in terminating VF.

8. **(b)** Synchronized cardioversion delivers the energy during the R wave. This will avoid the T wave and reduce the likelihood of precipitating VF. The energy may be slightly delayed after depressing the buttons, since the synchronizing circuit needs to identify the R wave prior to discharge.

9. **(d)** Because of the synchronizing circuit of the defibrillator, it avoids the T wave and thus reduces the likelihood of causing ventricular fibrillation. Since it also uses a lower amount of energy initially, it can also reduce the chances of direct myocardial damage.

10. **(b)** Identification of the "hemodynamically unstable" patient is imperative to proper management. It is necessary to make the decision to treat the patient with electrical therapy rather than drugs initially. The four main indicators are chest pain, hypotension, pulmonary edema, and altered orientation. These findings identify the patient who is extremely unstable as a result of the tachycardia, and termination of the rhythm is imperative.

11. **(b)** A risk of synchronized cardioversion is the development of ventricular fibrillation. Should this occur during patient management, you should immediately turn off the synchronizing circuit and charge the machine to 200 joules to deliver an asynchronous countershock. Normal patient management would then occur, depending upon the resultant rhythm.

12. **(b)** AEDs are not used in pediatric cardiac arrests because they cannot deliver the small amounts of energy necessary for these patients. Additionally, since the primary cause of arrest in pediatric patients is respiratory in nature, ventricular fibrillation is an uncommon occurrence.

13. **(b)** This is a false statement for a number of reasons. Implantation of an automatic implantable cardioverter/defibrillator (AICD) does not preclude possible malfunction due to poor batteries, inaccurate sensing of the rhythm, or exhaustion of the preprogrammed number of countershocks. Therefore, you should administer electrical therapy, as appropriate, to these patients. Remember to avoid placing your paddle directly over the AICD mechanism.

14. **(a)** Transcutaneous pacing is the preferred treatment for symptomatic bradycardias. It is quick, doesn't interfere with other interventions, and is highly effective. It may also be considered for asystole and tachydysrhythmias, but these rhythms typically respond better to drugs first. Therefore, pacing in these individuals is indicated for problems that are refractory to other therapies.

15. **(e)** Not only is it important to assure that the pacer is creating a QRS complex, it is obviously necessary for the QRS complex to create a pulse (hence blood flow). The presence of a blood pressure is not a reliable indicator in the patient who already had a pressure before pacing, and the patient may complain of pain from the electrical impulse whether or not it captures.

Chapter 7—Pharmacological Therapy

1. **(c)** Any patient experiencing any type of cardiovascular emergency should initially receive oxygen to help prevent cellular hypoxia. Additional drug therapy (e.g., atropine, nitroglycerin) will be based upon the specific needs or management regimen of the cardiac abnormality. While a sodium chloride IV infusion is appropriate, it should be the 0.9% concentration, rather than the 0.45%, which is actually hypotonic.

2. **(b)** Atropine is known as a vagolytic (or parasympatholytic) drug. As such, it exerts its action by decreasing the degree of vagal stimulation on the heart by inhibiting the actions of acetylcholine (the neurotransmitter of the parasympathetic nervous system). If vagal tone is blocked, the degree of sympathetic tone present should have a more pronounced effect, causing an increase in the heart rate.

3. **(d)** Epinephrine is known to be a relatively equal stimulator of both beta and alpha sites. During cardiac arrest, however, there is profound vasodilation due to hypoxia and the failure of the vasomotor center. Epinephrine administration in this situation will help restore vascular constriction which will increase the systolic pressure generated with compressions. In turn, this will increase cerebral and coronary perfusion.

4. **(a)** Stimulation of alpha adrenergic receptor sites results in smooth muscle contraction. Since the vasculature is composed of smooth muscle, this results in vasoconstriction. Beta stimulation is either beneficial to the heart by increasing its activity (beta 1 stimulation), or promotes smooth muscle relaxation and peripheral vasodilation (beta 2 stimulation). Dopaminergic stimulation results in renal and mesenteric vasodilation. "Synaptic" is not a type of adrenergic stimulation.

5. **(a)** Atropine is a parasympatholytic drug. It will block the vagal tone and allow the sympathetic nervous system stimulation to have a pronounced effect. Since pupillary dilation is caused by sympathetic stimulation, it is an expected side effect of atropine administration. The other listed drugs do not affect the pupils.

6. **(d)** Lidocaine is a ventricular antidysrhythmic drug which exerts its beneficial action by diminishing the activity of ischemic or irritated ventricular ectopic sites. It achieves this by depressing retrograde conduction in re-entry pathways, as well as by diminishing the increased action potential in ischemic tissue, both of which cause dysrhythmias from disturbances in automaticity. Calcium channel blockers (verapamil and diltiazem, not lidocaine) are the types of drugs that interfere with calcium ion movement across cellular membranes.

7. **(d)** In clinical trials, lidocaine and bretylium have been shown to have similar ventricular antidysrhythmic properties. However, bretylium carries with it undesirable side effects that lidocaine does not, including initial increased myocardial workload and subsequent hypotension. Lidocaine has minimal side effects at normal doses. Therefore, lidocaine is preferred as the initial agent for ventricular dysrhythmias.

8. **(a)** Both verapamil and diltiazem are calcium channel blockers, substances that interfere with calcium ionic movement across cellular membranes. This in turn slows conduction velocity and repolarization times and also diminishes the force of muscle contraction. Typically these drugs are used to slow tachycardic rates or to reduce vascular resistance.

9. **(a)** Since verapamil and diltiazem both interfere with calcium movement during the depolarization of a myocardial cell, they slow conduction and prolong the repolarization phase. This makes them beneficial in paroxysmal supraventricular tachycardia (PSVT) rhythms where rate control will help restore the patient to a more normal cardiovascular status. This drug class would be detrimental for the patient with bradycardia, hypotension, or pulmonary edema; it would only aggravate these conditions due to its vasodilitory and cardiosuppressive effects.

10. **(c)** Procainamide's action is most similar to the action of lidocaine. Although their exact actions are slightly different, they are both useful drugs in the management of ventricular irritability. Adenosine and

verapamil are primarily for tachydysrhythmic rates, and atropine will increase myocardial activity by diminishing the degree of vagal tone.

11. **(d)** Adenosine is the preferred drug for patients with symptomatic tachydysrhythmias from Wolff-Parkinson-White (WPW) syndrome. Adenosine has a short half-life and does not increase the conduction velocity in the accessory pathway as verapamil does. It is well documented that a WPW patient who receives calcium channel blockers (verapamil or diltiazem) will most likely experience a deterioration of the dysrhythmia. Morphine is used as an analgesic or vasodilator and is not indicated to control tachydysrhythmic rates.

12. **(d)** Diltiazem is the most dissimilar since it is used to control atrial dysrhythmias or hypertension. Magnesium sulfate, lidocaine, and procainamide are used to control ventricular irritability and have no appreciable effect on controlling atrial dysrhythmias. Additionally, among antidysrhythmics, diltiazem is classified as a drug used for rate control while magnesium, lidocaine, and procainamide are classified as drugs used for rhythm control.

13. **(c)** Since epinephrine is both an alpha and a beta receptor site stimulator, it may have applications in a variety of cardiac emergencies. For example, it is beneficial in the cardiac arrest patient since it increases vascular tone by alpha stimulation, which in turn increases perfusion pressures. Additionally, being a beta stimulator as well, it has been used to help correct bradydysrhythmic rates unresponsive to more traditional therapy such as atropine and pacing. This drug would be detrimental in the treatment of hypertension or ventricular irritability since it would only potentiate the irregularity through sympathetic stimulation. Epinephrine is not used for chest pain.

14. **(d)** Sodium bicarbonate administration is indicated in the cardiac arrest patient only after more appropriate therapy (CPR, intubation, drug therapy, defibrillations, etc.) has failed to generate a response. Since the cardiac arrest patient will eventually develop metabolic acidosis, it is indicated only after 10–20 minutes of arrest management to help buffer the increased hydrogen ions. Hypotension is not affected by sodium bicarbonate. Respiratory acidosis is better controlled by increasing alveolar ventilation, and hyperkalemia (not hypokalemia) may be benefited by bicarbonate administration.

15. **(c)** Morphine is a narcotic agent which has the ability to reduce both preload and afterload by promoting vascular relaxation. This may be desirable to reduce intramyocardial wall tension and drop oxygen requirements in ischemic tissue during a myocardial infarction (MI). Dopamine is a sympathomimetic which can increase the blood pressure. Procainamide slows conduction velocity in the ventricles which may lead to hypotension, but not from vasodilation. Nitrous oxide is used primarily for its analgesic properties.

16. **(c)** Diltiazem is a calcium channel blocker which will slow the heart rate and reduce the force of contraction by hampering calcium movement across the cellular membrane during depolarization and contraction. These effects will depress the pumping action of the heart. Atropine, calcium chloride, and epinephrine will increase the pumping action by either increasing the heart rate by blocking vagal tone (atropine), or increasing the force of contraction by supplying additional calcium ions for muscle activity (calcium chloride), or stimulating beta receptor sites (epinephrine).

17. **(a)** At therapeutic doses, lidocaine (a ventricular antidysrhythmic) will have no depressive effect on the contractility of the myocardium. By contrast, diltiazem, a calcium channel blocker, will depress the activity of the heart by interfering with calcium movement. Propranolol and atenolol are both beta blockers, which inhibit the stimulation of beta 1 receptor sites, which in turn will also depress the activity of the myocardium.

18. **(b)** While all the choices are sympathomimetics with varying degrees of alpha stimulation, norepinephrine is primarily (>90%) an alpha site stimulator. Epinephrine is about a 50-50 stimulator of alpha and beta sites, and dopamine stimulates alpha sites primarily at higher infusion rates.

19. **(d)** By the same rationale as for Question 18, the sympathomimetic drugs (epinephrine, norepinephrine, and dopamine) are all vasoconstrictors. They will achieve this effect in varying degrees.

20. **(b)** Dobutamine, a synthetic sympathomimetic drug, has the ability to stimulate both beta and alpha sites according to a dose-dependent response. The major dissimilarity between dopamine and dobutamine is that dobutamine does not stimulate dopaminergic sites; however dobutamine, like dopamine, does increase renal output by increasing renal perfusion. Atropine is a parasympatholytic drug, isoproterenol is a sympathomimetic drug with primarily beta effects, and metaprolol is a beta blocker.

21. **(d)** Amrinone acts by (a) increasing stroke volume and (c) decreasing vascular resistance. Calcium channel blockers (verapamil and diltiazem) are the class of drugs that inhibit calcium ion movement.

22. **(a)** As discussed in the rationale for Question 21, amrinone increases stroke volume and reduces systemic vascular resistance. Both actions promote relief of increased pulmonary pressures and fluid backup in the lungs by increasing myocardial contraction and cardiac output. Amrinone does not affect heart rate and would exacerbate hypotension.

23. **(c)** Digitalis is a drug that slows conduction velocity through the AV node. Although this may interfere with cardiac output, it does not change vascular tone at therapeutic doses. The other drugs mentioned all promote vasodilation, which will diminish preload and systemic vascular resistance.

24. **(d)** Beta blockers decrease, not increase, blood pressure. They also decrease heart contractility and rate, so (a) and (c) are true. As a result, (b) is also true, since a myocardium not working as hard will require less oxygen.

25. **(d)** The problem in congestive heart failure (CHF) arises from a myocardium that cannot efficiently eject its given blood volume. As a result, increased venal hydrostatic pressure results in fluid back-up into the lungs and periphery. Administration of a drug that will increase venous capacitance (nitroglycerin or morphine) will reduce the preload. As a result, the volume of blood delivered to the left ventricle may be more manageable. Additionally, administering a diuretic such as furosemide (Lasix) will help remove excess fluid, also reducing preload. However, verapamil administration will decrease myocardial contractile force by slowing calcium movement, thus making the heart less effective and the CHF more severe.

26. **(b)** The initial dose of verapamil is 2.5 mg IVP. Oxygen is administered at rates from 1 to 15 lpm; the initial IV dose for adenosine is 6 mg, for diltiazem is 0.25 mg/kg.

27. **(b)** Oxygen is always the first drug administered to a patient with cardio-vascular instability. To ensure oxygenation, use a nonrebreather mask until blood gases dictate otherwise.

28. **(a)** The standard repeat (Class I) dose for epinephrine is at 1 mg. Higher doses should be considered if several attempts at the traditional dose fail.

29. **(d)** The maximum dose of atropine, when administered for unstable bradycardia, is 0.04 mg/kg. This is not the maximum dose for epineph-rine, isoproterenol, or dopamine, although all of these drugs may, at times, be used in the treatment of bradycardia. (See the bradycardia algorithm in Chapter 9.)

30. **(a)** Initially, lidocaine can be administered at a 1–1.5 mg/kg IV bolus. Bretylium is administered initially at 5–10 mg/kg, and procainamide at 20–30 mg/min.

31. **(c)** The initial dose of sodium bicarbonate is 1 milliequivalent per kilo-gram (1mEq/kg). Epinephrine and atropine can be initiated at 1 mg.

32. **(c)** When repeated during ventricular fibrillation, the proper dose of Bretylium is 10 mg/kg.

33. **(b)** The initial bolus range for verapamil is 2.5–5 mg IVP. Adenosine is 6 mg, and diltiazem is 0.25 mg/kg.

34. **(d)** None of the given drugs is administered at 10 mg initial bolus for PSVT. Adenosine is 6 mg, verapamil is 2.5–5 mg, and diltiazem is 0.25 mg/kg.

35. **(b)** 1 to 2 grams of magnesium sulfate should be diluted into the D_5W to achieve a therapeutic dose and concentration of the drug.

36. **(a)** Sodium bicarbonate is administered according to its unit of measure, milliequivalents per kilogram (mEq/kg). Lidocaine and bretylium are administered according to mg/kg.

37. **(a)** The initial dose of sodium bicarbonate is 1 mEq/kg.

38. **(d)** Morphine should be administered in 1–3-mg increments IV push, repeated at 5-minute intervals till the desired effect is achieved.

39. **(c)** The initial bolus should be at 8–16 mg/kg of a 10% solution. Responses (a) and (b) would be insufficient.

40. **(b)** The dose range for norepinephrine is 0.5–30 µg/kg per minute, initiat-ed at 0.5–1.0 µg/kg per minute, then titrated upwards to the desired effect. The traditional dose of epinephrine is 1 mg to a maximum high dose of 0.1 mg/kg every 3–5 minutes. The dose range for dopamine is 2–20 µg/kg per minute.

41. **(a)** The effects of dopamine are dose dependent. Lower doses of dopamine (2–5 µg/kg/min) allow for renal dopaminergic stimulation. Moderate doses (5–10 µg/kg/min) cause primarily cardiac beta effects, while high doses (10–20 µg/kg/min) cause alpha vasopressor responses.

42. **(d)** While similar in activity to dopamine, dobutamine does not actually stimulate dopaminergic receptor sites in the mesentery. Therefore, none of the listed doses is correct. Note, however, that dobutamine does increase renal output (as does dopamine), by increasing renal perfusion pressures.

43. **(c)** The maximum dose of dopamine is 20 µg/kg/min. Both epinephrine and isoproterenol infusion maximums are at 10 µg/min.

44. **(a)** The proper loading dose of amrinone is 0.75–1.0 mg/kg. A maintenance infusion is then warranted at 2–5 µg/kg/min, which can be titrated to a level of 10–15 µg/kg/min to maintain therapeutic blood levels.

45. **(c)** Digitalis can be given at a 10–15 µg/kg loading bolus. Bretylium is administered by mg/kg, and procainamide by mg/min (although the maximum procainamide dose is based on mg/kg).

46. **(b)** The proper sublingual dose of nitroglycerin is either 0.3 mg or 0.4 mg, repeated three times. As such, the maximum allowance would either be 0.9 mg or 1.2 mg respectively.

47. **(b)** When administering nitroglycerin via constant infusion, an appropriate range is 10–20 µg/min.

48. **(d)** Propranolol is administered initially at 1–3 mg IV push. Metoprolol and atenolol are administered initially at 5 mg. Esmolol is administered initially at 250-500 µg.

49. **(a)** Furosemide can be administered at 0.5–1 mg/kg initial dose, via IV push.

50. **(c)** Alteplase is the only thrombolytic typically administered in milligrams. The other three are measured according to units (U).

Chapter 8—Acute Coronary Syndromes

1. **(a)** Increased afterload with diminished preload would most effectively decrease cardiac output. In this situation, while the heart is receiving less blood to pump, it must also pump against a higher pressure. Therefore, the stroke volume will be lower with a subsequent diminishment in the overall cardiac output. Response (b) is incorrect because increased heart rate with unchanged stroke volume would increase cardiac output. Responses (c) and (d) are incorrect because decreased heart rate with increased stroke volume, or increased heart rate with decreased stroke volume will both amount to a cardiac output with no notable increase or decrease.

2. **(b)** The acute MI patient who presents with systemic hypotension and clear lung sounds is most likely suffering an infarction of the right ventricle. A right ventricular MI causes blood to back up in the periphery of the body and not the lungs. Consequently, the health care provider would note jugular vein distention (JVD), pedal edema, and clear lung sounds. Items (a) and (c) can be ruled out because the lungs are clear. In light of the systemic hypotension, a left ventricular infarction would most likely manifest itself with adventitious lung sounds as blood backs up into the lungs. Item (d) can be discounted because, essentially, the ventricles are responsible for the pumping of blood, and the presence of hypotension would seemingly indicate a problem with ventricular pumping.

3. **(c)** Anything that serves to decrease the heart's workload will also decrease its demand for oxygen. So a decrease in the pressure which the heart must pump against (afterload) will effectively decrease the workload and oxygen demand. An (a) increase in afterload, (b) increase in preload, and (d) increase in contractility all serve to increase the workload of the heart and ultimately raise its demand for oxygen.

4. **(d)** Administration of oxygen works to reverse ischemia and improve function to ischemic tissues of the heart. Item (a) is incorrect because infarction is irreversible. The cells are dead, and activity cannot be increased in the infarcted area. Item (b) is incorrect because reversal of damage to injured cells is very dependent upon time. While the delivery of oxygen can help reverse the damage to some injured cells, it will most likely not restore normal activity in all injured cells. Item (c) is incorrect because oxygen administration will not increase the workload of the heart but decrease it as the heart does not have to work as hard to deliver adequate quantities of oxygen to the body and itself.

5. **(a)** The patient suffering the greatest damage will be the patient with an occlusion of the left coronary artery. The higher the occlusion, the greater the number of cardiac cells effectively deprived of oxygenated blood. Items (b) and (c) are incorrect because the left descending and left circumflex coronary arteries are inferior to, and fed by, the left coronary artery. Item (d) is incorrect because the subclavian artery is not part of the coronary artery system.

6. **(c)** Aberrant conduction of electricity through ischemic and injured tissues is the correct choice. Electrical instability that produces dysrhythmias is the most common cause of death in the acute MI. Item (a) is incorrect, because myocardial wall rupture can occur but is rare in comparison to electrical dysrhythmias. Item (b) is incorrect because infarcted tissue does not conduct electricity at all. Item (d) is incorrect for reasons related to item (a): Aneurysms can lead to myocardial wall weakening and rupture but, like the ruptures themselves, are relatively rare.

7. **(b)** Of the choices given, the indication that most supports an evaluation of acute myocardial infarction would be the presence of ST elevation in two contiguous leads. Item (a) can be discounted. Remember, an acute MI can occur in the absence of chest pain, and chest pain can have a non-cardiac cause. Also eliminate (c) because hypotension can have many causes other than MI. Finally, (d) does not show elevation in two contiguous leads; therefore, it is not the most appropriate answer.

8. **(d)** The provider must suspect an anterior wall MI. The ST elevation in leads V_3 and V_4 and the shortness of breath, even without chest pain, would seemingly indicate myocardial ischemia occurring in the anterior wall. (a) COPD should be placed low on the diagnostic list because the ST elevation noted indicates myocardial ischemia. Item (b) is incorrect because the location of the ST elevation in leads V3 and V4 does not indicate right coronary artery occlusion (this would show up in leads II, III, and aVF). Rule out (c) by remembering that myocardial infarctions can occur without the symptom of chest pain.

9. **(a)** While the other choices would lead the practitioner to suspect an MI, confirmation of an acute MI is definitively made by the changing of serum enzymes and the development of pathologic Q waves.

10. **(c)** Based upon the presented information, it would appear that the patient is suffering from a right ventricular wall MI. In the presence of such an infarct, oxygen and aggressive fluid therapy should be initiated in an attempt to stretch the right ventricular wall for a greater contractile

response (Starling's Law). This will hopefully increase cardiac output and decrease the chance of severe hypotension and reduced coronary artery perfusion. While the administration of (a) oxygen is correct, it does not represent the best (most complete) choice of the listed items. Items (b) and (d) are incorrect because nitroglycerin is a vasodilator. Vasodilation should be strictly avoided, in that this will decrease the amount of fluid returning to the right sided pump and further worsen the situation. Also, beta blockers would serve to decrease the cardiac output by decreasing the heart rate and contractility and should therefore not be employed.

11. **(a)** Even though thrombolytic therapy dissolves the obstructing clot, the rough atherosclerotic surface upon which the clot formed is still intact. Upon this surface, blood can collect and form another thrombus. Therefore, the administration of heparin with its anticoagulatory effects would prove beneficial in preventing reformation and in keeping this artery open and patent. Heparin does nothing to (b) lower the preload or (c) decrease the myocardial workload. Also, heparin is an anticoagulant and exerts no action that serves to prevent (d) hemorrhage elsewhere in the body.

12. **(d)** In the presence of an acute MI, warning dysrhythmias such as PVCs usually occur in relation to an underlying abnormality. Therefore, correcting this abnormality will most likely abolish the dysrhythmia. To accomplish this, the provider must give interventions such as oxygen, nitroglycerin, morphine, etc. a first shot at correcting abnormalities such as hypoxemia or a high state of circulating catecholamines. If these interventions do not abolish the rhythm, only then should specific pharmacological therapy such as lidocaine be initiated. To serve these purposes, item (d) represents the most correct answer.

13. **(a)** Because this patient has a low pulse oximeter reading, high flow oxygen administered by a nonrebreather is prudent. Item (b) is incorrect in that 4 liters per minute is inappropriate for delivery by a simple face mask. Also, in light of this patient's presentation, low flow oxygen will not do the trick. For the same reason, item (c) is not applicable. Item (d) is also incorrect. Never withhold oxygen from a patient who needs it! Even in the setting of COPD, a patient with a myocardial infarction needs supplemental oxygen. In the short term emergent setting, the respiratory drive will most likely not be affected.

14. **(b)** Nitroglycerin causes vasodilation, which can effectively bottom out the blood pressure along with coronary artery perfusion. If cardiac arrest ensues secondary to the administration of nitroglycerin, relative hypovolemia is most likely the culprit. Therefore, fluid should be administered to bring the coronary perfusion back up to an acceptable level. (a) While placing the patient supine with the legs elevated is a good technique to return blood to the heart, defibrillation should not occur in the presence of PEA. (c) Dopamine may be indicated to raise the blood pressure, but not until fluid therapy is well underway to correct the underlying problem of hypovolemia. (d) CPR is appropriate but would be ineffective as the sole therapy since it would do nothing to correct the underlying problem.

15. **(b)** The female patient with the transmural MI and cerebrovascular accident (CVA, or stroke) 11 months ago would be the most eligible for

thrombolytic therapy. A CVA in general is only a relative contraindication for the administration of thrombolytic therapy. Only when the CVA has occurred within the last 6 months is thrombolytic therapy absolutely contraindicated. (a) Diastolic pressure of greater than 110 mmHg, (c) head trauma, and (d) pregnancy are all absolute contraindications to the use of thrombolytic therapy.

16. **(d)** Ventricular fibrillation occurs with the highest incidence within the first hour of infarction. The remaining dysrhythmias do occur, but with a lower incidence.

17. **(d)** The best choice for management would be item (d). In the cardiogenic shock patient, aggressive airway control via intubation should be attempted, followed by oxygen, dopamine, and norepinephrine if needed. (a) This item is not the best choice in that the airway is not protected and an adequate passage for oxygen is questionable. Items (b) and (c) utilize nitroglycerin, which will cause vasodilation and worsen shock.

18. **(b)** Oxygen is the most important drug in the management of the acute MI, because the infarcting heart is oxygen-starved. Oxygen is the drug that is administered first and is indicated in any type of myocardial infarction. While the other medications all play an active role in the treatment of the acute MI, none of them is as universally indicated as is oxygen.

19. **(a)** This patient appears to be in pulmonary edema. Oxygen is always the initial drug of choice for any cardiovascular emergency. As discussed, oxygen can help alleviate chest pain and assist in preventing further infarct that may well worsen the pulmonary edema. While the remaining choices all have application in pulmonary edema, they are not initial interventions, as oxygen is.

Chapter 9-Acute Stroke

1. **(d)** An acute ischemic stroke is caused by an interruption in cerebral blood flow that will result in necrosis of tissues distal to the site of interruption. A TIA is a temporary occlusion of a cerebral vessel caused usually by an embolus which the body dissolves, which is why the effects resolve within 24 hours. Finally, a massive acute stroke is capable of causing cardiac arrest, especially if it involves or encroaches on the brain stem.

2. **(a)** A TIA is sometimes referred to as a "warning stroke," because many victims of a TIA will eventually experience an actual acute ischemic stroke. Identifying a TIA is important so additional diagnostic tests can be performed to assess the likelihood of an acute ischemic stroke.

3. **(a)** An acute stroke or TIA can potentially occur in any portion of the brain or stem that receives blood flow. The presenting signs and symptoms will vary according to the area affected.

4. **(d)** On the Glasgow Coma Scale, 2 points would be awarded for eye opening to pain; 5 points for localizing the noxious stimulus and moving it away; and 2 points for incomprehensible sounds. The total would be 9.

5. **(a)** Reduction of ICP is an important component of acute stroke management. Without it, ICP may continue to rise and cause additional

complications, including death. Hyperventilation has been shown to initially reduce ICP by promoting cerebral vasoconstriction by eliminating excessive carbon dioxide. IV therapy and anticonvulsants have no action that will decrease ICP. Trendelenburg position may actually be harmful since it will inhibit venous drainage from the brain.

6. **(b)** An abrupt onset of a severe headache is most typical of a hemorrhagic etiology of stroke. An occlusive stroke, thrombotic or embolic, may present with a headache; however, the onset is usually not as abrupt and the intensity not as severe. The patient typically complains of a "pistol shot" headache or "the worst headache in my life".

7. **(c)** Cheyne-Stokes respirations usually occur when bilateral cerebral hemisphere damage has occurred due to a large hemorrhagic stroke. Central neurogenic hyperventilation results from early herniation or damage to the pons or lower midbrain. Apneustic breathing occurs from lower pontine lesions seen in basilar artery occlusion. Biot's breathing occurs when the medulla is compressed.

8. **(a)** The doll's eye maneuver provides an indication of the integrity of the brainstem. An indication of an intact brainstem is when the eyes remain focused upward when the head is turned; the eyes do not move in the direction of the turned head.

9. **(b)** Thrombolytics must be administered within 3 hours following the onset of signs and symptoms of an acute ischemic stroke.

10. **(c)** Aggressive hypertension management should be considered in the hemorrhagic patient when the blood pressure exceeds 220 mmHg systolic and 120 mmHg diastolic. The hypertension in an embolic and thrombotic stroke typically decreases within a couple of hours after the onset. Reducing the blood pressure in an occlusive stroke may subsequently reduce the cerebral perfusion pressure.

Chapter 10—Putting It All Together: The Algorithms

1. **(c)** A class IIb drug or intervention is one that is not well supported by scientific evidence, however is accepted as standard practice. It is considered possibly helpful and poses no harm to the patient. A Class I intervention is always indicated and is considered useful and effective. Class IIa interventions are considered useful and effective. A Class III intervention is not supported by scientific evidence and is considered inappropriate and possibly harmful.

2. **(a)** Bretylium can not be administered down the endotracheal tube. Lidocaine, epinephrine, atropine, and naloxone are all acceptable drugs that can be administered endotracheally.

3. **(d)** Epinephrine administered at 0.1 mg/kg IV push every 3 to 5 minutes is considered a high dose regimen. The intermediate dose is 2 to 5 mg IV push repeated every 3 to 5 minutes. The escalating dose is 1 mg, 3 mg, 5 mg IV push administered 3 minutes apart.

4. **(b)** Administration of sodium bicarbonate is a Class III (inappropriate and possibly harmful) recommendation in a patient suspected to be in

hypoxic lactic acidosis. The treatment of choice in this case is intubation and aggressive alveolar ventilation with supplemental oxygen. Sodium bicarbonate is a Class IIa recommendation in the tricyclic antidepressant overdose patient and a Class IIb recommendation in the patient in prolonged cardiac arrest who is intubated. It is assumed that a patient who is intubated has adequate alveolar ventilation. It is a Class I recommendation in the hyperkalemic patient.

5. **(a)** Immediately upon identifying ventricular fibrillation on the monitor, your priority is to defibrillate. Defibrillation terminates ventricular fibrillation. Medications, endotracheal intubation, chest compressions, and ventilation are all adjuncts to defibrillation and are contributing factors to how successful the defibrillation might be.

6. **(b)** Upon identification of asystole on the monitor, it is necessary to check another lead to ensure that the patient is still not in ventricular fibrillation. Ventricular fibrillation waves may be more prominent in one lead and very fine in another. Defibrillating the asystolic patient can unnecessarily lead to and increase in parasympathetic tone and worsen the resuscitation efforts. Chest decompression should be considered in a patient in pulseless electrical activity who is suspected of having a tension pneumothorax. Asystole is not an indication for sodium bicarbonate administration.

7. **(c)** The treatment of choice to terminate ventricular fibrillation is defibrillation. Defibrillation should not be delayed for any other interventions. You start at the energy level that was last effective in terminating the rhythm, which was 360 joules in this case. The lidocaine bolus and endotracheal intubation will follow the defibrillation.

8. **(a)** Bretylium is administered as a 5 mg/kg bolus repeated every 5 minutes at 10 mg/kg to a total maximum cumulative dose of 30 mg/kg.

9. **(b)** Immediately following the administration of a medication while treating the patient in ventricular fibrillation, you should perform CPR for 30 to 60 seconds then defibrillate at 360 joules. The sequence is drug–shock. The drug is thought to reach the core circulation after a 1 to 2 minute period; however, defibrillation should not be delayed for that period of time.

10. **(d)** Possible etiologies of pulseless electrical activity include hypovolemia, hypoxemia, hypoventilation, cardiac tamponade, tension pneumothorax, hypothermia, massive pulmonary embolism, drug overdose, hyperkalemia, acidosis, and massive myocardial infarction.

11. **(b)** Needle thoracentesis or needle decompression is the treatment of choice for the patient in pulseless electrical activity (PEA) secondary to a tension pneumothorax. Administration of medications, fluids, or transcutaneous pacing will not correct the etiology of the PEA.

12. **(c)** The total maximum cumulative dose of atropine in asystole is 0.04 mg/kg. Therefore, the total cumulative dose for a 70 kg patient would be 2.8 mg. A total maximum cumulative dose for the symptomatic bradycardic patient is 0.03 mg/kg.

13. **(a)** Provided the patient is not exhibiting any signs of having (nor is suspected of having) fluid overload, a fluid bolus of 250 to 500 ml of normal saline is recommended. If the fluid bolus does not reverse the hypotension, or the patient is potentially fluid-overloaded, the administration of

dopamine, norepinephrine and other inotropic and vasopressor agents would be considered a first choice intervention.

14. **(b)** Unless the patient is hypotensive or exhibiting signs and symptoms of hemodynamic instability, leave the rhythm untreated. Supraventricular tachycardias are commonly a result of high amounts of circulating catecholamines following resuscitation.

15. **(c)** Transcutaneous pacing is the intervention of choice in the third-degree heart block patient. Administration of lidocaine can abolish the ventricular rhythm and lead to ventricular asystole and subsequent cardiac arrest. Atropine has little effect on the ventricle; thus it is of no real value in the third-degree block. An epinephrine infusion would follow unsuccessful transcutaneous pacing and dopamine infusion.

16. **(c)** If the external pacer fails to capture, it is necessary to proceed to other pharmacologic interventions. (You will have administered atropine before attempting the pacing.) The next drug of choice is a dopamine infusion beginning at 5 ug/kg/minute and titrating it to the heart rate and blood pressure. If the dopamine fails to work, initiate an epinephrine infusion at 2 to 10 ug/minute.

17. **(b)** The initial treatment of choice for a stable supraventricular tachycardia (SVT) patient is vagal maneuvers. If these fail to convert the rhythm, then adenosine should be administered, followed by verapamil. If still no conversion occurs, consider the administration of digoxin, beta blockers, diltiazem, and synchronized cardioversion.

18. **(a)** This patient obviously deteriorated from a stable SVT to an unstable SVT. The treatment of choice for the unstable SVT patient is synchronized cardioversion. You can consider sedation prior to cardioverting.

19. **(b)** Management of torsades de pointes is significantly different than that of other ventricular type rhythms. The treatment of choice for the patient in torsades de pointes is overdrive electrical pacing. The second-line treatment of choice is administration of magnesium sulfate at 1 to 2 grams IV. Isoproterenol can be used to overdrive the ventricular rate in an attempt to abolish the dysrhythmia. Ventricular antiarrhythmic agents are not a standard treatment for torsades de pointes.

20. **(c)** Since the total cumulative bolus dose of lidocaine was 2.0 mg/kg, the infusion should be set at 3 mg/minute. If the total bolus dose was 1 mg/kg, the infusion is set at 2 mg/minute. A total cumulative bolus dose of 3 mg/kg will require an infusion rate of 4 mg/minute.

Chapter 11—Case Studies: Application Exercises

1. **(a)** The first step upon identifying an unconscious patient is to assure that you have help on the way. Research has indicated that if you start patient care, you rarely stop to get help. Assuring that help is on the way takes precedence over any clinical actions. If you are in a hospital situation, be sure to alert the code team. If you are in an out-of-hospital situation, call the local emergency access number.

2. **(d)** The best, easiest, safest, and fastest method of opening the airway in the non-trauma patient is the head tilt, chin lift. An oropharyngeal airway and endotracheal tube are used to manage the airway after the initial techniques are employed. The chin lift without head tilt is generally used to open the airway in trauma patients.

3. **(c)** The first defibrillatory shock must be delivered within 90 seconds of the arrival of an AED.

4. **(d)** The definitive treatment for any patient in ventricular fibrillation is defibrillation. The possibility of successful defibrillation is very time dependent and should be done immediately. Defibrillation takes precedence over getting help, performing CPR, airway management, and ventilation.

5. **(b)** You should immediately confirm tube placement by auscultating the chest and epigastrium after inflation of the endotracheal tube cuff. Pulse oximetry is an unreliable indication of proper tube placement in the patient in cardiac arrest and takes a few minutes to show a change. After confirmation of tube placement, secure the tube and insert a bite block.

6. **(c)** It takes 30–60 seconds for a medication to reach the central circulation during CPR. You should follow any medication administration by a fluid bolus and elevation of the extremity.

7. **(d)** Adenosine is a supraventricular antidysrhythmic and is not indicated in the treatment of ventricular fibrillation.

8. **(a)** Epinephrine is given in any case of cardiac arrest to increase myocardial and cerebral blood flow during CPR. Lidocaine is indicated for ventricular fibrillation and pulseless ventricular tachycardia. Atropine is indicated for bradycardia and/or asystolic rhythms. Sodium bicarbonate is indicated for the specific treatment of hyperkalemia, or profound metabolic acidosis.

9. **(d)** Cardiac tamponade is a complication of chest trauma. The main signs are distended neck veins, muffled heart tones, bilaterally equal lung sounds, hypotension, and decreased QRS amplitude.

10. **(b)** Asystole typically represents the endpoint of resuscitation efforts. The survival rate of patients in asystole is very low. Continued resuscitation of patients in asystole who do not respond to epinephrine and pacing is considered futile. High dose epinephrine, sodium bicarbonate, and fluid resuscitation are not indicated in the routine management of asystolic patients unless you suspect specific etiologies.

11. **(c)** The initial supplemental oxygen therapy for the suspected acute MI patient is guided by the level of respiratory distress. Patients in no or minor distress receive low flow oxygen by nasal cannula; patients in moderate respiratory distress should receive medium flow oxygen; and patients in severe respiratory distress should receive high flow oxygen. Following the initial supplemental oxygen therapy, blood gasses, and pulse oximetry are used to assist in titrating oxygen needs in the MI patient.

12. **(a)** The most important factor in decreasing morbidity and mortality from myocardial infarction is the time to reperfusion, not the method of reperfusion.

13. **(c)** The external pacer should be set at 80 beats per minute and the output gradually increased until mechanical capture is accomplished.

14. **(d)** The treatment for any unstable tachycardia is immediate, synchronized cardioversion. The use of pharmacological therapy is *not* initially indicated in unstable patients.

15. **(b)** Verapamil is the second line medication for the treatment of supraventricular tachydysrythmias. Lidocaine, procainamide, and bretylium are ventricular antidysrythmics.

Chapter 12—Special Resuscitation Situations

1. **(e)** A massive hemorrhage can precipitate cardiac arrest from a loss of circulating volume; this in turn reduces perfusion pressures necessary for organ (including the brain and heart) function. Spinal cord injury above C-5 can affect the phrenic nerve which provides innervation of the diaphragm. This paralysis causes hypoxia which can lead to arrest. Tamponade causes a mechanical pressure on the heart which inhibits diastolic filling. Since the heart can only pump as much as it receives, this reduction can also cause arrest. All of these mentioned injures are also common causes of PEA.

2. **(a)** Spinal immobilization is mandatory for any trauma patient until x-rays prove otherwise. Intubation is also necessary but may be achieved orotracheally. IV therapy should be with a volume expander (normal saline or Ringer's lactate), and oxygen therapy should be maximized at 15 liters per minute.

3. **(b)** 20 ml/kg is the proper bolus amount for fluid replacement. This can be repeated as appropriate; just ensure you do not accidentally cause fluid overload or pulmonary edema.

4. **(b)** It is important to recognize patients for whom full resuscitative measures would be futile in order to avoid an unwarranted waste of health care resources. In arrest patients with full body burns, resuscitation is almost always futile. The other listed causes of arrest may be reversible with appropriate treatment.

5. **(d)** While there are many changes in the pregnant female's body, the cardiovascular changes are most likely to interfere with shock recognition. Early signs of shock include tachypnea and tachycardia, and these may go unrecognized since those findings would be expected in the pregnant female. The care provider has to rely heavily on the mechanism of injury to guide initial treatment.

6. **(d)** While all the conditions listed can potentially cause arrest, maternal cardiac arrest is the number one cause of fetal death. Thus, treatment should be aggressive in restoring and maintaining the mother's cardiovascular hemodynamics. Remember that two lives are at risk.

7. **(c)** While lying supine, the gravid uterus puts excessive pressure on the inferior vena cava. Since this can markedly drop cardiac preload, hypotension ensues. Treatment includes displacement of the uterus to the left by rolling the patient to the left 15–20 degrees.

8. **(d)** The treatment of a maternal cardiac arrest will follow the same algorithms and drug dosages as the non-pregnant cardiac arrest. This includes the provision of electrical therapy when appropriate.

9. **(b)** Often, immediately after a lightning strike, the patient is found to be apneic and asystolic. However, the heart recovers more quickly and may restore cardiac activity in the absence of spontaneous respirations. For these patients, then, positive pressure ventilation (with or without intubation) is imperative. The patient will have a better chance of survival if the blood stays oxygenated while the heart stabilizes itself. Failing to do so will lead to a hypoxic arrest.

10. **(c)** The provision of electrical therapy in the victims of a lightning strike is the same as in the normal arrest. The initial defibrillation will start out at 200 joules and progress by steps to 360 joules.

11. **(a)** All of the injuries listed are possible as a result of a lightning strike. But respiratory arrest from brain stem depression is the most likely cause of death. Persistent ventricular fibrillation is most likely to be a result of the hypoxia that results from apnea. Trauma and burns are also possible from the strike but usually do not cause as extensive damage as once thought.

12. **(a)** Since the electricity of a lightning strike can cause violent muscular contractions or cause the patient to be thrown, spinal immobilization is a good preventative measure till x-rays can rule out associated fractures or spinal injury.

13. **(b)** As a response to hypothermia, the body will begin to slow down its cardiac, respiratory, and metabolic activity. Peripheral vasoconstriction occurs to preserve body heat and to assist in redirecting blood to vital organs.

14. **(a)** As in any patient care situation, the primary concern is your personal safety. An injured health care provider is of no use to the patient and becomes a burden to the other care providers by being added to the injured/sick list. In any rescue or patient contact, only proceed if you are adequately prepared and equipped to help—without falling victim to the same problem as the patient.

15. **(a)** Because the hypothermic patient has sluggish perfusion to the extremities, movement of IV drugs to the core circulation may be delayed and they may accumulate to toxic levels in the extremities before being "dumped" on the heart as rewarming begins. For this reason, it is recommended that drug administration be delayed until internal rewarming increases the core temperature above 30°C. Because the heart is less responsive to the medications when cold, with a core temp > 30°C, the standard repeat times for the medications should be lengthened. Although a hypothermic heart is less responsive to drugs, the drugs do not become "ineffective." They should not be doubled, since increasing the dosage does not make them "more effective."

16. **(a)** Any patient in cardiac arrest should be intubated with an endotrachael tube to secure and control the airway. There is no specific contraindication to intubation for the cardiac arrest patient. Defibrillation, antidote treatment, and NG tube placement are not used on *all* toxicologic arrest patients since those treatments are administered only when appropriate. For example, if the arrested patient is never in V-fib, defibrillation should not be performed.

17. **(e)** Poison Control Centers are a valuable asset to the management of any poisoning or overdose. They have a constantly updated databank which holds the current treatment plans and specific antidotes when appropriate. They also provide tracking of current trends and perform follow-up on patients during recovery. They are accessible in every large community 24 hours a day, usually by a toll free number.

Chapter 13—Special Treatment Considerations

1. **(d)** The postresuscitation period following cardiac arrest refers to the state of cerebral hypoperfusion that occurs despite the return of spontaneous cardiac output. Regardless of the varied causes, attention needs to be directed to those factors that help limit the postresuscitation syndrome initially and, consequently, influence survivability. The prefix *post-*, meaning "afterward," is your clue that this is not a syndrome that precedes cardiac arrest; it is not related to chest pain. The syndrome occurs whether or not the patient is otherwise hypotensive. Although it may precipitate seizures, this syndrome is not characterized by seizures.

2. **(e)**—a, b, and c are all correct. The goal in limiting the effects of the postresuscitation syndrome is to improve cerebral blood flow and to maintain a balance between the brain's demand for oxygenated blood and the available supply. The necessary steps include glucose regulation to avoid the detrimental effects of hyperglycemia; hyperventilation to help reduce cerebral edema after the arrest and improve oxygenation of the brain cells; and temperature regulation to prevent either hyperthermia (which increases metabolic activity) or hypothermia (which reduces metabolic demand but increases blood viscosity).

3. **(b)** Should a seizure occur during the fragile postresuscitation period, it needs to be terminated, since it can greatly increase cerebral blood flow demands due to the increased metabolic activity. In this instance, seizures are best treated by administering diazepam (Valium) or barbiturates. However, since seizures are not a common occurrence during this phase, automatic prophylactic therapy is not warranted. Lastly, a decision to withhold anticonvulsant medication because of possible ill effects is also not warranted since the seizure is capable of precipitating a cardiac arrest.

4. **(a)** Arterial cannulation is the method of choice when repeated assessments are needed from arterial blood. Arterial puncture is simply the process of passing a needle into the artery to obtain just one sampling. The disadvantage to this is the necessity of making repeated sticks for further sampling. The saphenous vessel is a vein and cannot be used to monitor arterial pressure. If intravascular access is warranted, initiation of an IV through a peripheral vessel is preferred. Finally, pulmonary artery cannulation is actually performed to assess deoxygenated venous blood.

5. **(d)** Adjuncts for artificial circulation assist in the improvement of cardiac output and core perfusion during cardiac arrest, provided the adjuncts are used correctly. The net effects in using one of these devices are the elimination of rescuer fatigue (which also means more personnel available for other tasks) and the reduction in inappropriate compressions due to rescuer error.

In conjunction, these considerations stand to improve the hemodynamics of the cardiac output during compressions.

6. **(a)** The safest and most reliable method of assessing the adequacy of compressions now recommended for clinical practice is palpating the carotid pulse. The femoral pulse should be avoided since you may actually feel venous backflow caused by increased intrathoracic pressure from the chest compressions, rather than arterial flow. Monitoring end tidal CO_2 readings shows promise as a means of assessing CPR effectiveness, but research on its usefulness in clinical practice is still being conducted. And lastly, pulse oximetry is usually not an option for a person in cardiac arrest since the perfusion pressures generated during CPR are not great enough to perfuse the distal capillary beds of the extremities.

7. **(b)** False. In light of the increasing understanding of the causes and effects of cardiac arrest and postresuscitation syndrome, more and more therapeutic modalities to improve patient outcome are being tested. So far, technologies and methods have been developed to help improve brain perfusion and *prevent* some of the ill effects of postresuscitation syndrome. Unfortunately, however, no drug has yet been identified as capable of *reversing* postresuscitation brain damage.

Index

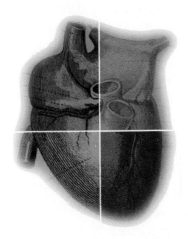

A

Aberrant conduction, 111

Acidosis, 292

Acute ischemic stroke (*see* stroke)

Acute myocardial infarction (acute coronary syndromes) (*see* Myocardial: infarction)

Adenosine, 196-7, 305

Advanced Cardiac Life Support, 5

Advance directives, 8-9

Aerobic metabolism, 168

Afterload, 225

Agonal breathing, 122

Airway:
    combitube, 24, 35, 68
    esophageal gastric tube, 35
    esophageal obturator, 35, 63-68
    nasopharyngeal, 37, 41-43, 265
    obstruction, 4, 33
    opening the, 18-19
    oropharyngeal, 20, 37, 38-41, 265
    pharyngeotracheal lumen, 24, 35, 68

Algorithm, 284
    acute myocardial infarction, 240
    asystole, 295
    automated external defibrillation, 152
    bradycardia, 300
    electrical (synchronized) cardioversion, 154
    hypotension/shock/acute pulmonary edema, 253
    hypothermia, 357
    suspected stroke, 279
    pulseless electrical activity algorithm, 293
    tachycardia, 304
    universal, 287
    ventricular fibrillation /pulseless ventricular tachycardia, 289

Alteplase, 210

Amrinone, 180-81

Anaerobic metabolism, 168

Analgesics, 203, 247

Anisteplase, 210

Antecubital vein, 26, 97

Antianginals, 203

Anticholinergic syndrome, 194

Anticipation, 7

Anticoagulant, 278, 367

Antidysrhythmics, 183

Antihypertensives, 207

Apneustic breathing, 266

Arrhythmia, 116 (*see also* dysrhythmia)

Arterial blood gasses, 170

Arterial puncture, 369

Arytenoid cartilage, 55

Aseptic technique, 95

Aspiration, 21

Aspirin, 244, 275

Asynchronous cardioversion, 141

Asystole, 122, 148
    algorithm, 295

Atenolol, 183

Atherosclerosis, 228

Atherosclerotic plaque, 228

Atrial fibrillation, 116, 302, 303, 305

Atrial flutter, 119, 302, 303, 305

Atrioventricular node, 104, 122

Atropine, 27, 192-96, 286, 292, 294, 301

Automated external defibrillator, 5, 17, 22, 148-52
    algorithm, 152
    components, 148-49
    fully automated, 149
    maintenance, 156
    use in pediatric patients, 155
    procedure, 149-51
    semi automated, 149

Automatic implantable cardioverter/defibrillator, 156

Automatic transport ventilator, 81-82

Automaticity, 104

Autonomic nervous system, 104

AV block:
    first degree, 122
    second degree, type I, 127
    second degree, type II, 127, 301
    third degree, 124, 301

B

Bag-valve-mask ventilation, 19, 25

Bag-valve devices, 76-80

Barbiturate, 277

Basic Cardiac Life Support (BCLS), 5

Benzodiazepine, 277

Beta blockers, 182-83, 208, 247-48
    overdose, 292
    in atrial fibrillation/flutter, 305

Biots breathing, 266

Body substance isolation precautions, 24

Bradyasystolic rhythms, 292

Bradycardia, 108, 233, 254
    absolute, 299, 301
    algorithm, 300
    in AMI, 250-51
    postresuscitation, 296, 298
    relative, 299, 301

Brain attack, 261, 262, 271

Breathing, 19-21, 25
    agonal, 122
    apneustic, 266
    Biots, 266
    central neurogenic hyperventilation, 266
    Cheyne-Stokes, 266

Bretylium Tosylate, 189-91, 290, 291, 306

Bundle branch block, 111

C

Calcium channel blockers, 197-200
    overdose, 292
    in atrial fibrillation/flutter, 305

Calcium chloride, 213-15

Cannulation
    arterial, 368
    intravenous, 94
    pulmonary artery, 368

Capnometry, 371

Cardiac output, 225-26

Cardiac pacing, 157-63
    in asystole, 294
    complications, 160
    components, 157
    contraindications, 160
    equipment, 158-59
    indications, 158-59
    in Torsades de Pointes, 307

Cardiac tamponade, 292

Cardiogenic shock, 254-55

Cardiopulmonary bypass, 370

Cardiopulmonary resuscitation, 16-18, 142, 156, 285
    active compression-decompression, 370
    chest compressions, 21
    high frequency, 369
    interposed abdominal compressions, 369
    simultaneous ventilation-compression, 369
    vest, 370

Cardioversion, 303, 305
    synchronous, 306
    unsynchronous, 306

Carotid sinus massage, 303

Central neurogenic hyperventilation, 266

Cerebral blood flow, 275, 277, 365

Cerebral perfusion, 297

Cerebral resuscitation, 3, 365-68

Cerebral vascular accident, 262
    (*see also* Stroke)

Cesarean section, 352, 353

Chain of survival, 6

Chest compressions, 21 (*see also* Cardiopulmonary resuscitation)

Chest pain, 230

Chest x-ray, 25, 56, 242

Cheyne-Stokes respiratory pattern, 266

Chin-lift maneuver, 19, 58

Chronotropic effects, 171

Circulation, 21, 26-27

Combitube, 24, 68

Compensatory pause, 132

Competence, 8

Conduction blocks, 251-52 (*see also* AV blocks)

Contractility, 225

Continuum of care, 5

Corniculate cartilage, 55

Coronary artery disease, 230

CPR *see* Cardiopulmonary resuscitation

CPR board, 17

Crash cart, 16, 20

Cricoid pressure, 21, 24-25, 50, 55, 58, 76, 82 (*see also* Sellick's maneuver)

Cricothyrotomy, 35, 73-74
    needle, 35
    surgical, 33, 73

Critique, 8

Crowing, 34

Cuneiform cartilage, 55

Cyanosis, central, 35

D

Defibrillator:
    automated, 5, 17, 22

Defibrillator (*continued*)
  components, 142-43
  maintenance, 156
  manual, 22
  semi-automated, 22

Defibrillation, 5, 21-23, 141-48, 286, 290
  in asystole, 294
  in hypothermia, 155
  implanted automatic, 290
  procedure, 146-47

Dentures, 19

Depolarization, 104-5

Dextrose, 273

Diazepam, 278

Differential diagnosis, 14, 28

Digital intubation, 59-61

Digitalis glycosides, 200-202
  overdose, 292

Diltiazem, 197-200

Diuretics, 206, 255

Dobutamine, 179-80

Do-not-attempt-resuscitation, 9

Do-not-resuscitate, 9

Dopamine, 177-79, 202, 301

Doppler ultrasound, 292, 371

Drug overdose, 292, 294

Durable power of attorney, 9

Dysrhythmias, 116
  warning, 249

E

ECG *see* electrocardiogram

Ectopic beats, 127

Edema, 231

Electrical therapy, 141

Electrocardiogram, 103, 105-7
  leads, 105-6
  monitor, 23, 27, 241-42
  12 lead, 235

Electrode:
  size, 143-44
  position, 144

Electrocution, 294

Electro-mechanical dissociation, 292

Electrophysiology, 103-5

Emergency Medical Technician-Basic, 5

End-tidal carbon dioxide, 25, 56, 273

Endotracheal intubation, 23, 24-25, 35, 44-59
  advantages, 44
  complications, 57
  digital, 59-61
  equipment, 45-51
  evaluating the patient, 45
  indications, 44
  nasal, 58
  oral technique, 51-57
  transillumination, 61-63

Endotracheal tube, 24, 48

Endotracheal tube aspirator, 25

Entry, 7

Epiglottis, 35, 47, 55

Epinephrine, 27, 171-74, 202, 290, 301
  intermediate dose, 286
  escalating dose, 286
  high dose, 286

Escape beats, 127

Esmolol, 183

Esophageal detector, 56

Esophageal gastric tube airway, 35, 66

Esophageal obturator airway, 35, 63-66

F

Fibrillation, 116

Fibrillatory dysrhythmias, 116

Fibrillatory waves, 116

Face mask, 87

Face mask with reservoir, 87

Family notification, 8

Femoral pulses, 371

First degree AV block, 122

Flow-restricted oxygen-powered ventilation device:
    complications, 81
    features, 80
    manually triggered, 80
    technique, 81

Flutter waves, 119

Furosemide, 206-7, 255

G

Gag reflex, 34, 37

Gastric distention, 20-21, 24, 43, 78

Glascow Coma Scale, 267

Glossoepiglottic ligament, 47

Glottic opening, 47, 55

Glucose, 367

Gurgling, 34

H

Head-tilt, chin-lift, 19, 33, 35-36, 37, 76

Heart:
    as a pump, 223-26
    cardiac output, 225-26
    left-side pump, 224-25
    right-side pump, 224

Heparin, 246-47, 278

Hollow needles, 96

Hyperkalemia, 286, 292, 307

Hypertension, 252, 266, 275-76

Hyperventilation, 265, 274, 277, 292

Hypoperfusion, 6

Hypotension, 252, 267
    algorithm, 253
    postresuscitation, 296, 297

Hypothermia, 155, 292, 294, 354-58

Hypoventilation, 292, 366

Hypovolemia, 292

Hypoxia, 6, 292

Hypoxic drive, 170

I

Idioventricular rhythms, 292

Inotropic effects, 171

Infection control precautions, 15

Internodal pathways, 104

Intra-aortic balloon pump, 255

Intracerebral hemorrhage, 263

Intracranial pressure, 277

Intravenous:
    access, 241
    cannulas, 96
    cannulation, 94
    line, 26, 94
        central, 94-95
        peripheral, 94-95, 96-99

Isoproterenol, 176-77, 202, 301, 307

J

Jaw thrust, 19, 35-37, 58, 76

Joules, 143

Jugular vein, 97, 99

L

Labetalol, 276

Laryngeal edema, 35

Laryngoscope, 46
    blade, 24, 46-47
    handle, 24

Laryngoscopy, 21, 35

Left-side pump, 224-25

Level of responsiveness, 15

Lidocaine, 27, 184-87, 277, 290, 291, 301, 305, 306

Lighted stylet, 61-63

Lightening strikes 353-54

Living will, 8-9

Lorazepam, 278

Lung sounds, 255

M

Magnesium sulfate, 191-92, 248, 291, 307

Mannitol, 278

Manual in-line stabilization, 79

McGill forceps, 21, 35, 50

Metabolic acidosis, 367

Metaprolol, 183

Morphine sulfate, 203-4, 243-44, 255

Mouth-to-mask ventilation, 19, 75
  advantage, 75
  technique, 76

Mouth-to-mouth ventilation, 74

Mouth-to-nose ventilation, 74

Myocardial:
  infarction, 222-23, 226, 292
    algorithm, 240
    assessment, 231-36
    management, 237-56
    pathophysiology, 226-31
    right ventricular, 301
    transmural, 228
    silent, 231
    subendocardial, 228-29
    and ventricular dysrhythmias, 250
  injury, 226-27
  ischemia, 226-27
  working cells, 105

N

Naloxone (Narcan), 27, 244, 273

Nasal cannula, 85-86

Nasal intubation, 58

Nasopharyngeal airway, 37, 41-43, 78, 265
  complications, 43
  indications, 41
  sizing, 41
  technique for insertion, 42

Near drowning, 354-55

Nimodipine, 272

Nitroglycerin, 205-6, 208, 242-43, 255
  patches, 290

Nitroprusside, 255

No-CPR order, 9

Non-compensatory pause, 130

Norcuron, 277

Norepinephrine, 174-75

Normal saline, 26

Normal sinus rhythm, 111

O

Oropharyngeal airway, 20, 37, 38-41, 78, 265
  complications, 40-41
  indications, 38
  sizing, 38
  technique for insertion, 39

Oxygen, 85, 168, 170, 241

P

P-wave, 107, 109, 111

Pacemaker, 290

Pacemaker cells, 104

Pancuronium, 277

Parasympatholytic, 193

Paroxysmal supraventricular tachycardia, 119, 305

Pathologic Q-Waves, 235

Pentobarbital, 278

Percutaneous transluminal coronary angioplasty, 248-49, 255

Pericardiocentesis, 292, 351

Pharyngeotracheal-lumen airway, 24, 35, 67

Phased-response approach, 7

Phenobarbital, 278

Phenytoin, 278

Phone first, 16, 22

Pneumothorax, 25, 81

Pocket mask, 20, 25

Poison control centers, 358

Positive end-expiratory pressure, 366

Postresuscitation management, 296-98

P-R interval, 109, 111

Precordial thump, 288

Pregnancy, 351-53

Preliminary (presurvey) actions, 13-18

Preload, 225

Premature atrial contractions, 130

Premature beats, 127

Premature junctional contractions, 130

Premature ventricular contractions, 130-31, 233
   in AMI, 249-50
   bigeminy, 134
   couplets, 133
   multi focal, 133
   postresuscitation, 298
   salvos, 133
   trigeminy, 134
   unifocal, 133

Primary survey, 13, 18

Pseudo-EMD, 292

Procainamide, 187-89, 291, 305, 306

Propanolol, 183

Pulmonary embolism, 292

Pulseless electrical activity, 292-94
   algorithm, 293

Purkinje fibers, 104

Q

QRS complex, 107, 109-10
   narrow, 110
   wide, 111, 122

Quick look, 290

R

Rate, 108-9

Rate Control, 192-202

Recovery position, 286

Reentry dysrhythmias, 119

Regularity, 109-10

Regurgitation, 21

Resuscitation, 7

Rhythm control, 184-92

Right-side pump, 224

S

Secondary survey, 13, 23

Second degree AV block:
   Type I, 127
   Type II, 127, 301

Sedation, 277, 367

Seizure, 278, 367

Sellick's maneuver, 50, 277 (*see also* Cricoid pressure)

Semi-automated external defibrillation, 22

Sinoatrial node, 104

Sinus bradycardia, 114

Sinus dysrhythmias, 115

Sinus tachycardia, 113

Smart defibrillator, 148

Sniffing position, 54, 55

Snoring, 34

Sodium bicarbonate, 211-13, 286

Sodium nitroprusside, 207-8

Sodium pentothal, 277

Sonorous respiration, 34

Spinal immobilization, 350, 356

ST segment depression, 235

ST segment elevation, 235

Standby pacing, 160

Starling's law, 225, 255, 301

Streptokinase, 211

Stridor, 35

Stroke:
  acute ischemic, 262-65
  initial assessment, 265-70
    differential diagnosis,
      269-72
  Treatment, 271-79

Stroke volume, 225

Stylet, 24, 49

Subarachnoid hemorrhage, 262

Succinylcholine, 277

Suction, 24
  oropharyngeal, 83
  tracheobronchial, 83-85

Sudden cardiac death, 142

Supine hypotension syndrome,
  352

Supraventricular tachycardia, 302

Survey:
  primary, 13, 18
  secondary, 13, 23

Synchronized cardioversion,
  153-55
  algorithm, 154
  indications, 153
  procedures, 153-55

Sympatholytics, 181-82

Sympathomimetic, 171, 202

T

T-wave, 107

Tachycardia, 108, 254
  algorithm, 304
  in AMI, 251
  narrow complex, 302
  postresuscitation, 296, 298
  wide complex, 302

Team leader, 23, 316

Tension pneumothorax, 292

Therapeutic classifications, 285

Thiamine, 273

Third degree AV block, 124, 301
  (*see also* AV block)

Thrombolytics, 208-11, 223,
  244-46

Thrombus, 228

Ticlodipine, 275

Tongue, 35

Torsades de Pointes, 306

Tracheostomy, 74

Transcutaneous pacing, 157-59,
  301

Transfer, 8

Transient ischemic attack (TIA),
  262-65 (*see also* Stroke)

Transillumination intubation,
  61-63

Transtracheal catheter ventilation,
  35, 71-72

Traumatic cardiac arrest, 348-51

Trendelenburg position, 99, 305

Tricyclic antidepressants, 286,
  358
  overdose, 292

U

Universal algorithm, 286-88

Urokinase, 211

V

Vagal maneuvers, 305

Vallecula, 47

Veins:
   antecubital, 26, 97
   dorsal hand, 97
   forearm, 97
   jugular, 97, 99
   saphenous, 97
   wrist, 97

Ventilation:
   automatic transport
      ventilator, 81-82
   bag-valve-device, 76-78
   mouth-to-mask, 19, 75-76
   mouth-to-mouth, 74
   mouth-to-nose, 74

Ventricular escape rhythms, 292

Ventricular failure, 233, 254,
   255

Ventricular fibrillation, 21, 116,
   118, 141, 142, 229, 288-91
   algorithm, 289

   primary, 250
   secondary, 250

Ventricular tachycardia, 21, 122,
   142, 302
   pulseless, 306
   stable, 306
   unstable, 306

Venturi mask, 88

Verapamil, 197-200, 305

Vocal cords, 47, 55

W

Watt-seconds, 143

Wenckebach, 127

Y

Yankauer, 83

Notes

Notes

Notes

Notes

Notes

Notes

Notes